Injury & Trauma Sourcebook

Learning Disabilities Sourcebook, 3rd Edition

Leukemia Sourcebook

Liver Disorders Sourcebook

Medical Tests Sourcebook, 4th Edition

Men's Health Concerns Sourcebook, 3rd Edition

Mental Health Disorders Sourcebook, 4th Edition

Mental Retardation Sourcebook

Movement Disorders Sourcebook, 2nd Edition

Multiple Sclerosis Sourcebook

Muscular Dystrophy Sourcebook

Obesity Sourcebook

Osteoporosis Sourcebook

Pain Sourcebook, 3rd Edition

Pediatric Cancer Sourcebook

Physical & Mental Issues in Aging Sourcebook

Podiatry Sourcebook, 2nd Edition

Pregnancy & Birth Sourcebook, 3rd Edition

Prostate & Urological Disorders Sourcebook

Prostate Cancer Sourcebook

Rehabilitation Sourcebook

Respiratory Disorders Sourcebook, 2nd Edition

Sexually Transmitted Diseases Sourcebook, 4th Edition

Sleep Disorders Sourcebook, 3rd Edition

Smoking Concerns Sourcebook

Sports Injuries Sourcebook, 4th Edition

Stress-Related Disorders Sourcebook, 2nd Edition

Stroke Sourcebook, 2nd Edition

Surgery Sourcebook, 2nd Edition

Thyroid Disorders Sourcebook

Transplantation Sourcebook

Traveler's Health Sourcebook

Urinary Tract & Kidney Diseases & Disorders Sourcebook, 2nd Edition

Vegetarian Sourcebook

Women's Health Concerns Sourcebook, 3rd Edition

Workplace Health & Safety Sourcebook

Worldwide Health Sourcebook

Teen Health Series

Abuse & Violence Information for Teens

Accident & Safety Information for Teens

Alcohol Information for Teens, 2nd Edition

Allergy Information for Teens

Asthma Information for Teens, 2nd Edition

Body Information for Teens

Cancer Information for Teens, 2nd Edition

Complementary & Alternative Medicine Information for Teens

Diabetes Information for Teens, 2nd Edition

Diet Information for Teens, 3rd Edition

Drug Information for Teens, 3rd Edition

Eating Disorders Information for Teens, 2nd Edition

Fitness Information for Teens, 2nd Edition

Learning Disabilities Information for Teens

Mental Health Information for Teens, 3rd Edition

Pregnancy Information for Teens, 2nd Edition

Sexual Health Information for Teens, 3rd Edition

Skin Health Information for Teens, 2nd Edition

Sleep Information for Teens

Sports Injuries Information for Teens, 2nd Edition

Stress Information for Teens

Suicide Information for Teens, 2nd Edition

Tobacco Information for Teens, 2nd Edition

Medical
Tests
SOURCEBOOK

Fourth Edition

Health Reference Series

Fourth Edition

Medical Tests

SOURCEBOOK

Basic Consumer Health Information about Preventive Care Guidelines, Routine Health Screenings, Home-Use Tests, Blood, Stool, and Urine Tests, Genetic Testing, Biopsies, Endoscopic Exams, and Imaging Tests, Such as X-Ray, Ultrasound, Computed Tomography (CT), and Nuclear and Magnetic Resonance Imaging (MRI) Exams

Along with Facts about Diagnostic Tests for Allergies, Cancer, Diabetes, Heart and Lung Disease, Infertility, Osteoporosis, Sleep Problems, and Other Specific Conditions, a Glossary of Related Terms, and Directories of Additional Resources

Edited by
Joyce Brennfleck Shannon

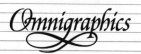

155 W. Congress, Suite 200, Detroit, MI 48226

Bibliographic Note

Because this page cannot legibly accommodate all the copyright notices, the Bibliographic Note portion of the Preface constitutes an extension of the copyright notice.

Edited by Joyce Brennfleck Shannon

Health Reference Series

Karen Bellenir, *Managing Editor*

David A. Cooke, MD, FACP, *Medical Consultant*

Elizabeth Collins, *Research and Permissions Coordinator*

Cherry Edwards, *Permissions Assistant*

EdIndex, Services for Publishers, *Indexers*

* * *

Omnigraphics, Inc.

Matthew P. Barbour, *Senior Vice President*

Kevin M. Hayes, *Operations Manager*

* * *

Peter E. Ruffner, *Publisher*

Copyright © 2011 Omnigraphics, Inc.

ISBN 978-0-7808-1151-5

Library of Congress Cataloging-in-Publication Data

Medical tests sourcebook : basic consumer health information about preventive care guidelines, routine health screenings, home-use tests, blood, stool, and urine tests, genetic testing, biopsies, endoscopic exams, and imaging tests, such as x-ray, ultrasound, computed tomography (CT), and nuclear and magnetic resonance imaging (MRI) exams; along with facts about diagnostic tests for allergies, cancer, diabetes, heart and lung disease, infertility, osteoporosis, sleep problems, and other specific conditions, a glossary of related terms, and directories of additional resources / edited by Joyce Brennfleck Shannon. -- 4th ed.
  p. cm. -- (Health reference series)
Includes bibliographical references and index.
Summary: "Provides basic consumer health information about laboratory, imaging, and other types of medical testing for disease screening, diagnosis, and monitoring, along with information and guidelines for preventive care testing in children and adults. Includes index, glossary of related terms, and other resources"-- Provided by publisher.
ISBN 978-0-7808-1151-5 (hardcover : alk. paper) 1. Diagnosis--Popular works. 2. Diagnosis, Laboratory--Popular works. 3. Medicine, Popular. I. Shannon, Joyce Brennfleck.
RC71.3.M45 2011
616.07'5--dc23

2011026847

This book is printed on acid-free paper meeting the ANSI Z39.48 Standard. The infinity symbol that appears above indicates that the paper in this book meets that standard.

Printed in the United States

Table of Contents

Visit www.healthreferenceseries.com to view *A Contents Guide to the Health Reference Series*, a listing of more than 16,000 topics and the volumes in which they are covered.

Part III: Imaging Tests

Part IV: Catheterization, Endoscopic, and Electrical Tests and Assessments

Part V: Screening and Assessments for Specific Conditions and Diseases

Part VI: Home and Self-Ordered Tests

Part VII: Additional Help and Information

Preface

About This Book

Informed decisions about health and the treatment of disease are guided by the wealth of information discovered though medical screening and diagnostic tests. Screening tests identify risk factors for specific disorders, while diagnostic tests find markers of disease or dysfunction. Medical tests assist in diagnosing the causes of symptoms, making treatment decisions, and assessing treatment effectiveness. When faced with decisions about health, consumers need to understand the benefits and limitations of medical tests and how test results guide treatment and lifestyle choices.

Medical Tests Sourcebook, Fourth Edition provides updated information about exams, tests, and other screening, diagnostic, and disease-monitoring procedures. It discusses preventive care guidelines and the screening tests used for such specific conditions as allergies, cancer, celiac disease, cardiovascular disorders, diabetes, kidney and thyroid dysfunction, and others. Details about laboratory blood tests, biopsies, throat cultures, toxicology screens, urinalysis, and genetic tests are also presented. Imaging tests, such as x-ray, ultrasound, computed tomography, and magnetic resonance, nuclear, and thermal imaging are described, and facts are offered about electrical, endoscopic, and home use tests. The book concludes with a glossary of related terms, a list of online health screening tools, and directories of breast and cervical cancer early detection programs and other resources for more information.

How to Use This Book

This book is divided into parts and chapters. Parts focus on broad areas of interest. Chapters are devoted to single topics within a part.

Part I: Screening and Preventive Care Tests are used to identify individuals with specific risk factors for which the timely provision of medical care or other interventions can help avoid or reduce health consequences. These include high blood pressure, high cholesterol, and certain genetic characteristics. Information is included about regular health exams, newborn screening tests, and preventive screening recommendations for all ages.

Part II: Laboratory Tests begins with an overview of lab tests. It identifies the features that distinguish quality services and provides help for understanding lab reports. Information about commonly used diagnostic and preventive care tests is provided along with details about tests of body fluids, such as those that analyze blood, urine, and spinal fluid. Specific biopsies and cultures are also explained.

Part III: Imaging Tests describes the many types of imaging available and the accompanying risks associated with exposure to radiation emissions. Imaging tests include radiography (x-rays), contrast studies, ultrasound exams, computed tomography (CT) scans, magnetic resonance imaging (MRI), nuclear imaging, and thermal imaging. Mammograms, neurological imaging, and new imaging techniques are also discussed.

Part IV: Catheterization, Endoscopic, and Electrical Tests and Assessments describes tests that use scopes, cameras, and electrical data. Cardiac catheterization, endoscopy, and laparoscopy enable physicians to see the structure of the heart, esophagus, colon, and other areas inside the body. Electrical tests provide data about the functioning of the cardiovascular, brain, and nervous systems.

Part V: Screening and Assessments for Specific Conditions and Diseases explains tests used to identify and monitor conditions such as allergy, cancer, celiac disease, cystic fibrosis, diabetes, heart disease, infectious disease, kidney disease, lung disease, sleep disorders, and endocrine dysfunction. Information is also provided about hearing assessments, vision tests, and prenatal and infertility tests.

Part VI: Home and Self-Ordered Tests discusses products that offer consumers a private option for the initial screening of fecal occult blood, drug abuse, human immunodeficiency virus (HIV), and other health concerns. The pros and cons of each test are given, and consumers are cautioned to use only tests approved by the U. S. Food and Drug Administration. All questions about home or self-ordered test results should be discussed with a health care provider.

Part VII: Additional Help and Information provides a glossary of terms related to medical tests and a list of online health screening tools. Directories of early detection programs for breast and cervical cancer and other resources for people undergoing medical tests are also included.

Bibliographic Note

This volume contains documents and excerpts from publications issued by the following U.S. government agencies: Agency for Healthcare Research and Quality (AHRQ); Centers for Disease Control and Prevention (CDC); Centers for Medicare and Medicaid Services (CMS); Genetics Home Reference; National Cancer Institute (NCI); NCI Visuals Online; National Eye Institute (NEI); National Heart, Lung, and Blood Institute (NHLBI); National Human Genome Research Institute; National Institute of Allergy and Infectious Diseases (NIAID); National Institute of Biomedical Imaging and Bioengineering (NIBIB); National Institute of Diabetes and Digestive and Kidney Diseases (NIDDK); National Institute on Deafness and Other Communication Disorders (NIDCD); National Institute of Neurological Disorders and Stroke (NINDS); National Kidney Disease Educational Program (NKDEP); National Institutes of Health (NIH); NIH Osteoporosis and Related Bone Diseases National Resource Center (NORBD); Office on Women's Health; United States (U.S.) Department of Health and Human Services (HHS); and the U.S. Food and Drug Administration (FDA).

In addition, this volume contains copyrighted documents from the following organizations: A.D.A.M., Inc.; Alzheimer Disease Cooperative Study; American College of Clinical Thermology; American Association for Clinical Chemistry; American Speech-Language-Hearing Association; American Society for Gastrointestinal Endoscopy; American Society of Echocardiography; American Society of Radiologic Technologists; Glaucoma Research Foundation; Health Physics Society; Imaginis Corporation; Joint Commission; Muscular Dystrophy Association of the United States; National Newborn Screening and Genetics Resource Center; Nemours Foundation; Society of Nuclear Medicine; and University of Maryland Medical Center.

Acknowledgements

In addition to the listed organizations and agencies who have contributed to this *Sourcebook*, special thanks go to managing editor Karen Bellenir, research and permissions coordinator Liz Collins, and prepress services provider WhimsyInk for their help and support.

About the Health Reference Series

The *Health Reference Series* is designed to provide basic medical information for patients, families, caregivers, and the general public. Each volume takes a particular topic and provides comprehensive coverage. This is especially important for people who may be dealing with a newly diagnosed disease or a chronic disorder in themselves or in a family member. People looking for preventive guidance, information about disease warning signs, medical statistics, and risk factors for health problems will also find answers to their questions in the *Health Reference Series*. The *Series*, however, is not intended to serve as a tool for diagnosing illness, in prescribing treatments, or as a substitute for the physician/patient relationship. All people concerned about medical symptoms or the possibility of disease are encouraged to seek professional care from an appropriate health care provider.

A Note about Spelling and Style

Health Reference Series editors use *Stedman's Medical Dictionary* as an authority for questions related to the spelling of medical terms and the *Chicago Manual of Style* for questions related to grammatical structures, punctuation, and other editorial concerns. Consistent adherence is not always possible, however, because the individual volumes within the *Series* include many documents from a wide variety of different producers and copyright holders, and the editor's primary goal is to present material from each source as accurately as is possible following the terms specified by each document's producer. This sometimes means that information in different chapters or sections may follow other guidelines and alternate spelling authorities. For example, occasionally a copyright holder may require that eponymous terms be shown in possessive forms (Crohn's disease *vs.* Crohn disease) or that British spelling norms be retained (leukaemia *vs.* leukemia).

Locating Information within the Health Reference Series

The *Health Reference Series* contains a wealth of information about a wide variety of medical topics. Ensuring easy access to all the fact sheets, research reports, in-depth discussions, and other material contained within the individual books of the *Series* remains one of our highest priorities. As the *Series* continues to grow in size and scope, however, locating the precise information needed by a reader may become more challenging.

A Contents Guide to the Health Reference Series was developed to direct readers to the specific volumes that address their concerns. It presents an extensive list of diseases, treatments, and other topics of general interest compiled from the Tables of Contents and major index headings. To access *A Contents Guide to the Health Reference Series*, visit www.healthreferenceseries.com.

Medical Consultant

Medical consultation services are provided to the *Health Reference Series* editors by David A. Cooke, MD, FACP. Dr. Cooke is a graduate of Brandeis University, and he received his MD degree from the University of Michigan. He completed residency training at the University of Wisconsin Hospital and Clinics. He is board-certified in Internal Medicine. Dr. Cooke currently works as part of the University of Michigan Health System and practices in Ann Arbor, MI. In his free time, he enjoys writing, science fiction, and spending time with his family.

Our Advisory Board

We would like to thank the following board members for providing guidance to the development of this *Series*:

- Dr. Lynda Baker
  Associate Professor of Library and Information Science,
  Wayne State University, Detroit, MI

- Nancy Bulgarelli
  William Beaumont Hospital Library, Royal Oak, MI

- Karen Imarisio
  Bloomfield Township Public Library, Bloomfield Township, MI

- Karen Morgan
  Mardigian Library, University of Michigan-Dearborn,
  Dearborn, MI

- Rosemary Orlando
  St. Clair Shores Public Library, St. Clair Shores, MI

Health Reference Series Update Policy

The inaugural book in the *Health Reference Series* was the first edition of *Cancer Sourcebook* published in 1989. Since then, the *Series* has been enthusiastically received by librarians and in the medical community. In order to maintain the standard of providing high-quality health information for the layperson the editorial staff at Omnigraphics felt it was necessary to implement a policy of updating volumes when warranted.

Medical researchers have been making tremendous strides, and it is the purpose of the *Health Reference Series* to stay current with the most recent advances. Each decision to update a volume is made on an individual basis. Some of the considerations include how much new information is available and the feedback we receive from people who use the books. If there is a topic you would like to see added to the update list, or an area of medical concern you feel has not been adequately addressed, please write to:

Editor
Health Reference Series
Omnigraphics, Inc.
155 W. Congress, Suite 200
Detroit, MI 48226
E-mail: editorial@omnigraphics.com

Part One

Screening and Preventive Care Tests

Chapter 1

Regular Health Exams Are Important

Schedule an appointment with your health care provider to discuss what preventive health services you need and when you need them. You and your health care provider determine what health services and screenings are best for you.

Why Are Check-Ups Important?

Regular health exams and tests can help find problems before they start. They also can help find problems early, when your chances for treatment and cure are better. By getting the right health services, screenings, and treatments, you are taking steps that help your chances for living a longer, healthier life. Your age, health and family history, lifestyle choices (such as what you eat, how active you are, whether you smoke), and other important factors impact what and how often you need services and screenings.

Check-Up Checklist: Things to Do before Your Next Check-Up

Getting check-ups is one of many things you can do to help stay healthy and prevent disease and disability.

1. Make the appointment to see your health care provider.

This chapter includes excerpts from "Regular Check-Ups Are Important," Centers for Disease Control and Prevention (CDC), January 27, 2011; and, "Check-Up Checklist," CDC, January 29, 2010.

3

2. Review the instructions on how to prepare for certain tests.

3. Do the usual paperwork.

Done, right? Not quite. Before your next check-up, make sure you do the following.

Review Your Family Health History

Are there any new conditions or diseases that have occurred in your close relatives since your last visit? If so, let your health care provider know. Family history might influence your risk of developing heart disease, stroke, diabetes, or cancer. Your provider will assess your risk of disease based on your family history and other factors. Your provider may also recommend things you can do to help prevent disease, such as exercising more, changing your diet, or using screening tests to help detect disease early.

Find Out if You Are Due for Any General Screenings or Vaccinations

Have you had the recommended screening tests based on your age, general health, family history, and lifestyle? Check with your health care provider to see if it is time for any vaccinations, follow-up exams, or tests. For example, it might be time for you to get a Pap test, mammogram, prostate cancer screening, colon cancer screening, sexually transmitted disease screening, blood pressure check, tetanus shot, eye check, or other screening.

Write a List of Issues and Questions to Take with You

Review any existing health problems and note any changes:

- Have you noticed any body changes, including lumps or skin changes?

- Are you having pain, dizziness, fatigue, problems with urine or stool, or menstrual cycle changes?

- Have your eating habits changed?

- Are you experiencing depression, anxiety, trauma, distress, or sleeping problems?

If so, note when the change began, how it's different from before, and any other observation that you think might be helpful.

Be honest with your provider. If you haven't been taking your medication as directed, exercising as much, or anything else, say so. You may be at risk for certain diseases and conditions because of how you live, work, and play. Your provider develops a plan based partly on what you say you do. Help ensure that you get the best guidance by providing the most up-to-date and accurate information about you.

Be sure to write your questions down beforehand. Once you're in the office or exam room, it can be hard to remember everything you want to know. Leave room between questions to write down your provider's answers.

Consider Your Future

Are there specific health issues that need addressing concerning your future? Are you thinking about having infertility treatment, losing weight, taking a hazardous job, or quitting smoking? Discuss any issues with your provider so that you can make better decisions regarding your health and safety.

Chapter 2

Questions about Medical Tests

Asking questions about medical tests—which ones you need, which ones you don't, and what the results tell you—can help you stay healthy and alert your doctor to the signs of a medical problem. A wide array of medical tests is available today that can detect disease or illness at an early stage, when many conditions can be treated effectively. Your physician should not prescribe tests that you do not need, but you should get the tests that are right for your age, gender, and medical history.

Maybe you do not know why you need a particular test or do not understand how it will help you. Here are some questions about medical tests that the Agency for Healthcare Research and Quality (AHRQ) developed to help you talk to your doctor.

Ask your doctor the following:

- How is the test done?

- What kind of information will the test provide?

- Is this test the only way to find out that information?

- What are the risks and benefits of having this test?

- How accurate is the test?

- What do I need to do to prepare for the test?

Excerpted from "Navigating the Health Care System, Asking Questions about Medical Tests" by Dr. Carolyn Clancy, Agency for Healthcare Research and Quality (AHRQ), February 5, 2008.

- Will the test be uncomfortable?

- How long will it take to get the results, and how will I get them?

- What is the next step after the test?

Your doctor should be able to tell you when the results of your medical test will be ready. Do not assume that everything is fine if you do not hear from your doctor. Tests results can get lost or people can think someone else gave you the results. No news is not necessarily good news. In fact, a study conducted at Harvard Medical School found that up to 33% of doctors did not always notify patients about abnormal test results. If you do not hear from your doctor, call to get your results.

It is also possible that your test results are incorrect. If you, or your doctor, think the test results may not be right, retake the test. A second test can confirm or rule out a diagnosis.

It is also a good idea to get information on the lab your doctor uses to analyze test results. For example, you may want to know if your doctor uses a lab because he or she has a business arrangement with them or if a health insurance company requires your doctor to use a certain lab. You can find out if a lab is accredited by or has a seal of approval from groups such as the College of American Pathologists or the Joint Commission. Both groups require labs to meet certain standards, which are linked to better-quality services.

If you need a mammogram, which is a test to detect breast cancer, make sure the test is performed at a facility that is approved by the Food and Drug Administration (FDA). You can ask this when you make your appointment, or you can call 800-4-CANCER (800-432-6337) to find out the names and locations of approved facilities in your area.

By asking your doctor questions about medical tests and your test results, you will have the information that you need to make smart decisions about your health care.

Chapter 3

Newborn Screening Tests

About Newborn Screening

Newborn screening is the practice of testing every newborn for certain harmful or potentially fatal disorders that aren't otherwise apparent at birth. Many of these are metabolic disorders (often called inborn errors of metabolism) that interfere with the body's use of nutrients to maintain healthy tissues and produce energy. Other disorders that screening can detect include problems with hormones or the blood.

In general, metabolic and other inherited disorders can hinder an infant's normal physical and mental development in a variety of ways. And parents can pass along the gene for a certain disorder without even knowing that they are carriers. With a simple blood test, doctors often can tell whether newborns have certain conditions that could

This chapter begins with "Newborn Screening Tests," June 2009, reprinted with permission from www.kidshealth.org. Copyright © 2009 The Nemours Foundation. This information was provided by KidsHealth, one of the largest resources online for medically reviewed health information written for parents, kids, and teens. For more articles like this one, visit www.KidsHealth.org, or www.TeensHealth.org. The chapter continues with an excerpt from "Traditional 'Heel Stick' Test Is Not an Effective Screening Tool for CMV in Newborns," National Institute on Deafness and Other Communication Disorders (NIDCD), April 13, 2010; and concludes with "National Newborn Screening Status Report," © 2011 National Newborn Screening and Genetics Resource Center (NNSGRC). Reprinted with permission. For additional information, contact the NNSGRC at 1912 W. Anderson Lane, Suite 210, Austin, TX 78757, 512-454-6419, or visit their website at http://genes-r-us .uthscsa.edu.

eventually cause problems. Even though these conditions are considered rare and most babies are given a clean bill of health, early diagnosis and proper treatment can make the difference between lifelong impairment and healthy development.

Newborn Screening: Past, Present, and Future

In the early 1960s, scientist Robert Guthrie, PhD, developed a blood test that could determine whether newborns had the metabolic disorder phenylketonuria (PKU). People with PKU lack an enzyme needed to process the amino acid phenylalanine, which is necessary for normal growth in kids and for normal protein use throughout life. However, if too much phenylalanine builds up, it damages the brain tissue and can eventually cause substantial developmental delay.

If kids born with PKU are put on a special diet right away, they can avoid the developmental delay the condition caused in past generations and lead normal lives. Since the development of the PKU test, researchers have developed additional blood tests that can screen newborns for other disorders that, unless detected and treated early, can cause physical problems, developmental delay, and in some cases, death.

Most states, the District of Columbia, Puerto Rico, and the U.S. Virgin Islands now have their own mandatory newborn screening programs (in some states, such as Wyoming and Maryland, the screening is not mandatory). Because the federal government has set no national standard, screening requirements vary from state to state, as determined by individual state public health departments.

Almost all states now screen for more than 30 disorders. One screening technique, the tandem mass spectrometry (or MS/MS), can screen for more than 20 inherited metabolic disorders with a single drop of blood.

Almost all states offer expanded MS/MS screening on every baby. However, there's some controversy over whether the new technology has been tested adequately. Also, some experts want more evidence that early detection of every disease tested for will actually offer babies long-term benefit. Equally important, parents may not want to know ahead of time that their child will develop a serious condition when there are no medical treatments or dietary changes that can improve the outcome. And some questions about who will pay (states, insurance companies, or parents) for it have yet to be resolved.

The American Academy of Pediatrics (AAP) and the federal government's Health Resources and Services Administration formed a task force of experts to examine these issues and recommend next steps. Their report identified some flaws and inconsistencies in the current state-driven screening system and proposed the following:

- All state screening programs should reflect current technology.
- All states should test for the same disorders.
- Parents should be informed about screening procedures and have the right to refuse screening, as well as the right to keep the results private and confidential.
- Parents should be informed about the benefits and risks associated with newborn screening.

How States and Hospitals Decide Which Tests to Offer

Traditionally, state decisions about what to screen for have been based on weighing the costs against the benefits. Cost considerations include:

- the risk of false positive results (and the worry they cause),
- the availability of treatments known to help the condition,
- financial costs.

And states often face conflicting priorities when determining their budgets. For instance, a state may face a choice between expanding newborn screening and ensuring that all expectant mothers get sufficient prenatal care. Of course, this is little comfort to parents whose children have a disorder that could have been found through a screening test but wasn't. These questions have not yet all been decided, even though most states have acknowledged the recommendations and have expanded screening.

So what can you do? Your best strategy is to stay informed. Discuss this issue with both your obstetrician or health care provider and your future baby's doctor before you give birth. Know what tests are routinely done in your state and in the hospital where you'll deliver (some hospitals go beyond what's required by state law).

If your state isn't offering screening for the expanded panel of disorders, you may want to ask your doctors about supplemental screening, though you'll probably have to pay for additional tests yourself. If you're concerned about whether your infant was screened for certain conditions, ask your child's doctor for information about which tests were done and whether further tests are recommended.

Screening Tests

Newborn screening varies by state and is subject to change, especially given advancements in technology. However, the disorders listed here are the ones typically included in newborn screening programs.

Phenylketonuria (PKU): When this disorder is detected early, feeding an infant a special formula low in phenylalanine can prevent mental retardation. A low-phenylalanine diet will need to be followed throughout childhood and adolescence and perhaps into adult life. This diet cuts out all high-protein foods, so people with PKU often need to take a special artificial formula as a nutritional substitute. Incidence: One in 10,000 to 25,000.

Congenital hypothyroidism: This is the disorder most commonly identified by routine screening. Affected babies don't have enough thyroid hormone and so develop retarded growth and brain development. (The thyroid, a gland at the front of the neck, releases chemical substances that control metabolism and growth.)

If the disorder is detected early, a baby can be treated with oral doses of thyroid hormone to permit normal development. Incidence: One in 4,000.

Galactosemia: Babies with galactosemia lack the enzyme that converts galactose (one of two sugars found in lactose) into glucose, a sugar the body is able to use. As a result, milk (including breast milk) and other dairy products must be eliminated from the diet. Otherwise, galactose can build up in the system and damage the body's cells and organs, leading to blindness, severe mental retardation, growth deficiency, and even death.

Incidence: One in 60,000 to 80,000. Several less severe forms of galactosemia that may be detected by newborn screening may not require any intervention.

Sickle cell disease: Sickle cell disease is an inherited blood disease in which red blood cells mutate into abnormal "sickle" shapes and can cause episodes of pain, damage to vital organs such as the lungs and kidneys, and even death. Young children with sickle cell disease are especially prone to certain dangerous bacterial infections, such as pneumonia (inflammation of the lungs) and meningitis (inflammation of the brain and spinal cord).

Studies suggest that newborn screening can alert doctors to begin antibiotic treatment before infections occur and to monitor symptoms of possible worsening more closely. The screening test can also detect other disorders affecting hemoglobin (the oxygen-carrying substance in the blood).

Incidence: About one in every 500 African-American births and one in every 1,000 to 1,400 Hispanic-American births; also occurs with some frequency among people of Mediterranean, Middle Eastern, and South Asian descent.

Biotinidase deficiency: Babies with this condition don't have enough biotinidase, an enzyme that recycles biotin (a B vitamin) in the body. The deficiency may cause seizures, poor muscle control, immune system impairment, hearing loss, mental retardation, coma, and even death. If the deficiency is detected in time, however, problems can be prevented by giving the baby extra biotin. Incidence: One in 72,000 to 126,000.

Congenital adrenal hyperplasia: This is actually a group of disorders involving a deficiency of certain hormones produced by the adrenal gland. It can affect the development of the genitals and may cause death due to loss of salt from the kidneys. Lifelong treatment through supplementation of the missing hormones manages the condition. Incidence: One in 12,000.

Maple syrup urine disease (MSUD): Babies with MSUD are missing an enzyme needed to process three amino acids that are essential for the body's normal growth. When not processed properly, these can build up in the body, causing urine to smell like maple syrup or sweet, burnt sugar. These babies usually have little appetite and are extremely irritable.

If not detected and treated early, MSUD can cause mental retardation, physical disability, and even death. A carefully controlled diet that cuts out certain high-protein foods containing those amino acids can prevent this. Like people with PKU, those with MSUD are often given a formula that supplies the necessary nutrients missed in the special diet they must follow. Incidence: One in 250,000.

Tyrosinemia: Babies with this amino acid metabolism disorder have trouble processing the amino acid tyrosine. If it accumulates in the body, it can cause mild retardation, language skill difficulties, liver problems, and even death from liver failure. Treatment requires a special diet and sometimes a liver transplant. Early diagnosis and treatment seem to offset long-term problems, although more information is needed. Incidence: not yet determined. Some babies have a mild self-limited form of tyrosinemia.

Cystic fibrosis (CF): A genetic disorder that particularly affects the lungs and digestive system and makes kids who have it more vulnerable to repeated lung infections. There is no known cure—treatment involves trying to prevent serious lung infections (sometimes with antibiotics) and providing adequate nutrition. Early detection may help doctors reduce the problems associated with CF, but the real impact of newborn screening has yet to be determined. Incidence: One in 2,000 Caucasian babies; less common in African-Americans, Hispanics, and Asians.

MCAD deficiency (medium chain acyl CoA dehydrogenase deficiency): Children with this fatty acid metabolism disorder are prone to repeated episodes of low blood sugar (hypoglycemia), which can cause seizures and interfere with normal growth and development. Treatment makes sure kids don't fast (skip meals) and supplies extra nutrition (usually by intravenous nutrients) when they're ill. Early detection and treatment can help affected children live normal lives.

Toxoplasmosis: A parasitic infection that can be transmitted through the mother's placenta to an unborn child. The disease-causing organism, which is found in uncooked or undercooked meat, can invade the brain, eye, and muscle, possibly resulting in blindness and mental retardation. The benefit of early detection and treatment is uncertain. Incidence: One in 1,000. But only one or two states screen for toxoplasmosis.

These aren't the only disorders that can be detected through newborn screening. Other conditions that are candidates for newborn screening include:

- Duchenne muscular dystrophy, a childhood form of muscular dystrophy that can be detected through a blood test;

- human immunodeficiency virus (HIV);

- neuroblastoma, a type of cancer that can be detected with a urine test.

Hearing Screening

Most, but not all, states require newborns' hearing to be screened before they're discharged from the hospital. If your baby isn't examined then, be sure that he or she does get screened within the first three weeks of life. Kids develop critical speaking and language skills in their first few years. A hearing loss that's caught early can be treated to help prevent interference with that development.

Should I request additional tests?

If you answer "yes" to any of these questions, talk to your doctor and perhaps a genetic counselor about additional tests:

- Do you have a family history of an inherited disorder?

- Have you previously given birth to a child who's affected by a disorder?

- Did an infant in your family die because of a suspected metabolic disorder?

- Do you have another reason to believe that your child may be at risk for a certain condition?

How Newborn Screening Is Performed

In the first two or three days of life, your baby's heel will be pricked to obtain a small blood sample for testing. Most states have a state or regional laboratory perform the analyses, although some use a private lab.

It's generally recommended that the sample be taken after the first 24 hours of life. Some tests, such as the one for PKU, may not be as sensitive if they're done too soon after birth. However, because mothers and newborns are often discharged within a day, some babies may be tested within the first 24 hours. If this happens, the American Association of Pediatricians (AAP) recommends that a repeat sample be taken no more than one to two weeks later. It's especially important that the PKU screening test be run again for accurate results. Some states routinely do two tests on all infants.

Getting the Results

Different labs have different procedures for notifying families and pediatricians of the results. Some may send the results to the hospital where your child was born and not directly to your child's doctor, which may mean a delay in getting the results to you. And although some states have a system that allows doctors to access the results via phone or computer, others may not. Ask your doctor how you'll get the results and when you should expect them.

If a test result comes back abnormal, try not to panic. This does not necessarily mean that your child has the disorder in question. A screening test is not the same as diagnostic test. The initial screening provides only preliminary information that must be followed up with more specific diagnostic testing.

If testing confirms that your child does have a disorder, your child's doctor may refer you to a specialist for further evaluation and treatment. Keep in mind that dietary restrictions and supplements, along with proper medical supervision, can often prevent most of the serious physical and mental problems that were associated with metabolic disorders in the past.

You also may wonder whether the disorder can be passed on to any future children. You'll want to discuss this with your doctor and perhaps a genetic counselor. Also, if you have other children who weren't screened for the disorder, consider having testing done. Again, speak with your doctor.

Know Your Options

Because state programs are subject to change, you'll want to find up-to-date information about your state's (and individual hospital's) program. Talk to your doctor or contact your state's department of health for more information.

Traditional 'Heel Stick' Test Is Not an Effective Screening Tool for Cytomegalovirus (CMV) in Newborns

A routine screening test for several metabolic and genetic disorders in newborns, the heel-stick procedure, is not effective in screening for cytomegalovirus (CMV) infection, a leading cause of hearing loss in children, according to research published in the April 14, 2010 on-line issue of the *Journal of the American Medical Association*. About 20,000–30,000 infants are born infected with CMV each year, 10%–15% of whom are at risk for eventually developing hearing loss.

The study, funded by the National Institute on Deafness and Other Communication Disorders (NIDCD), one of the National Institutes of Health, is part of a multicenter research project headed by the University of Alabama at Birmingham that is seeking to find the most effective screening test for CMV infection in newborns. The standard method for detecting CMV infection in newborns is labor-intensive and not conducive to a widespread screening program.

"The heel-stick test is a simple test that is already being used to screen for other diseases in newborns across the United States, so it seemed like a good candidate for a possible universal screening program for CMV," said James F. Battey, Jr., MD, PhD, director of the NIDCD. "However, these findings show us that, at least with current technologies, the heel-stick test should not be used as a primary newborn screening tool for CMV."

CMV is the most common infection passed from a mother to her unborn child. The vast majority of CMV-infected babies show no initial symptoms, and many babies will never develop health problems. But in some CMV-infected babies, serious problems can develop over time. Hearing loss is the most common deficit to emerge later on. The earlier doctors can identify CMV infection, the better they can monitor a child's hearing. If signs of hearing loss are present, appropriate intervention should be provided as soon as possible.

In this study, 20,448 babies were screened, 92 of whom were confirmed to have congenital CMV infection. The rapid culture method identified 91 of the 92 infants, for nearly 100% sensitivity. For the 11,422 infants who were screened with the single-primer PCR assay derived from dried blood spots, only 17 out of 60 infected children were identified—a 28.3% sensitivity. Of the 9,026 infants who were screened with the two-primer PCR method, 11 out of 32 infected children were identified, a sensitivity of 34.4%.

"In order to be included as part of a screening test, the minimum sensitivity should be at least 95%," said Suresh Boppana, MD, a co-principal investigator on the study with Karen Fowler, PhD, both of whom are with the University of Alabama at Birmingham. "Our findings indicate that dried blood spot PCR (polymerase chain reaction) will only detect 30–40% of babies with CMV infection. More than half of babies who are infected would be missed."

The researchers are now assessing whether analysis of saliva samples using real-time PCR technology can do a better job than dried blood spots when compared with the rapid culture method. They believe that the use of saliva may be beneficial since babies with congenital CMV infection are known to have a lot of virus in their saliva, compared to the blood, where amounts can vary depending on when the infant was infected during development. In addition, saliva samples require minimal processing and are noninvasive.

National Newborn Screening Status Report

The *U.S. National Screening Status Report* lists the status of newborn screening in the United States [see Tables 3.1, 3.2, and 3.3].

Additional Conditions/Abbreviations and Names

BIO: Biotinidase

CAH: Congenital adrenal hyperplasia

CF: Cystic fibrosis

CH: Congenital hypothyroidism

GALT: Transferase deficient galactosemia (Classical)

HB S/A: S-βeta thalassemia

HB S/C: Sickle-C disease

HB S/S: Sickle cell anemia

HEAR: Hearing screening

SCID: Severe Combined Immunodeficiency

Table 3.1. National Newborn Screening Core[1] Conditions (left side) Dot "•" indicates that screening for the condition is universally required by law or rule and fully implemented; A = universally offered but not yet required; B = offered to select populations, or by request; C = testing required but not yet implemented;

State	Hearing	Endocrine		Hemoglobin		
	HEAR	CH	CAH	Hb S/S	Hb S/A	Hb S/C
Alabama	•	•	•	•	•	•
Alaska	•	•	•	•	•	•
Arizona	A	•	•	•	•	•
Arkansas	•	•	•	•	•	•
California	B	•	•	•	•	•
Colorado	•	•	•	•	•	•
Connecticut	•	•	•	•	•	•
District of Columbia (DC)	•	•	•	•	•	•
Delaware	•	•	•	•	•	•
Florida	•	•	•	•	•	•
Georgia	A	•	•	•	•	•
Hawaii	•	•	•	•	•	•
Idaho	A	•	•	•	•	•
Illinois	•	•	•	•	•	•
Indiana	•	•	•	•	•	•
Iowa	•	•	•	•	•	•
Kansas	•	•	•	•	•	•
Kentucky	A	•	•	•	•	•
Louisiana	•	•	•	•	•	•
Maine	A	•	•	•	•	•
Maryland	•	•	•	•	•	•
Massachusetts	•	•	•	•	•	•
Michigan	•	•	•	•	•	•
Minnesota	•	•	•	•	•	•

Table 3.1. Right side *(Table continues on next two pages)*

D = likely to be detected (and reported) as a by-product of multiple reaction monitoring (MRM) screening tandem mass spectrometry (MS/MS) targeted by law or rule.

Other				Additional Conditions Included in Screening Panel (universally required unless otherwise indicated)
BIO	GALT	CF	SCID	
•	•	•		
•	•	•		
•	•	•		
•	•	•		
•	•	•	A	HHH; PRO; EMA ; OTC, MTHFR (D)
•	•	•		
•	•	•		HH; HIV[2]; NKH
•	•	•		G6PD
•	•	•		
•	•	•		
•	•	•		
•	•	•		
•	•	•		
•	•	•		Pompe, Gaucher, Fabry (B) CPS (D), NKH, 5-OXO, HIV[2]
•	•	•		
•	•	•		
•	•	•		
•	•	•		
•	•	•	A	
•	•	•		HHH; CPS (D)
•	•	•		EMA
•	•	•	A	TOXO; HHH, CPS (D)
•	•	•	C	
•	•	•		

Table 3.1. Left side (*continued from previous pages*)

State	Hearing	Endocrine		Hemoglobin		
	HEAR	CH	CAH	Hb S/S	Hb S/A	Hb S/C
Mississippi	•	•	•	•	•	•
Missouri	•	•	•	•	•	•
Montana	•	•	•	•	•	•
Nebraska	A	•	•	•	•	•
Nevada	A	•	•	•	•	•
New Hampshire	A	•	•	•	•	•
New Jersey	•	•	•	•	•	•
New Mexico	•	•	•	•	•	•
New York	•	•	•	•	•	•
North Carolina	•	•	•	•	•	•
North Dakota	A	•	•	•	•	•
Ohio	•	•	•	•	•	•
Oklahoma	•	•	•	•	•	•
Oregon	A	•	•	•	•	•
Pennsylvania	•	•	•	•	•	•
Rhode Island	•	•	•	•	•	•
South Carolina	•	•	•	•	•	•
South Dakota	A	•	•	•	•	•
Tennessee	•	•	•	•	•	•
Texas	B	•	•	•	•	•
Utah	•	•	•	•	•	•
Vermont	•	•	•	•	•	•
Virginia	•	•	•	•	•	•
Washington	A	•	•	•	•	•
West Virginia	•	•	•	•	•	•
Wisconsin	A	•	•	•	•	•
Wyoming	•	•	•	•	•	•

[1]Terminology consistent with ACMG report–Newborn Screening: Towards a Uniform Screening Panel and System. *Genet Med. 2006; 8*(5) Suppl: S12–S252.

Table 3.1. Right side (*continued from previous pages*)

Other				Additional Conditions Included in Screening Panel (universally required unless otherwise indicated)
BIO	GALT	CF	SCID	
•	•	•		5-OXO; CPS; HHH
•	•	•		
•	•	•		
•	•	•		5-OXO; HHH; NKH (A)
•	•	•		
•	•	•		TOXO
•	•	•		
•	•	•		
•	•	•	•	HIV; HHH; Krabbe disease
•	•	•		
•	•	•		HHH; NKH
•	•	•		
C	•	•		
•	•	•		
•	•	•		5-OXO; CPS; G6PD; HHH; NKH (B)
•	•	•		
•	•	•		
•	•	•		5-OXO; EMA; HHH; NKH
•	•	•		HHH; NKH
•	•	•	B	
•	•	•		
•	•	•		
•	•	•		
•	•	•		
•	•	•		
•	•	•	•	
•	•	•		

[2]Newborn screened for HIV only if mother was not screened during pregnancy.

Table 3.2. National Newborn Screening Core[1] Conditions–Metabolic (left side). Dot "•" indicates that screening for the condition is universally required by law or rule and fully implemented; A = universally offered but not yet required; B = offered to select populations, or by request;

State	Fatty Acid Disorders				
	CUD	LCHAD	MCAD	TFP	VLCAD
Alabama	•	•	•	•	•
Alaska	•	•	•	•	•
Arizona	•	•	•	•	•
Arkansas	•	•	•	•	•
California	•	•	•	•	•
Colorado	•	•	•	•	•
Connecticut	•	•	•	•	•
District of Columbia	•	•	•	•	•
Delaware	•	•	•	•	•
Florida	•	•	•	•	•
Georgia	•	•	•	•	•
Hawaii	•	•	•	•	•
Idaho	•	•	•	•	•
Illinois	•	•	•	•	•
Indiana	•	•	•	•	•
Iowa	•	•	•	•	•
Kansas	•	•	•	•	•
Kentucky	•	•	•	•	•
Louisiana	•	•	•	•	•
Maine	•	•	•	•	•
Maryland	•	•	•	•	•
Massachusetts	•	•	•	D	•
Michigan	•	•	•	•	•
Minnesota	•	•	•	•	•
Mississippi	•	•	•	•	•
Missouri	•	•	•	•	•

Newborn Screening Tests

Table 3.2. Right side *(Table continues on next two pages)*
C = testing required but not yet implemented; **D** = likely to be detected
(and reported) as a by-product of multiple reaction monitoring (MRM)
screening tandem mass spectrometry (MS/MS) targeted by law or rule.

Organic Acid Disorders									Amino Acid Disorders					
GA-I	HMG	IVA	3-MCC	Cbl-A,B	BKT	MUT	PROP	MCD	ASA	CIT	HCY	MSUD	PKU	TYR-I
•	•	•	•	D	•	•	•	•	•	•	•	•	•	•
•	•	•	•	•	•	•	•	•	•	•	•	•	•	•
•	•	•	•	•	•	•	•	•	•	•	•	•	•	•
•	•	•	•	•	•	•	•	•	•	•	•	•	•	•
•	•	•	•	•	•	•	•	•	•	•	•	•	•	•
•	•	•	•	•	•	•	•	•	•	•	•	•	•	•
•	•	•	•	•	•	•	•	•	•	•	•	•	•	•
•	•	•	•	•	•	•	•	•	•	•	•	•	•	•
•	•	•	•	•	•	•	•	•	•	•	•	•	•	•
•	•	•	•	•	•	•	•	•	•	•	•	•	•	•
•	•	•	•	•	•	•	•	•	•	•	•	•	•	•
•	•	•	•	•	•	•	•	•	•	•	•	•	•	•
•	•	•	•	•	•	•	•	•	•	•	•	•	•	•
•	•	•	•	•	•	•	•	•	•	•	•	•	•	•
•	•	•	•	•	•	•	•	•	•	•	•	•	•	•
•	•	•	•	•	•	•	•	•	•	•	•	•	•	•
•	•	•	•	•	•	•	•	•	•	•	•	•	•	•
•	•	•	•	•	•	•	•	•	•	•	•	•	•	•
•	•	•	•	•	•	•	•	•	•	•	•	•	•	•
•	•	•	•	•	•	•	•	•	•	•	•	•	•	•
•	•	•	D	•	•	•	•	D	•	•	•	•	•	•
•	•	•	•	•	•	•	•	•	•	•	•	•	•	•
•	•	•	•	•	•	•	•	•	•	•	•	•	•	•
•	•	•	•	•	•	•	•	•	•	•	•	•	•	•
•	•	•	•	•	•	•	•	•	•	•	•	•	•	•

Table 3.2. Left side *(continued from previous pages)*

State	CUD	LCHAD	MCAD	TFP	VLCAD
			Fatty Acid Disorders		
Montana	•	•	•	•	•
Nebraska	•	•	•	•	•
Nevada	•	•	•	•	•
New Hampshire	•	•	•	•	•
New Jersey	•	•	•	•	•
New Mexico	•	•	•	•	•
New York	•	•	•	•	•
North Carolina		•	•	•	•
North Dakota	•	•	•	•	•
Ohio	•	•	•	•	•
Oklahoma	•	•	•	•	•
Oregon	•	•	•	•	•
Pennsylvania	•	•	•	•	•
Rhode Island	•	•	•	•	•
South Carolina	•	•	•	•	•
South Dakota	•	•	•	•	•
Tennessee	•	•	•	•	•
Texas	•	•	•	•	•
Utah	•	•	•	•	•
Vermont	•	•	•	•	•
Virginia	•	•	•	•	•
Washington	•	•	•	•	•
West Virginia	•	•	•	•	•
Wisconsin	•	•	•	•	•
Wyoming	•	•	•	•	•

[1]Terminology consistent with ACMG report–Newborn Screening: Towards a Uniform Screening Panel and System. *Genet Med. 2006; 8*(5) Suppl: S12–S252.

Table 3.2. Right side *(continued from previous pages)*

Organic Acid Disorders									Amino Acid Disorders					
GA-I	HMG	IVA	3-MCC	Cbl-A,B	BKT	MUT	PROP	MCD	ASA	CIT	HCY	MSUD	PKU	TYR-I
•	•	•	•	•	•	•	•	•	•	•	•	•	•	•
•	•	•	•	•	•	•	•	•	•	•	•	•	•	•
•	•	•	•	•	•	•	•	•	•	•	•	•	•	•
•	•	•	•	•	•	•	•	•	•	•	•	•	•	•
•	•	•	•	•	•	•	•	•	•	•	•	•	•	•
•	•	•	•	•	•	•	•	•	•	•	•	•	•	•
•	•	•	•	•	•	•	•	•	•	•	•	•	•	•
•	•	•	•	•	•	•	•	•	•	•	•	•	•	•
•	•	•	•	•	•	•	•	•	•	•	•	•	•	•
•	•	•	•	•	•	•	•	•	•	•	•	•	•	•
•	•	•	•	•	•	•	•	•	•	•	•	•	•	•
•	•	•	•	•	•	•	•	•	•	•	•	•	•	•
•	•	•	•	•	•	•	•	•	•	•	•	•	•	•
•	•	•	•	•	•	•	•	•	•	•	•	•	•	•
•	•	•	•	•	•	•	•	•	•	•	•	•	•	•
•	•	•	•	•	•	•	•	•	•	•	•	•	•	•
•	•	•	•	•	•	•	•	•	•	•	•	•	•	•
•	•	•	•	•	•	•	•	•	•	•	•	•	•	•
•	•	•	•	•	•	•	•	•	•	•	•	•	•	•
•	•	•	•	•	•	•	•	•	•	•	•	•	•	•
•	•	•	D	•	•	•	•	•	•	•	•	•	•	•
•	•	•	•	•	•	•	•	•	•	•	•	•	•	•
•	•	•	•	•	•	•	•	•	•	•	•	•	•	•
•	•	•	•	•	•	•	•	•	•	•	•	•	•	•

Other Disorders

5-OXO: 5-oxoprolinuria (pyroglutamic aciduria)

CPS: Carbamoylphosphate synthetase

EMA: Ethylmalonic encephalopathy

G6PD: Glucose 6 phosphate dehydrogenase

HHH: Hyperammonemia/ornithinemia/citrullinemia (Ornithine transporter defect)

HIV: Human immunodeficiency virus

NKH: Nonketotic hyperglycinemia

PRO: Prolinemia

TOXO: Toxoplasmosis

Deficiency/Disorder Abbreviations and Names (Optional Nomenclature) for Table 3.2

3-MCC: 3-Methylcrotonyl-CoA carboxylase

ASA: Argininosuccinate aciduria

BKT: Beta ketothiolase (mitochondrial acetoacetyl-CoA thiolase; short-chain ketoacyl thiolase; T2)

CBL A,B: Methylmalonic academia (Vitamin B12 disorders)

CIT I: Citrullinemia type I (Argininosuccinate synthetase)

CUD: Carnitine uptake defect (Carnitine transport defect)

GA-1: Glutaric acidemia type 1

HCY: Homocystinuria (cystathionine beta synthase)

HMG: 3-Hydroxy 3-methylglutaricaciduria (3-Hydroxy 3-methylglutaryl-CoA lyase)

IVA: Isovaleric acidemia (Isovaleryl-CoA dehydrogenase)

LCHAD: Long-chain L-3- hydroxyacyl-CoA dehydrogenase

MCAD: Medium-chain acyl-CoA dehydrogenase

MCD: Multiple carboxylase (Holocarboxylase synthetase)

MSUD: Maple syrup urine disease (branched-chain ketoacid dehydrogenase)

MUT: Methylmalonic Acidemia (methylmalonyl-CoA mutase)

PKU Phenylketonuria/hyperphenylalaninemia

PROP: Propionic acidemia (Propionyl-CoA carboxylase)

TFP: Trifunctional protein deficiency

TYR-1: Tyrosinemia Type 1

VLCAD: Very long-chain acyl-CoA dehydrogenase

Deficiency/Disorder Abbreviations and Names (Optional Nomenclature) for Table 3.3

2M3HBA: 2-Methyl-3-hydroxybutyric aciduria

2MBG: 2-Methylbutyryl-CoAdehydrogenase

3MGA: 3-Methylglutaconicaciduria

ARG: Argininemia (Arginase deficiency)

BIOPT-BS: Defects of biopterin cofactor biosynthesis

BIOPT-REG: Defects of biopterin cofactor regeneration

CACT: Carnitine acylcarnitine translocase

CBL-C,D: Methylmalonic academia (Cbl C,D)

CIT-II: Citrullinemia type II

CPT-Ia: Carnitine palmitoyltransferase I

CPT-II: Carnitine palmitoyltransferase II

De-Red: Dienoyl-CoA reductase

GA-II: Glutaric academia Type II

GALE: Galactose epimerase

GALK: Galactokinase

H-PHE: Benign hyperphenylalaninemia

IBG: Isobutyryl-CoA dehydrogenase

M/SCHAD: Medium/Short chain L-3-hydroxyacyl-CoA dehydrogenase

MAL: Malonic academia (Malonyl-CoA decarboxylase)

MCKAT: Medium-chain ketoacyl-CoA thiolase

MET: Hypermethioninemia

SCAD: Short-chain acyl-CoA dehydrogenase

TYR-II: Tyrosinemia type II

TYR-III: Tyrosinemia type III

Table 3.3. National Newborn Screening Secondary Target[1] Conditions (left side)

Dot "•" indicates that screening for the condition is universally required by law or rule and fully implemented; **A** = universally offered but not yet required; **B** = offered to select populations, or by request;

State	Fatty Acid Disorders								Organic Acid Disorders					
	CACT	CPT-Ia	CPT-II	DE-RED.	GA-II	MCKAT	M/SCHAD	SC AD	2M3HBA	2MBG	3MGA	Cbl-C,D	IBG	MAL
Alabama	•		•		•				•	•	•	•		
Alaska	•	•	•		•			•	•	•	•	•	•	•
Arizona	D	D	D	D					D		D	D		
Arkansas														
California	•	•	•		•		•	•	•	•	•	•	•	•
Colorado	•	•			•		•	•		•	•			•
Connecticut	•	•	•	•	•			•				•		•
District of Columbia	•	•	•	•	•	•	•	•	•	•	•	•	•	•
Delaware	•		•		•	D		•	D	•	D	•	•	
Florida	•	•	•		•			•						
Georgia	D	D	D		D	D	D	D	D	D	D	D	D	D
Hawaii	•	•	•		•			•	•	•	•	•	•	•
Idaho	•	•	•		•			•	•	•	•	•	•	•
Illinois	•	D	•	D	•	D	•	•	D	•	•	•	•	•
Indiana	•	•	•	•	•	•	•	•	•	•	•	•	•	•
Iowa	•	•	•		•	•	•	•	•	•	•	•	•	•
Kansas														
Kentucky	A	A	A		A			•	A	A	A	A	A	A
Louisiana														
Maine	D	D	•		•			•		D	D	•	D	
Maryland	•	•	•	•	•	•	•	•	•	•	•	•	•	•
Massachusetts	D	D	A	A	D	D	A	D	D	D	D	•	D	A
Michigan	•	•	•	•	•	•	•	•	•	•	•	•	•	•
Minnesota	•	•	•	•	•	•	•	•	•	•	•	•	•	•

Table 3.3. Right side *(Table continues on next two pages)*
C = testing required but not yet implemented; **D** = likely to be detected (and reported) as a by-product of multiple reaction monitoring (MRM) screening tandem mass spectrometry (MS/MS) targeted by law or rule.

Amino Acid Disorders								Other Metabolic		Hbg
ARG	BIOPT-BS	BIOPT-RG	CIT-II	H-PHE	MET	TYR-II	TYR-III	GALE	GALK	Variant Hbg's
	•	•	•	•	•	•	•			•
•	B	B	•	•	•	•	D	B	B	•
			D	D		D	D			D
										•
•	•	•	•	•	•	•				•
•			•	•	•	•	•			•
•			•	•	•	•	•	•	•	•
•	A	A	•	•	•	•	•	•	•	•
•	D	D	•	•	•	•	•	•	•	•
				•		•				
A			D	D	D	D	D	B	B	•
•	B	B	•	•	•	•		B	B	•
•	B	B	•	•	•	•		B	B	•
•	D	D	D	•	•	•	•			•
•	•	•	•	•	•	•	•			•
•	•	•	•	•	•	•	•			•
			•							•
A	D	D	A	•	A	A	A			•
			•							•
•			•	•	D	•	D	•	•	•
•	B	B	•	•	•	•	•	•	•	•
•	D	D	A	D	D	D	D	D	D	•
•	•	•	•	•	•	A	A			•
•	•	•	•	•	•	•	•	•	•	•

Table 3.3. Left side *(continued from previous pages)*

State	Fatty Acid Disorders								Organic Acid Disorders					
	CACT	CPT-Ia	CPT-II	DE-RED.	GA-II	MCKAT	M/SCHAD	SC AD	2M3HBA	2MBG	3MGA	Cbl-C,D	IBG	MAL
Mississippi	•	•	•	A	•	A	•	•	A	•	•	•	•	•
Missouri	•	•	•	•	•	•	•	•	•	•	•	•	•	•
Montana	D		D	D	D	D	D	D	D	D	D	D	D	
Nebraska	D	D	D	D	D	D	D	D	D	D	D	D	D	D
Nevada	•	•	•		•			•	•	•	•	•	•	•
New Hampshire	D	D	•		•					D	D	D		
New Jersey	•	•	•	•	•	•	•	•	•	•	•	•	•	•
New Mexico	A	D	A		A			A	D	D	A	A	D	D
New York	•	•	•	•	•	•	•	•	•	•	•	•	•	•
North Carolina	•		•					•			•		•	
North Dakota	•	•	•	•	•	•	•	•	•	•	•	•		•
Ohio	•		•					•		•			•	
Oklahoma	•	•	•		•	D		•	•	•	•	•	•	•
Oregon	•	D	•		•			•	D	D	•		D	D
Pennsylvania	B	B	B	B	B		B	B		B	B	B	B	B
Rhode Island		D												
South Carolina	•	•	•	•	•	•	•	•	•	•	•	•	•	•
South Dakota	•	•	•		•	•	•	•	•	•	•	•	•	•
Tennessee	•	•	•	•	•	D		•	•	•	•	•	•	•
Texas	D	D	D	C	D	C	C	C	D	D	D	D	C	C
Utah	•	•	•		•	D		•	•	•	D	•		D
Vermont	D	D	D		D					D	D	•		
Virginia	D	D	D		D	D			D	D	D	D		
Washington	D		D		D	D			D	D	D	D		
West Virginia	D	D	D	D	D	D	D	D	D	D	D	D	D	D
Wisconsin	•		•	•	•	•	•	•	•	•	•	•	•	
Wyoming	A	A	A	A	A	A	A	A	A	A	A	A	A	A

[1]Terminology consistent with ACMG report–Newborn Screening: Towards a Uniform Screening Panel and System. *Genet Med. 2006; 8*(5) Suppl: S12–S252.

Table 3.3. Right side *(continued from previous pages)*

Amino Acid Disorders								Other Metabolic		Hbg
ARG	BIOPT-BS	BIOPT-RG	CIT-II	H-PHE	MET	TYR-II	TYR-III	GALE	GALK	Variant Hbg's
•	A	A	•	•	•	•	A	•	•	•
•	•	•	•	•	•	•	•			•
	D	D	D	•	D	D	D			•
D	D	D	D	•	D	D	D	•	•	•
•	B	B	•	•	•	•		B	B	A
•	D	D	D	•	D			•	•	•
•	•	•	•	•	•	•	•	•	•	•
D	B	B	A	A	A	A	D	B	B	•
•		•	•	•	•	•	•			•
•	•	•	•	•	•	•	•			•
•		•	•	•	•	•	•			•
•	•	•	•	•	•	•	•			•
D	B	B	•	•	•	•	D	B	B	•
B	B	B	B	•	B	B	B	•	•	•
			•					•	•	•
•	•	•	•	•	•	•	•	•	•	•
•	•	•	•	•	•	•	•			•
•	•	•	•	•	•	•	•	•	•	•
C	D	D	D	•	D	D	D			•
•	•	•	•	•	•	•	•			•
D			•	•	D	D	D	•	•	•
	D	D	D	D	D	D	D	D	D	•
	D	D	•	D	D					•
D	D	D	D	•	D	D	D	•	•	•
	•	•	•	•	•	•	•			•
A			A	•	A	A	B			•

Chapter 4

Preventive Care for Children and Adolescents

Chapter Contents

Section 4.1

Recommended Screening Tests for Children and Adolescents

Excerpted from "The Guide to Clinical Preventative Services, 2010–2011,"
Agency for Healthcare Research and Quality (AHRQ), August 2011.

The U.S. Preventative Services Task Force (USPSTF) is an independent panel of non-federal experts in prevention and evidence-based medicine and is composed of primary care providers (such as internists, pediatricians, family physicians, gynecologists/obstetricians, nurses, and health behavior specialists).

The USPSTF conducts scientific evidence reviews of a broad range of clinical preventive health care services (such as screening, counseling, and preventive medications) and develops recommendations for primary care clinicians and health systems.

The U.S. Preventive Services Task Force (USPSTF) assigns one of five letter grades to each of its recommendations (A, B, C, D, or I).

- **A:** The USPSTF recommends the service. There is high certainty that the net benefit is substantial.

- **B:** The USPSTF recommends the service. There is high certainty that the net benefit is moderate or there is moderate certainty that the net benefit is moderate to substantial.

- **C:** The USPSTF recommends against routinely providing the service. There may be considerations that support providing the service in an individual patient. There is at least moderate certainty that the net benefit is small.

- **D:** The USPSTF recommends against the service. There is moderate or high certainty that the service has no net benefit or that the harms outweigh the benefits.

- **I statement:** The USPSTF concludes that the current evidence is insufficient to assess the balance of benefits and harms of the service. Evidence is lacking, of poor quality, or conflicting, and the balance of benefits and harms cannot be determined.

Following are recommendations made by the USPSTF for children and adolescents.

Screening for Congenital Hypothyroidism

The U.S. Preventive Services Task Force (USPSTF) recommends screening for congenital hypothyroidism (CH) in newborns. *Grade: A Recommendation.*

This recommendation applies to all infants born in the United States. Premature, very low birth weight, and ill infants may benefit from additional screening because these conditions are associated with decreased sensitivity and specificity of screening tests.

Screening for CH is mandated in all 50 states and the District of Columbia, though methods of screening vary. There are two main methods used in the U.S.: Primary thyroid-stimulating hormone (TSH) with backup (thyroxine) T4; and primary T4 with backup TSH. A few states use both tests in initial screening. Families should be provided with appropriate information about newborn screening tests, including the benefits and harms of screening. They should be aware of the potential of a false-positive test, and the process required for definitive testing. Nationally, only one in 25 positive screening tests are confirmed to be CH. Normal newborn screening results for CH should not preclude appropriate evaluation of infants presenting with clinical signs and symptoms suggestive of hypothyroidism.

Infants should be tested between two and four days of age. Infants discharged from hospitals before 48 hours of life should be tested immediately before discharge. Specimens obtained in the first 24–48 hours of age may be falsely elevated for TSH regardless of the screening method used.

Primary care clinicians should ensure that infants with abnormal screens receive confirmatory testing and begin appropriate treatment with thyroid hormone replacement within two weeks after birth. Children with positive confirmatory testing in whom no permanent cause of CH is found (such as lack of thyroid tissue on thyroid ultrasound or thyroid scan), should, at some time point after the age of three years, undergo a 30-day trial of reduced or discontinued thyroid hormone replacement therapy to determine if the hypothyroidism is permanent or transient.

Screening for Phenylketonuria

The U.S. Preventive Services Task Force (USPSTF) recommends screening for phenylketonuria (PKU) in newborns. *Grade: A Recommendation.*

This recommendation applies to newborns. Screening for PKU is mandated in all 50 states, though methods of screening vary. There are three principal methods used for PKU screening in the United States: the Guthrie Bacterial Inhibition Assay (BIA), automated fluorometric assay, and tandem mass spectrometry. Screening tests are most accurate if performed after 24 hours of life but before the infant is seven days old.

It is essential that phenylalanine restrictions be instituted shortly after birth to prevent the neurodevelopmental effects of PKU. Infants who are tested within the first 24 hours after birth should receive a repeat screening test by two weeks of age. Premature infants and those with illnesses should be tested at or near seven days of age, but in all cases before newborn nursery discharge.

Screening for Sickle Cell Disease in Newborns

The U.S. Preventive Services Task Force (USPSTF) recommends screening for sickle cell disease in newborns. *Grade: A Recommendation.*

Screening for sickle cell disease in newborns is mandated in all 50 states and the District of Columbia. Most states use either thin-layer isoelectric focusing (IEF) or high performance liquid chromatography (HPLC) as the initial screening test. Both methods have extremely high sensitivity and specificity for sickle cell anemia. Specimens must be drawn prior to any blood transfusion due to the potential for a false negative result as a result of the transfusion. Extremely premature infants may have false-positive results when adult hemoglobin is undetectable.

All newborns should undergo testing regardless of birth setting. In general, birth attendants should make arrangements for samples to be obtained, and the first physician to see the child at an office visit should verify screening results. Confirmatory testing should occur no later than two months of age.

Universal Screening for Hearing Loss in Newborns

The U.S. Preventive Services Task Force (USPSTF) recommends screening for hearing loss in all newborn infants. *Grade: B Recommendation.*

The patient population considered here includes all newborn infants. Screening programs should be conducted by using a 1- or 2-step validated protocol. A frequently used protocol requires a 2-step screening process, which includes otoacoustic emissions (OAEs) followed by auditory brainstem response (ABR) in those who failed the first test.

Equipment should be well maintained, staff should be thoroughly trained, and quality-control programs should be in place to reduce avoidable false-positive test results. Programs should develop protocols to ensure that infants with positive screening test results receive appropriate audiologic evaluation and follow-up after discharge. Newborns delivered at home, birthing centers, or hospitals without hearing screening facilities should have some mechanism for referral for newborn hearing screening, including tracking of follow-up.

All infants should have hearing screening before one month of age. Those infants who do not pass the newborn screening should undergo audiologic and medical evaluation before three months of age for confirmatory testing. Because of the elevated risk of hearing loss in infants with risk indicators, an expert panel made a recommendation in 2000 that these children should undergo periodic monitoring for three years.

Screening for Visual Impairment in Children Younger than Age Five Years

The U.S. Preventive Services Task Force (USPSTF) recommends screening to detect amblyopia, strabismus, and defects in visual acuity in children age 3–5 years. *Grade: B Recommendation.*

Various screening tests are used in primary care to identify visual impairment in children, including: Visual acuity test, stereo-acuity test, cover-uncover test, Hirschberg light reflex test, auto-refraction, and photoscreening.

Various tests are used widely in the United States to identify visual defects in children, and the choice of tests is influenced by the child's age. During the first year of life, strabismus can be assessed by the cover test and the Hirschberg light reflex test. Screening children younger than age three years for visual acuity is more challenging than screening older children and typically requires testing by specially trained personnel. Newer automated techniques can be used to test these children.

Screening and Treatment for Major Depressive Disorder in Children and Adolescents

The U.S. Preventive Services Task Force (USPSTF) recommends screening of adolescents (12–18 years of age) for major depressive disorder (MDD) when systems are in place to ensure accurate diagnosis, psychotherapy (cognitive/behavioral or interpersonal), and follow-up. *Grade: B Recommendation.*

This USPSTF recommendation addresses screening for MDD in adolescents (12–18 years of age) and children (7–11 years of age) in the general population. There is a spectrum of depressive disorders. This report focuses only on screening for MDD and does not address screening for various less-severe depressive disorders.

Instruments developed for primary care (Patient Health Questionnaire for Adolescents [PHQ-A] and the Beck Depression Inventory-Primary Care Version [BDI-PC]) have been used successfully in adolescents. There are limited data describing the accuracy of using MDD screening instruments in younger children (7–11 years of age).

Screening for Obesity in Children and Adolescents

The U.S. Preventive Services Task Force (USPSTF) recommends that clinicians screen children aged six years and older for obesity and offer them or refer them to comprehensive, intensive behavioral interventions to promote improvement in weight status. *Grade: B Recommendation.*

This recommendation statement applies to children and adolescents aged 6–18 years. The USPSTF is using the following terms to define categories of increased body mass index (BMI): overweight is defined as an age- and gender-specific BMI between the 85th and 95th percentiles, and obesity is defined as an age- and gender-specific BMI at greater than or equal to the 95th percentile. The USPSTF did not find sufficient evidence for screening children younger than six years.

In 2005, the USPSTF found adequate evidence that BMI was an acceptable measure for identifying children and adolescents with excess weight. BMI is calculated from the measured weight and height of an individual.

No evidence was found regarding appropriate intervals for screening. Height and weight, from which BMI is calculated, are routinely measured during health maintenance visits.

Section 4.2

Body Mass Index
Screening for Weight Problems

This section includes "About BMI for Children and Teens," Centers for Disease Control and Prevention (CDC), February 15, 2011; Figure 4.1 is from "2 to 20 years: Boys Body Mass Index-for-Age Percentiles," CDC, October 16, 2000; and Figure 4.2 is from "2 to 20: Girls Body Mass Index-for-Age Percentiles," CDC, October 16, 2000.

Body mass index (BMI) is a number calculated from a child's weight and height. BMI is a reliable indicator of body fatness for most children and teens. BMI does not measure body fat directly, but research has shown that BMI correlates to direct measures of body fat, such as underwater weighing and dual energy x-ray absorptiometry (DXA). BMI can be considered an alternative for direct measures of body fat. Additionally, BMI is an inexpensive and easy-to-perform method of screening for weight categories that may lead to health problems.

For children and teens, BMI is age- and sex-specific and is often referred to as BMI-for-age.

What is a BMI percentile?

After BMI is calculated for children and teens, the BMI number is plotted on the Centers for Disease Control and Prevention (CDC) BMI-for-age growth charts (for either girls or boys) to obtain a percentile ranking. Percentiles are the most commonly used indicator to assess the size and growth patterns of individual children in the United States. The percentile indicates the relative position of the child's BMI number among children of the same sex and age. The growth charts show the weight status categories used with children and teens (underweight, healthy weight, overweight, and obese).

How is BMI used with children and teens?

BMI is used as a screening tool to identify possible weight problems for children. CDC and the American Academy of Pediatrics (AAP) recommend the use of BMI to screen for overweight and obesity in children beginning at two years old.

For children, BMI is used to screen for obesity, overweight, healthy weight, or underweight. However, BMI is not a diagnostic tool. For example, a child may have a high BMI for age and sex, but to determine if excess fat is a problem, a health care provider would need to perform further assessments. These assessments might include skinfold thickness measurements, evaluations of diet, physical activity, family history, and other appropriate health screenings.

Table 4.1. BMI for Age-Weight Status Categories with the Corresponding Percentiles

Weight Status Category	Percentile Range
Underweight	Less than the 5th percentile
Healthy weight	5th percentile to less than the 85th percentile
Overweight	85th to less than the 95th percentile
Obese	Equal to or greater than the 95th percentile

How is BMI calculated and interpreted for children and teens?

Calculating and interpreting BMI involves the following steps:

1. Before calculating BMI, obtain accurate height and weight measurements.

2. Calculate the BMI and percentile.

    *   To calculate BMI: weight in pounds divided by height in inches divided (again) by height in inches and multiplied by 703.

    *   Or, use the "Child and Teen BMI Calculator" available online at http://apps.nccd.cdc.gov/dnpabmi.

3. Review the calculated BMI-for-age percentile and results. The BMI-for-age percentile is used to interpret the BMI number because BMI is both age- and sex-specific for children and teens. These criteria are different from those used to interpret BMI for adults—which do not take into account age or sex. Age and sex are considered for children and teens for two reasons: The amount of body fat changes with age (BMI for children and teens is often referred to as BMI-for-age); and the amount of body fat differs between girls and boys. The CDC BMI-for-age growth charts for girls and boys take into account these differences and allow translation of a BMI number into a percentile for a child's or teen's sex and age.

4. Find the weight status category for the calculated BMI-for-age percentile as shown in the Table 4.1. These categories are based on expert committee recommendations.

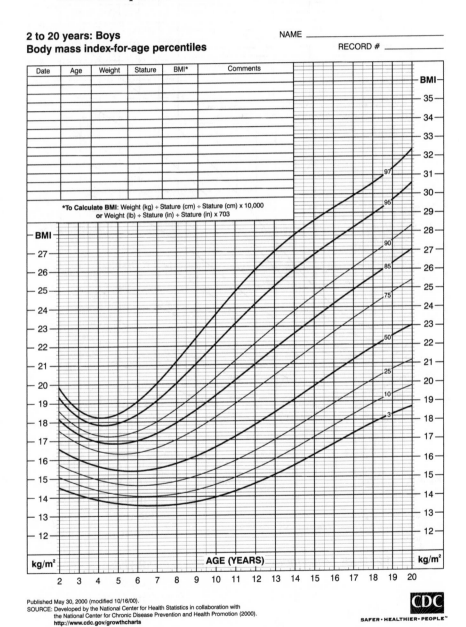

2 to 20 years: Boys
Body mass index-for-age percentiles

NAME _____

RECORD # _____

*To Calculate BMI: Weight (kg) ÷ Stature (cm) ÷ Stature (cm) x 10,000
or Weight (lb) ÷ Stature (in) ÷ Stature (in) x 703

Published May 30, 2000 (modified 10/16/00).
SOURCE: Developed by the National Center for Health Statistics in collaboration with
the National Center for Chronic Disease Prevention and Health Promotion (2000).
http://www.cdc.gov/growthcharts

CDC
SAFER · HEALTHIER · PEOPLE™

Figure 4.1. *Body Mass Index-for-Age Percentiles for Boys*

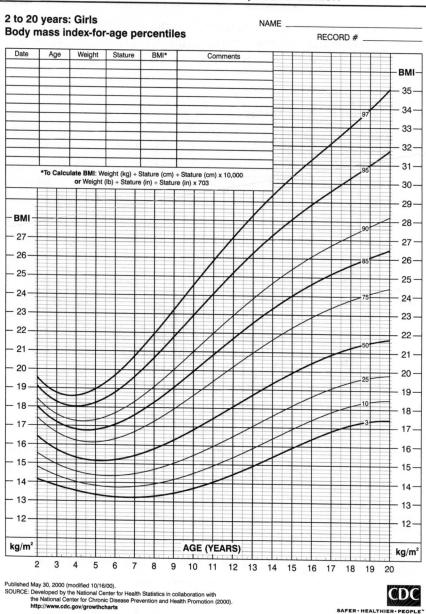

2 to 20 years: Girls
Body mass index-for-age percentiles

NAME _____

RECORD # _____

*To Calculate BMI: Weight (kg) ÷ Stature (cm) ÷ Stature (cm) x 10,000
or Weight (lb) ÷ Stature (in) ÷ Stature (in) x 703

Published May 30, 2000 (modified 10/16/00).
SOURCE: Developed by the National Center for Health Statistics in collaboration with
the National Center for Chronic Disease Prevention and Health Promotion (2000).
http://www.cdc.gov/growthcharts

Figure 4.2. *Body Mass Index-for-Age Percentiles for Girls*

Chapter 5

Prevention Care and Screening Test Guidelines for Adults

Chapter Contents

Section 5.1

Men's Health Screening Recommendations

This section includes excerpts from "Men: Stay Healthy at Any Age," Agency for Healthcare Research and Quality (AHRQ), September 2010; and excerpts from "Screening Tests and Immunizations Guidelines for Men," Office on Women's Health, March 18, 2010.

Get the Screenings You Need

Screenings are tests that look for diseases before you have symptoms. Blood pressure checks and tests for high cholesterol are examples of screenings. You can get some screenings, such as blood pressure readings, in your doctor's office. Others such as colonoscopy, a test for colorectal cancer, need special equipment, so you may need to go to a different office. After a screening test, ask when you will see the results and who you should talk to about them.

Common Screening Recommendations for Men

Abdominal aortic aneurysm: If you are between the ages of 65 and 75 and have ever been a smoker, talk to your doctor or nurse about being screened for abdominal aortic aneurysm (AAA). AAA is a bulging in your abdominal aorta, the largest artery in your body. An AAA may burst, which can cause dangerous bleeding and death.

Colorectal cancer: Have a screening test for colorectal cancer starting at age 50. If you have a family history of colorectal cancer, you may need to be screened earlier. Several different tests can detect this cancer. Your doctor can help you decide which is best for you.

Depression: Your emotional health is as important as your physical health. Talk to your doctor or nurse about being screened for depression especially if during the last two weeks you have felt down, sad, or hopeless, or you have felt little interest or pleasure in doing things.

Diabetes: Get screened for diabetes if your blood pressure is higher than 135/80 or if you take medication for high blood pressure. Diabetes (high blood sugar) can cause problems with your heart, brain, eyes, feet, kidneys, nerves, and other body parts.

High blood pressure: Starting at age 18, have your blood pressure checked at least every two years. High blood pressure is 140/90 or higher. High blood pressure can cause strokes, heart attacks, kidney and eye problems, and heart failure.

High cholesterol: If you are 35 or older, have your cholesterol checked. If the following are true, have your cholesterol checked starting at age 20:

- You use tobacco.

- You are obese.

- You have diabetes or high blood pressure.

- You have a personal history of heart disease or blocked arteries.

- A man in your family had a heart attack before age 50, or a woman relative had one before age 60.

Human immunodeficiency virus (HIV): Talk with your health care team about HIV screening if any of these apply to you:

- You have had unprotected sex with multiple partners.

- You have sex with men.

- You use or have used injection drugs.

- You exchange sex for money or drugs or have sex partners who do.

- You have or had a sex partner who is HIV-infected or injects drugs.

- You are being treated for a sexually transmitted disease.

- You had a blood transfusion between 1978 and 1985.

- You have any other concerns.

Syphilis: Ask your doctor or nurse whether you should be screened for syphilis.

Overweight and obesity: The best way to learn if you are overweight or obese is to find your body mass index (BMI). You can find your BMI by entering your height and weight into a BMI calculator, such as the one available at: http://www.nhlbisupport.com/bmi. A BMI between 18.5 and 25 indicates a normal weight. Persons with a BMI of 30 or higher may be obese. If you are obese, talk to your doctor or nurse about seeking intensive counseling and getting help with changing your

Table 5.1. Medical Screening Tests for Men

Screening Tests	Ages 18–39	Ages 40–49	Ages 50–64	Ages 65 and Older
General Health: Full checkup, including weight and height	Discuss with your doctor or nurse.	Discuss with your doctor or nurse.	Discuss with your doctor or nurse.	Discuss with your doctor or nurse.
HIV test	Get this test at least once to find out your HIV status. Ask your doctor if and when you need the test again.	Get this test at least once to find out your HIV status. Ask your doctor if and when you need the test again.	Get this test at least once to find out your HIV status. Ask your doctor if and when you need the test again.	Discuss with your doctor.
Heart Health: Blood pressure test	At least every 2 years	At least every 2 years	At least every 2 years	At least every 2 years
Cholesterol test	Start at age 20, discuss with your doctor or nurse.	Discuss with your doctor or nurse.	Discuss with your doctor or nurse.	Discuss with your doctor or nurse.
Diabetes: Blood glucose or A1c test		Start at age 45, then every 3 years	Every 3 years	Every 3 years
Prostate Health: Digital rectal exam (DRE)		Discuss with your doctor or nurse.	Discuss with your doctor or nurse.	Discuss with your doctor or nurse.
Prostate-specific antigen (PSA) test		Discuss with your doctor or nurse.	Discuss with your doctor or nurse.	Discuss with your doctor or nurse.
Reproductive Health: Testicular exam	Discuss with your doctor or nurse.	Discuss with your doctor or nurse.	Discuss with your doctor or nurse.	Discuss with your doctor or nurse.
Sexually transmitted infection (STI) tests	Both partners should get tested for STIs, including HIV, before initiating sexual intercourse.	Both partners should get tested for STIs, including HIV, before initiating sexual intercourse.	Both partners should get tested for STIs, including HIV, before initiating sexual intercourse.	Both partners should get tested for STIs, including HIV, before initiating sexual intercourse.

Table 5.1. *continued*

Screening Tests	Ages 18–39	Ages 40–49	Ages 50–64	Ages 65 and Older
Colorectal Health (use 1 of these 3 methods): Fecal occult blood test			Yearly	Yearly. Older than age 75, discuss with your doctor.
Flexible sigmoidoscopy (with fecal occult blood test)			Every 5 years	Every 5 years. Older than age 75, discuss with your doctor.
Colonoscopy			Every 10 years	Every 10 years. Older than age 75, discuss with your doctor.
Eye and Ear Health: Comprehensive eye exam	Discuss with your doctor.	Get a baseline exam at age 40, then every 2–4 years or as your doctor advises.	Every 2–4 years until age 55, then every 1–3 years until age 65, or as your doctor advises	Every 1–2 years
Hearing test	Starting at age 18, then every 10 years	Every 10 years	Every 3 years	Every 3 years
Skin Health: Mole exam	Monthly mole self-exam; by a doctor as part of a routine full checkup starting at age 20.	Monthly mole self-exam; by a doctor as part of your routine full checkup.	Monthly mole self-exam; by a doctor as part of your routine full checkup.	Monthly mole self-exam; by a doctor as part of your routine full checkup.
Oral Health: Dental exam	Routinely; discuss with your dentist.	Routinely; discuss with your dentist.	Routinely; discuss with your dentist.	Routinely; discuss with your dentist.
Mental Health Screening	Discuss with your doctor or nurse.	Discuss with your doctor or nurse.	Discuss with your doctor or nurse.	Discuss with your doctor or nurse.

47

Table 5.2. Medical Screening Tests for Women

Screening tests	Ages 19–39	Ages 40–49	Ages 50–64	Ages 65 and older
General health: Full checkup, including weight and height. Ask your doctor or nurse about health topics such as: overweight and obesity, tobacco use, alcohol use, depression, thyroid (TSH) testing, skin and mole exam	Discuss with your doctor or nurse.	Discuss with your doctor or nurse.	Discuss with your doctor or nurse.	Discuss with your doctor or nurse.
HIV test	At least once to find out your HIV status. Ask your doctor or nurse if and when you need the test again.	At least once to find out your HIV status. Ask your doctor or nurse if and when you need the test again.	At least once to find out your HIV status. Ask your doctor or nurse if and when you need the test again.	Discuss with your doctor or nurse.
Heart health: Blood pressure test	At least every 2 years	At least every 2 years	At least every 2 years	At least every 2 years
Cholesterol test	Start at age 20, discuss with your doctor or nurse.	Discuss with your doctor or nurse.	Discuss with your doctor or nurse.	Discuss with your doctor or nurse.
Bone health: Bone mineral density test			Discuss with your doctor or nurse.	At least once. Talk to your doctor or nurse about repeat testing.
Diabetes: Blood glucose or A1c test	Discuss with your doctor or nurse	Start at age 45, then every 3 years.	Every 3 years	Every 3 years
Breast health: Mammogram (x-ray of breast)		Every 1–2 years. Discuss with your doctor or nurse.	Every 1–2 years. Discuss with your doctor or nurse.	Every 1–2 years. Discuss with your doctor or nurse.
Clinical breast exam	Discuss with your doctor or nurse.	Discuss with your doctor or nurse.	Discuss with your doctor or nurse.	Discuss with your doctor or nurse.

Table 5.2. *continued*

Screening tests	Ages 19–39	Ages 40–49	Ages 50–64	Ages 65 and older
Reproductive health: Pap test	Every 2 years starting at age 21. Women 30 and older, every 3 years.	Every 3 years	Every 3 years	Discuss with your doctor or nurse.
Pelvic exam	Yearly beginning at age 21. Younger than 21 and sexually active, discuss with your doctor or nurse.	Yearly	Yearly	Yearly
Chlamydia test	Yearly until age 24 if sexually active. Age 25 and older, get this test if you have new or multiple partners.	Get this test if you have new or multiple partners.	Get this test if you have new or multiple partners.	Get this test if you have new or multiple partners.
Sexually transmitted infection (STI) tests	Discuss with your doctor or nurse.	Discuss with your doctor or nurse.	Discuss with your doctor or nurse.	Discuss with your doctor or nurse.
Colorectal health: Many tests can screen for colorectal cancer.			Talk to your doctor or nurse about which test is best for you and how often you need it.	Talk to your doctor or nurse about which test is best for you and how often you need it.
Eye and ear health: Comprehensive eye exam	Discuss with your doctor or nurse.	Get a baseline exam at age 40, then every 2–4 years or as your doctor advises.	Every 2–4 years until age 55, then every 1–3 years until age 65, or as your doctor advises.	Every 1–2 years
Hearing screening	Every 10 years	Every 10 years	Every 3 years	Every 3 years
Oral health: Dental and oral cancer exam	Routinely; discuss with your dentist.	Routinely; discuss with your dentist.	Routinely; discuss with your dentist.	Routinely; discuss with your dentist.

behaviors to lose weight. Overweight and obesity can lead to diabetes and cardiovascular disease.

Screening Tests for Men by Age Groups

Table 5.1 provides guidelines only. Your doctor or nurse will personalize the timing of each test to meet your health care needs.

Section 5.2

Women's Health Screening Recommendations

This section includes excerpts from "Women: Stay Healthy at Any Age," Agency for Healthcare Research and Quality (AHRQ), September 2010; and, excerpts from "General Screenings and Immunizations for Women," Office on Women's Health, February 28, 2011.

Get the Screenings You Need

Screenings are tests that look for diseases before you have symptoms. Blood pressure checks and mammograms are examples of screenings. You can get some screenings, such as blood pressure readings, in your doctor's office. Others, such as mammograms, need special equipment, so you may need to go to a different office. After a screening test, ask when you will see the results and who to talk to about them.

Common Screening Recommendations Tests for Women

Breast cancer: Ask your health care team whether a mammogram is right for you based on your age, family history, overall health, and personal concerns.

Cervical cancer: Have a Pap smear every 1–3 years if you are 21 to 65 years old and have been sexually active. If you are older than 65 and recent Pap smears were normal, you do not need a Pap smear. If you have had a hysterectomy for a reason other than cancer, you do not need a Pap smear.

Chlamydia and other sexually transmitted diseases: Sexually transmitted diseases can make it hard to get pregnant, may affect your baby, and can cause other health problems. Have a screening test for Chlamydia if you are 24 or younger and sexually active. If you are older than 24, talk to your health care team about being screened for Chlamydia. Ask your doctor or nurse whether you should be screened for other sexually transmitted diseases.

Colorectal cancer: Have a screening test for colorectal cancer starting at age 50. If you have a family history of colorectal cancer, you may need to be screened earlier. Several different tests can detect this cancer. Your health care team can help you decide which is best for you.

Depression: Your emotional health is as important as your physical health. Talk to your health care team about being screened for depression, especially if during the last two weeks: You have felt down, sad, or hopeless; and/or, you have felt little interest or pleasure in doing things.

Diabetes: Get screened for diabetes if your blood pressure is higher than 135/80 or if you take medication for high blood pressure. Diabetes (high blood sugar) can cause problems with your heart, brain, eyes, feet, kidneys, nerves, and other body parts.

High blood pressure: Starting at age 18, have your blood pressure checked at least every two years. High blood pressure is 140/90 or higher. High blood pressure can cause stroke, heart attack, kidney and eye problems, and heart failure.

High cholesterol: Starting at age 20, have your cholesterol checked regularly if the following applies:

- You use tobacco.
- You are obese.
- You have diabetes or high blood pressure.
- You have a personal history of heart disease or blocked arteries.
- A man in your family had a heart attack before age 50, or a woman relative had one before age 60.

Human immunodeficiency virus (HIV): Talk with your health care team about HIV screening if any of these apply to you:

- You have had unprotected sex with multiple partners.

51

- You have injected drugs.

- You exchange sex for money or drugs or have sex partners who do.

- You have or had a sex partner who is HIV-infected, bisexual, or injects drugs.

- You are being treated for a sexually transmitted disease.

- You had a blood transfusion between 1978 and 1985.

- You have any other concerns.

Osteoporosis (bone thinning): Have a screening test at age 65 to make sure your bones are strong. If you are younger than 65, talk to your health care team about whether you should be tested.

Overweight and obesity: The best way to learn if you are overweight or obese is to find your body mass index (BMI). You can find your BMI by entering your height and weight into a BMI calculator, such as the one available at: http://www.nhlbisupport.com/bmi. A BMI between 18.5 and 25 indicates a normal weight. Persons with a BMI of 30 or higher may be obese. If you are obese, talk to your doctor or nurse about seeking intensive counseling and help with changing your behaviors to lose weight. Overweight and obesity can lead to diabetes and cardiovascular disease.

Screening Tests for Women by Age Groups

Table 5.2 provides guidelines only. Your doctor or nurse will personalize the timing of each test to meet your health care needs. Check with your insurance plan to find out which tests are covered.

Chapter 6

Common Screenings in Your Doctor's Office

Chapter Contents

Section 6.1

Assessing Weight and Health Risk

Excerpted from "Assessing Your Weight and Health Risk,"
National Heart, Lung, and Blood Institute (NHLBI), 2010.

Assessment of weight and health risk involves using three key measures:

1. Body mass index (BMI)

2. Waist circumference

3. Risk factors for diseases and conditions associated with obesity

Body Mass Index (BMI)

BMI is a useful measure of overweight and obesity. It is calculated from your height and weight. BMI is an estimate of body fat and a good gauge of your risk for diseases that can occur with more body fat. The higher your BMI, the higher your risk for certain diseases such as heart disease, high blood pressure, type 2 diabetes, gallstones, breathing problems, and certain cancers.

Although BMI can be used for most men and women, it does have some limits:

- It may overestimate body fat in athletes and others who have a muscular build.

- It may underestimate body fat in older persons and others who have lost muscle.

Use the BMI calculator (http://www.nhlbisupport.com/bmi/bmicalc .htm), or BMI tables (http://www.nhlbi.nih.gov/guidelines/obesity/ bmi_tbl.htm), to estimate your body fat. The BMI calculator is also available in a mobile application. This tool provides results right on your iphone along with links to healthy weight resources (http://apps .usa.gov/bmi-app).

The BMI score means the following:

- BMI below 18.5 is underweight

- BMI of 18.5–24.9 is normal

- BMI of 25.0–29.9 is overweight

- BMI of 30.0 and above indicates obesity

Waist Circumference

Measuring waist circumference helps screen for possible health risks that come with overweight and obesity. If most of your fat is around your waist rather than at your hips, you're at a higher risk for heart disease and type 2 diabetes. This risk goes up with a waist size that is greater than 35 inches for women or greater than 40 inches for men. To correctly measure your waist, stand and place a tape measure around your middle, just above your hipbones. Measure your waist just after you breathe out. Table 6.1 provides you with an idea of whether your BMI combined with your waist circumference increases your risk for developing obesity-associated diseases or conditions.

Table 6.1. Classification of Overweight and Obesity by BMI, Waist Circumference, and Associated Disease Risks

	BMI(kg/m^2)	Obesity Class	Disease Risk* Relative to Normal Weight and Waist Circumference	
			Men 102 cm (40 in) or less / Women 88 cm (35 in) or less	Men over 102 cm (40 in) / Women over 88 cm (35 in)
Underweight	less than 18.5			
Normal	18.5–24.9			
Overweight	25.0–29.9		Increased	High
Obesity	30.0–34.9	I	High	Very High
	35.0–39.9	II	Very High	Very High
Extreme Obesity	40.0 +	III	Extremely High	Extremely High

*Disease risk for type 2 diabetes, hypertension, and cardiovascular disease.
+Increased waist circumference also can be a marker for increased risk, even in persons of normal weight.

Section 6.2

High Blood Pressure Screening

Excerpted from "High Blood Pressure," National Heart,
Lung, and Blood Institute (NHLBI), November 2008.

High blood pressure (HBP) is a serious condition that can lead
to coronary heart disease, heart failure, stroke, kidney failure, and
other health problems. Blood pressure is the force of blood pushing
against the walls of the arteries as the heart pumps out blood. If this
pressure rises and stays high over time, it can damage the body in
many ways.

Overview

About one in three adults in the United States has HBP. HBP itself
usually has no symptoms. You can have it for years without knowing
it. During this time, though, it can damage the heart, blood vessels,
kidneys, and other parts of your body. This is why knowing your blood
pressure numbers is important, even when you are feeling fine. If your
blood pressure is normal, you can work with your health care team to
keep it that way. If your blood pressure is too high, you need treatment
to prevent damage to your body's organs.

Blood Pressure Numbers

Blood pressure numbers include systolic and diastolic pressures.
Systolic blood pressure is the pressure when the heart beats while
pumping blood. Diastolic blood pressure is the pressure when the
heart is at rest between beats. You will most often see blood pressure
numbers written with the systolic number above or before the diastolic,
such as 120/80 mmHg. (The mmHg is millimeters of mercury—the
units used to measure blood pressure.)

Table 6.2 shows normal numbers for adults. It also shows which numbers put you at greater risk for health problems. Blood pressure tends
to go up and down, even in people who have normal blood pressure. If
your numbers stay above normal most of the time, you're at risk.

Table 6.2. Categories for Blood Pressure Levels in Adults (in mmHg, or millimeters of mercury)

Category	Systolic (top number)		Diastolic (bottom number)
Normal	Less than 120	and	Less than 80
Prehypertension	120–139	or	80–89
High blood pressure			
Stage 1	140–159	or	90–99
Stage 2	160 or higher	or	100 or higher

The ranges in the table apply to most adults (aged 18 and older) who do not have short-term serious illnesses.
All levels above 120/80 mmHg raise your risk, and the risk grows as blood pressure levels rise.

Your systolic and diastolic numbers may not be in the same blood pressure category. In this case, the more severe category is the one you are in. For example, if your systolic number is 160 and your diastolic number is 80, you have stage 2 HBP. If your systolic number is 120 and your diastolic number is 95, you have stage 1 HBP.

If you have diabetes or chronic kidney disease, HBP is defined as 130/80 mmHg or higher. HBP numbers also differ for children and teens.

Other Names for High Blood Pressure

- High blood pressure (HBP) also is called hypertension.

- When HBP has no known cause, it may be called essential hypertension, primary hypertension, or idiopathic hypertension.

- When another condition causes HBP, it is sometimes called secondary high blood pressure or secondary hypertension.

- In some cases of HBP, only the systolic blood pressure number is high. This condition is called isolated systolic hypertension (ISH). Many older adults have this condition. ISH can cause as much harm as HBP in which both numbers are too high.

Knowing your blood pressure numbers is important, even when you are feeling fine. If your blood pressure is normal, you can work with your health care team to keep it that way. If your numbers are too high, you can take steps to lower them and control your blood pressure. This helps reduce your risk for complications.

How Is High Blood Pressure Diagnosed?

Your doctor will diagnose high blood pressure (HBP) using the results of blood pressure tests. These tests will be done several times to make sure the results are correct. If your numbers are high, your doctor may have you return for more tests to check your blood pressure over time. If your blood pressure is 140/90 mmHg or higher over time, your doctor will likely diagnose you with HBP. If you have diabetes or chronic kidney disease, a blood pressure of 130/80 mmHg or higher is considered HBP. The HBP ranges in children are different.

How Is Blood Pressure Tested?

A blood pressure test is easy and painless. This test is done at a doctor's office or clinic. To prepare for the test:

- Do not drink coffee or smoke cigarettes for 30 minutes prior to the test. These actions may cause a short-term rise in your blood pressure.

- Go to the bathroom before the test. Having a full bladder can change your blood pressure reading.

- Sit for five minutes before the test. Movement can cause short-term rises in blood pressure.

To measure your blood pressure, your doctor or nurse will use some type of a gauge, a stethoscope (or electronic sensor), and a blood pressure cuff. Most often, you will sit or lie down with the cuff around your arm as your doctor or nurse checks your blood pressure. If he or she does not tell you what your blood pressure numbers are, you should ask.

Diagnosing High Blood Pressure in Children and Teens

Doctors measure blood pressure in children and teens the same way they do in adults. Your child should have routine blood pressure checks starting at three years of age. Blood pressure normally rises with age and body size. Newborn babies often have very low blood pressure numbers, while older teens have numbers similar to adults. The ranges for normal blood pressure and HBP are generally lower for youth than for adults. These ranges are based on the average blood pressure numbers for age, gender, and height. To find out whether a child has HBP, a doctor will compare the child's blood pressure numbers to average numbers for his or her age, height, and gender.

Section 6.3

Cholesterol Screening for Adults and Children

This section includes excerpts from "High Blood Cholesterol," National Heart, Lung, and Blood Institute (NHLBI), September 2008, and an excerpt from "September Is National Cholesterol Education Month," Centers for Disease Control and Prevention (CDC), August 25, 2010.

To understand high blood cholesterol, it is important to know more about cholesterol.

- Cholesterol is a waxy, fat-like substance that is found in all cells of the body. Your body needs some cholesterol to work the right way. Your body makes all the cholesterol it needs.

- Cholesterol is also found in some of the foods you eat.

- Your body uses cholesterol to make hormones, vitamin D, and substances that help you digest foods.

Blood is watery, and cholesterol is fatty. Just like oil and water, the two do not mix. To travel in the bloodstream, cholesterol is carried in small packages called lipoproteins. The small packages are made of fat (lipid) on the inside and proteins on the outside. Two kinds of lipoproteins carry cholesterol throughout your body. It is important to have healthy levels of both:

- Low-density lipoprotein (LDL) cholesterol is sometimes called bad cholesterol. High LDL cholesterol leads to a buildup of cholesterol in arteries. The higher the LDL level in your blood, the greater chance you have of getting heart disease.

- High-density lipoprotein (HDL) cholesterol is sometimes called good cholesterol. HDL carries cholesterol from other parts of your body back to your liver. The liver removes the cholesterol from your body. The higher your HDL cholesterol level, the lower your chance of getting heart disease.

Everyone age 20 and older should have their cholesterol levels checked at least once every five years. You and your doctor can discuss how often you should be tested.

How is high blood cholesterol diagnosed?

High blood cholesterol is diagnosed by checking levels of cholesterol in your blood. It is best to have a blood test called a lipoprotein profile to measure your cholesterol levels. You will need to not eat or drink anything (fast) for 9–12 hours before taking the test.

The lipoprotein profile will give information about the following:

- Total cholesterol

- Low-density lipoprotein (LDL) bad cholesterol: the main source of cholesterol buildup and blockage in the arteries

- High-density lipoprotein (HDL) good cholesterol: the good cholesterol that helps keep cholesterol from building up in arteries

- Triglycerides: another form of fat in your blood

If it is not possible to get a lipoprotein profile done, knowing your total cholesterol and HDL cholesterol can give you a general idea about your cholesterol levels. Testing for total and HDL cholesterol does not require fasting. If your total cholesterol is 200 mg/dL or more, or if your HDL is less than 40 mg/dL, you will need to have a lipoprotein profile done.

Cholesterol levels are measured in milligrams (mg) of cholesterol per deciliter (dL) of blood.

Table 6.3. Total Cholesterol

Total Cholesterol Level	Total Cholesterol Category
Less than 200 mg/dL	Desirable
200–239 mg/dL	Borderline high
240 mg/dL and above	High

Table 6.4. LDL Cholesterol

LDL Cholesterol Level	LDL Cholesterol Category
Less than 100 mg/dL	Optimal
100–129 mg/dL	Near optimal/above optimal
130–159 mg/dL	Borderline high
160–189 mg/dL	High
190 mg/dL and above	Very high

Table 6.5. HDL Cholesterol

HDL Cholesterol Level	HDL Cholesterol Category
Less than 40 mg/dL	A major risk factor for heart disease
40–59 mg/dL	The higher, the better
60 mg/dL and above	Considered protective against heart disease

Triglycerides can also raise your risk for heart disease. If you have levels that are borderline high (150–199 mg/dL) or high (200 mg/dL or more), you may need treatment.

Can children and adolescents have high cholesterol?

Yes. High cholesterol can develop in early childhood and adolescence, and your risk increases as your weight increases. In the United States, more than one-fifth (20%) of youth aged 12–19 years have at least one abnormal lipid level. It is important for children over two years of age to have their cholesterol checked, if they are overweight/obese, have a family history of high cholesterol, a family history of heart disease, diabetes, high blood pressure, or certain chronic condition (chronic kidney disease, chronic inflammatory diseases, congenital heart disease, and childhood cancer survivorship).

Table 6.6 shows optimal lipid levels for children and adolescents (aged 2–18 years).

Table 6.6. Desirable Cholesterol Levels for Children and Adolescents

Total Cholesterol	Less than 170 mg/dL
Low LDL (bad) cholesterol	Less than 110 mg/dL
High HDL (good) cholesterol	35 mg/dL or higher
Triglycerides	Less than 150 mg/dL

Chapter 7

Genetic Testing

Chapter Contents

Section 7.1

Frequently Asked Questions about Genetic Testing

Excerpted from "Frequently Asked Questions about Genetic Testing," National Human Genome Research Institute, November 26, 2010.

Genetic research is leading to the development of more genetic tests that can be used for the diagnosis of genetic conditions. Genetic testing is available for infants, children, and adults. Genetic tests can be used to diagnose a disease in an individual with symptoms and to help measure risk of developing a disease. Adults can undergo preconception testing before deciding to become pregnant, and prenatal testing can be performed during a pregnancy. Results of genetic tests can help physicians select appropriate treatments for their patients.

What is genetic testing?

Genetic tests look for alterations in a person's genes or changes in the level or structure of key proteins coded for by specific genes. Genetic tests can also be used to look at levels of ribonucleic acid (RNA) that play a role in certain conditions. Abnormal results on these tests could mean that someone has a genetic disorder.

Types of genetic tests include:

- gene tests (individual genes or relatively short lengths of deoxyribonucleic acid (DNA) or RNA are tested),

- chromosomal tests (whole chromosomes or very long lengths of DNA are tested), and

- biochemical tests (protein levels or enzyme activities are tested).

What is a gene test?

Gene tests look for signs of a disease or disorder in DNA or RNA taken from a person's blood, other body fluids like saliva, or tissues. These tests can look for large changes, such as a gene that has a section missing or added, or small changes, such as a missing, added, or altered chemical base (subunit) within the DNA strand. Gene tests may also detect genes with too many copies, individual genes that are too active, genes that are turned off, or genes that are lost entirely.

Gene tests examine a person's DNA in a variety of ways. Some tests use DNA probes. A probe is a short string of DNA with base sequence complementary to (able to bind with) the sequence of an altered gene. Another type of gene test relies on DNA or RNA sequencing. This test directly compares the base-by-base sequence of DNA or RNA in a patient's sample to a normal version of the DNA or RNA sequence.

What is a biochemical test?

Biochemical tests look at the amounts or activities of key proteins. Since genes contain the DNA code for making proteins, abnormal amounts or activities of proteins can signal genes that are not working normally. These types of tests are often used for newborn screening.

What information can genetic testing give?

Genetic testing can do the following:

1. Give a diagnosis if someone has symptoms.

2. Show whether a person is a carrier for a genetic disease. Carriers have an altered gene, but will not get the disease. However, they can pass the altered gene on to their children.

3. Help expectant parents know whether an unborn child will have a genetic condition. This is called prenatal testing.

4. Screen newborn infants for abnormal or missing proteins that can cause disease. This is called newborn screening.

5. Show whether a person has an inherited disposition to a certain disease before symptoms start.

6. Determine the type or dose of a medicine that is best for a certain person. This is called pharmacogenetics.

What are reasons to get different types of genetic tests?

Diagnostic testing is used to confirm a diagnosis when a person has signs or symptoms that suggest a genetic disease. The particular genetic test used depends on the disease for which a person is tested, for example testing for Down syndrome or Duchenne muscular dystrophy.

Predictive testing can show which people have a higher chance of getting a disease before symptoms appear. For example, one type of predictive test screens for inherited genetic risk factors that make it more likely for someone to develop certain cancers, such as colon or breast cancer, or diseases that usually develop later in life, such as adult onset (type 2) diabetes. Someone with an inherited genetic risk factor may have an increased chance of getting a disease, although this does not mean that the person will certainly get the disease.

Presymptomatic is a type of predictive testing that can indicate which family members are at risk for a certain genetic condition already known to be present in their family. This type of testing is done with people who do not yet show symptoms of that disease.

Preconception/carrier testing can tell individuals if they have (carry) a gene alteration for a type of inherited disorder called an autosomal recessive disorder. Autosomal means that the altered gene is on one of the 22 chromosomes other than the sex chromosomes (X or Y chromosomes). Recessive means that the person with only one altered copy of the disease gene will not get the disease, but might pass the alteration to their children. If both parents are carriers, their children might inherit an alteration from each parent and get the disease. Examples of autosomal recessive disorders are cystic fibrosis and Tay-Sachs disease.

Prenatal testing is available to pregnant women during pregnancy. Some reasons to have genetic testing include these:

- Age of the mother. Women age 35 or older are at a higher risk for having a child with chromosomal abnormalities or other birth defects. However, some tests are recommended for all pregnant women, regardless of age.

- A family history of an inherited condition such as Duchenne muscular dystrophy.

- Ancestry or ethnic background indicating that the parents might have a higher chance of carrying an inherited disorder.

- Screening for common genetic disorders that may occur during pregnancy, such as Down syndrome or spina bifida.

Three diagnostic procedures are common in prenatal testing: ultrasound, amniocentesis, and chorionic villus sampling (CVS). Ultrasound uses the reflection of sound waves to create an overall picture of the developing fetus. Amniocentesis involves testing a sample of amniotic fluid from the womb surrounding the fetus. CVS involves taking a tiny sample of tissue from a region of the placenta that carries fetal cells rather than maternal cells.

Newborn screening is the most widespread type of genetic testing. It is an important public health program that can find disorders in newborns that might have long-term health effects.

Pharmacogenetic testing examines a person's genes to understand how drugs may move through the body and be broken down.

How do I decide whether to be tested?

People have many different reasons for being tested or not being tested. For many, it is important to know whether a disease can be prevented if a gene alteration causing a disease is found. Pharmacogenetic testing can indicate the best medicine or dose of a medicine for a certain person.

Section 7.2

Genetic Consultation

Excerpted from "Genetic Consultation,"
Genetics Home Reference, March 13, 2011.

What is a genetic consultation?

A genetic consultation is a health service that provides information and support to people who have, or may be at risk for, genetic disorders. During a consultation, a genetics professional meets with an individual or family to discuss genetic risks or to diagnose, confirm, or rule out a genetic condition.

Genetics professionals include medical geneticists (doctors who specialize in genetics) and genetic counselors (certified health care workers with experience in medical genetics and counseling). Other health care professionals such as nurses, psychologists, and social workers trained in genetics can also provide genetic consultations.

Why might someone have a genetic consultation?

Individuals or families who are concerned about an inherited condition may benefit from a genetic consultation. The reasons that a person might be referred to a genetic counselor, medical geneticist, or other genetics professional include:

- A personal or family history of a genetic condition, birth defect, chromosomal disorder, or hereditary cancer.

- Two or more pregnancy losses (miscarriages), a stillbirth, or a baby who died.

- A child with a known inherited disorder, a birth defect, mental retardation, or developmental delay.

- A woman who is pregnant or plans to become pregnant at or after age 35. (Some chromosomal disorders occur more frequently in children born to older women.)

- Abnormal test results that suggest a genetic or chromosomal condition.

- An increased risk of developing or passing on a particular genetic disorder on the basis of a person's ethnic background.

- People related by blood (for example, cousins) who plan to have children together. (A child whose parents are related may be at an increased risk of inheriting certain genetic disorders.)

A genetic consultation is also an important part of the decision-making process for genetic testing. A visit with a genetics professional may be helpful even if testing is not available for a specific condition, however.

What happens during a genetic consultation?

A genetic consultation provides information, offers support, and addresses a patient's specific questions and concerns. To help determine whether a condition has a genetic component, a genetics professional asks about a person's medical history and takes a detailed family history (a record of health information about a person's immediate and extended family). The genetics professional may also perform a physical examination and recommend appropriate tests.

If a person is diagnosed with a genetic condition, the genetics professional provides information about the diagnosis, how the condition is inherited, the chance of passing the condition to future generations, and the options for testing and treatment.

During a consultation, a genetics professional will:

• interpret and communicate complex medical information;

• help each person make informed, independent decisions about their health care and reproductive options;

• respect each person's individual beliefs, traditions, and feelings.

A genetics professional will not:

• tell a person which decision to make,

• advise a couple not to have children,

• recommend that a woman continue or end a pregnancy, or

• tell someone whether to undergo testing for a genetic disorder.

Section 7.3

Genetic Testing for Breast Cancer Risk

Excerpted from "BRCA1 and BRCA2: Cancer Risk and
Genetic Testing," National Cancer Institute (NCI), May 29, 2009.

What are BRCA1 (breast cancer susceptibility gene1) and BRCA2?

BRCA1 and BRCA2 are human genes that belong to a class of genes known as tumor suppressors. In normal cells, BRCA1 and BRCA2 help ensure the stability of the cell's genetic material (deoxyribonucleic acid [DNA]) and help prevent uncontrolled cell growth. Mutation of these genes has been linked to the development of hereditary breast and ovarian cancer.

The names BRCA1 and BRCA2 stand for breast cancer susceptibility gene 1 and breast cancer susceptibility gene 2, respectively.

Are genetic tests available to detect BRCA1 and BRCA2 mutations, and how are they performed?

Yes. Several methods are available to test for BRCA1 and BRCA2 mutations. Most of these methods look for changes in BRCA1 and

BRCA2 DNA. At least one method looks for changes in the proteins produced by these genes. Frequently, a combination of methods is used.

A blood sample is needed for these tests. The blood is drawn in a laboratory, doctor's office, hospital, or clinic and then sent to a laboratory that specializes in the tests. It usually takes several weeks or longer to get the test results. Individuals who decide to get tested should check with their health care provider to find out when their test results might be available.

Genetic counseling is generally recommended before and after a genetic test. This counseling should be performed by a health care professional who is experienced in cancer genetics. Genetic counseling usually involves a risk assessment based on the individual's personal and family medical history and discussions about the appropriateness of genetic testing, the specific test(s) that might be used and the technical accuracy of the test(s), the medical implications of a positive or a negative test result, the possibility that a test result might not be informative (an ambiguous result), the psychological risks and benefits of genetic test results, and the risk of passing a mutation to children.

How much does BRCA1 and BRCA2 mutation testing cost?

The cost for BRCA1 and BRCA2 mutation testing usually ranges from several hundred to several thousand dollars. Insurance policies vary with regard to whether or not the cost of testing is covered. People who are considering BRCA1 and BRCA2 mutation testing may want to find out about their insurance company's policies regarding genetic tests.

What does a positive BRCA1 or BRCA2 test result mean?

A positive test result generally indicates that a person has inherited a known harmful mutation in BRCA1 or BRCA2 and, therefore, has an increased risk of developing certain cancers, as described earlier. However, a positive test result provides information only about a person's risk of developing cancer. It cannot tell whether an individual will actually develop cancer or when. Not all women who inherit a harmful BRCA1 or BRCA2 mutation will develop breast or ovarian cancer.

A positive genetic test result may have important health and social implications for family members, including future generations. Unlike most other medical tests, genetic tests can reveal information not only about the person being tested but also about that person's relatives. Men and women who inherit harmful BRCA1 or BRCA2 mutations (whether they develop cancer themselves or not) may pass the mutations on to their sons and daughters. However, not all children of people who have a harmful mutation will inherit the mutation.

What does a negative BRCA1 or BRCA2 test result mean?

How a negative test result will be interpreted depends on whether or not someone in the tested person's family is known to carry a harmful BRCA1 or BRCA2 mutation. If someone in the family has a known mutation, testing other family members for the same mutation can provide information about their cancer risk. If a person tests negative for a known mutation in his or her family, it is unlikely that they have an inherited susceptibility to cancer associated with BRCA1 or BRCA2. Such a test result is called a true negative. Having a true negative test result does not mean that a person will not develop cancer; it means that the person's risk of cancer is probably the same as that of people in the general population.

In cases in which a family has a history of breast and/or ovarian cancer and no known mutation in BRCA1 or BRCA2 has been previously identified, a negative test result is not informative. It is not possible to tell whether an individual has a harmful BRCA1 or BRCA2 mutation that was not detected by testing (a false negative) or whether the result is a true negative. In addition, it is possible for people to have a mutation in a gene other than BRCA1 or BRCA2 that increases their cancer risk but is not detectable by the test(s) used.

What does an ambiguous BRCA1 or BRCA2 test result mean?

If genetic testing shows a change in BRCA1 or BRCA2 that has not been previously associated with cancer in other people, the person's test result may be interpreted as ambiguous (uncertain). One study found that 10% of women who underwent BRCA1 and BRCA2 mutation testing had this type of ambiguous result.

Because everyone has genetic differences that are not associated with an increased risk of disease, it is sometimes not known whether a specific DNA change affects a person's risk of developing cancer. As more research is conducted and more people are tested for BRCA1 or BRCA2 changes, scientists will learn more about these changes and cancer risk.

71

What are some of the benefits of genetic testing for breast and ovarian cancer risk?

There can be benefits to genetic testing, whether a person receives a positive or a negative result. The potential benefits of a negative result include a sense of relief and the possibility that special preventive checkups, tests, or surgeries may not be needed. A positive test result can bring relief from uncertainty and allow people to make informed decisions about their future, including taking steps to reduce their cancer risk. In addition, many people who have a positive test result may be able to participate in medical research that could, in the long run, help reduce deaths from breast cancer.

Chapter 8

Required Medical Screening of Immigrants to the United States

Medical Screening: General Information

The Division of Global Migration and Quarantine, of the Center for Disease Control and Prevention (CDC), provides the technical instructions and guidance to physicians conducting the medical examination for immigration. These instructions are developed in accordance with Section 212(a)(1)(A) of the Immigration and Nationality Act (INA), which states those classes of aliens ineligible for visas or admission based on health-related grounds. The health-related grounds include those aliens who have a communicable disease of public health significance, who fail to present documentation of having received vaccination against vaccine-preventable diseases (immigrants only), who have or have had a physical or mental disorder with associated harmful behavior, and who are drug abusers or addicts.

Who performs the medical examination?

Outside the United States, medical examinations are performed by physicians called panel physicians, who are selected by Department of State consular officials. In the United States, medical examinations are performed by physicians called civil surgeons, who are designated by district directors of the U.S. Citizenship and Immigration Services (USCIS).

Excerpted from "CDC Domestic Refugee Health Program: Frequently Asked Questions," Centers for Disease Control and Prevention (CDC), January 19, 2010.

73

A panel physician is a physician outside the United States who performs the medical examinations for refugees and individuals applying for an immigrant visa. These physicians are selected by Department of State consular officials.

A civil surgeon is a physician who performs medical examinations in the United States for aliens applying for adjustment of their immigration status to that of permanent resident. These physicians are designated by district directors of the U.S. Citizenship and Immigration Service.

Who is required to have a medical examination?

A medical examination is mandatory for all refugees coming to the United States and all applicants outside the United States applying for an immigrant visa. Aliens in the United States who apply for adjustment of their immigration status to that of permanent resident are also required to be medically examined. Aliens applying for nonimmigrant visas (temporary admission) may be required to undergo a medical examination at the discretion of the consular officer overseas or immigration officer at the U.S. port of entry, if there is reason to suspect that an inadmissible health-related condition exists. Asylees are not required to have a medical examination.

What is the required overseas medical screening for a refugee?

Overseas, U.S.-bound refugees must undergo a medical examination as part of the visa application process. The purpose of the medical examination is to identify the presence or absence of certain physical or mental disorders that could result in ineligibility for admission to (or exclusion from) the United States under the provisions of the Immigration and Nationality Act. Waivers of ineligibility are available for certain medical grounds of inadmissibility.

How long are laboratory results valid for?

The 1991 Technical Instructions for Medical Examination of Aliens do not address the validity of laboratory results. However, the physician who performs the exam is required to ensure that all medical tests are properly conducted and that test results are in fact those of the applicant and are current. A standard medical examination is valid for immigration purposes for one year from the date of the physician's signature.

What is the allowable time interval between the overseas examination (validity period) and U.S. arrival?

The allowable time interval between the completion of the overseas examination and U.S. arrival is 12 months. If the applicant has a Class A or tuberculosis (TB) classification, the interval is six months. For Hmong and Burmese refugees resettling from Thailand, the allowable time interval between the overseas examination and U.S. arrival is three months, regardless of whether the refugee has a TB classification. For Class B1 refugees, the 3-month interval begins when the culture results are reported; culture results are usually reported within eight weeks of sputum collection.

Part Two

Laboratory Tests

Chapter 9

Understanding
Laboratory Tests

Chapter Contents

Section 9.1

Introduction to Lab Tests

This section is excerpted from "Laboratory Tests,"
U.S. Food and Drug Administration (FDA), June 18, 2009.

Laboratory tests are medical procedures that involve testing samples of blood, urine, or other tissues or substances in the body.
Your doctor uses laboratory tests to help:

- identify changes in your health condition before any symptoms occur,

- diagnose a disease or condition before you have symptoms,

- plan your treatment for a disease or condition,

- evaluate your response to a treatment, and

- monitor the course of a disease over time.

How are lab tests analyzed?

After your doctor collects a sample from your body, it is sent to a laboratory. Laboratories perform tests on the sample to see if it reacts to different substances. Depending on the test, a reaction may mean you do have a particular condition or it may mean that you do not have the particular condition. Sometimes laboratories compare your results to results obtained from previous tests, to see if there has been a change in your condition.

What do lab tests show?

Lab tests show whether or not your results fall within normal ranges. Normal test values are usually given as a range, rather than as a specific number, because normal values vary from person to person. What is normal for one person may not be normal for another person.

Some laboratory tests are precise, reliable indicators of specific health problems, while others provide more general information that gives doctors clues to your possible health problems. Information obtained from laboratory tests may help doctors decide whether other tests or procedures are needed to make a diagnosis or to develop or revise a previous treatment plan. All laboratory test results must be interpreted within the context of your overall health and should be used along with other exams or tests.

What factors affect your lab test results?

Many factors can affect test results, including sex, age, race, medical history, general health, specific foods, drugs you are taking, how closely your follow preparatory instructions, variations in laboratory techniques, and variations from one laboratory to another.

Section 9.2

Identifying Quality Laboratory Services

"Helping You Identify Quality Laboratory Services,"
© The Joint Commission, 2010. Reprinted with permission.

Helping You Identify Quality Laboratory Services

Selecting quality health care services for yourself, a relative, or friend requires special thought and attention. The Joint Commission has prepared this information to help you make your selection. Knowing what to look for and what to ask will help you choose a laboratory that provides quality care and best meets your needs.

Although you may not always have the opportunity to choose the laboratory where your tests are processed, you can obtain some important information about the laboratory. By doing so, you will have confidence that your tests will be performed properly. Begin by asking your doctor why he/she selected the laboratory and then discuss specifics about the quality improvement processes the laboratory has in place.

General Questions

- What is the name and location of the laboratory?

- What criteria did your doctor use to choose the laboratory?
- Does the doctor have confidence in the accuracy of the test results?
- Does the laboratory notify the doctor if a specimen is incorrectly collected? What is the follow-up procedure?
- Has the doctor ever received an incorrect result from the laboratory? How did the doctor handle the situation?
- How are complaints about inaccurate test results handled?

Questions about Sample Collection

- Are you given instructions about how to prepare for the lab test (for example, no eating or drinking)?
- Does the laboratory give your doctor clear instructions about how to properly collect specimens? Is this information included in the office staff's orientation and training materials? Is it periodically updated?
- If you are collecting the specimen yourself, did you receive clear instructions?
- When the specimen was collected, did the technician use two identifiers to label the sample collection containers in your presence?

Questions about the Test Results

- How soon can you expect to learn the test results?
- How will you be informed of test results? Will you receive a personal phone call if there was an abnormal test result?
- Is there a number you can call if you have questions?

Quality Oversight

Is the laboratory accredited by a nationally recognized accrediting body such as The Joint Commission? Joint Commission accreditation means the organization voluntarily sought accreditation and met national health and safety standards. To find out if the laboratory you are considering is accredited by The Joint Commission:

Quality Check®
Phone: 630-792-5800
Website: http://www.qualitycheck.org

Quality Check provides Quality Reports that include information on the organization's overall performance level and how it compares to other organizations nationwide and statewide in specific performance areas.

To report information or concerns about accredited organizations:

Office of Quality Monitoring
Toll-Free: 800-994-6610
E-mail: complaint@jointcommission.org

Section 9.3

Deciphering Your Lab Report

This section includes "Deciphering Your Lab Report Overview," and information from "Reference Ranges and What They Mean," © 2011 American Association for Clinical Chemistry. Reprinted with permission. For additional information about clinical lab testing, visit the Lab Tests Online website at www.labtestsonline.org.

Overview

If you've had laboratory tests performed, you may have been given a copy of the report by the laboratory or your health care provider. If not, you may wish to request one from your physician. Once you get your report, however, it may not be easy for you to read or understand, leaving you with more questions than answers. This article points out some of the different sections that may be found on a typical lab report and explains some of the information that may be found in those sections.

Different laboratories generate reports that can vary greatly in appearance and in the order and kind of information included. Despite the differences in format and presentation, all laboratory reports must contain certain elements as mandated by federal legislation known as the Clinical Laboratory Improvement Amendments (CLIA). Your lab report may look very different than a sample report, but it will contain each of the elements required by CLIA. It may also contain additional items not specifically required but which the lab chooses to include to aid in the timely reporting, delivery, and interpretation of your results.

Some items included on lab reports deal with administrative or clerical information:

Patient name and identification number or a unique patient identifier and identification number: These are required for proper patient identification and to ensure that the test results included in the report are correctly linked to the patient on whom the tests were run.

Name and address of the laboratory location where the test was performed: Tests may be run in a physician office laboratory, a laboratory located in a clinic or hospital, and/or samples may be sent to a reference laboratory for analysis.

Date report printed: This is the date this copy of the report was printed. Often, the time that the report was printed will also be included. The date of printing may be different than the date the results were generated, especially on cumulative reports.

Test report date: This is the day the results were generated and reported to the ordering physician or to the responsible person. Tests may be run on a particular patient's samples on different dates. Since a patient may have multiple results of the same test from different days, it is important that the report includes this information for correct interpretation of results.

Name of doctor or legally authorized person ordering the test(s): This information enables the lab to forward your results to the person who requested the test(s). Sometimes a report will also include the name of other doctors requesting a copy of your report. For example, a specialist may order tests and request that a copy of the results be sent to your primary physician.

Other elements found on reports deal with the specimen that was collected and with the test itself:

Specimen source, when appropriate: Some tests can be performed on more than one type of sample. For example, protein can be measured in blood, urine, or cerebrospinal fluid, and the results from these different types of specimens can indicate very different things.

Date and time of specimen collection: Some test results may be affected by the day and time of sample collection. This information may help your doctor interpret the results. For example, blood levels of drugs are affected by the time a dose of the drug was last taken, so results of the test and its interpretation can be affected by when the sample was collected.

Laboratory accession number: Number(s) assigned to the sample(s) when it arrives at the laboratory. Some labs will have a single accession number for all your tests and other labs may have multiple accession numbers that help the lab identify the samples.

Name of the test performed: Test names are often abbreviated on lab reports. You may want to look for abbreviated test names or type the acronym into a search box to find information on specific tests.

Test results: Some results are written as numbers when a substance is measured in a sample as with a cholesterol level (quantitative). Other reports may simply give a positive or negative result as in pregnancy tests (qualitative). Still others may include text, such as the name of bacteria for the result of a sample taken from an infected site.

Abnormal test results: Lab reports will often draw attention to results that are abnormal or outside the reference range by setting them apart or highlighting them in some way. For example, H next to a result may mean that it is higher than the reference range. L may mean low and WNL usually means within normal limits.

Critical results: Those results that are dangerously abnormal must be reported immediately to the responsible person, such as the ordering physician. The laboratory will often draw attention to such results with an asterisk (*) or something similar and will usually note on the report the date and time the responsible person was notified.

Units of measurement (for quantitative results): The units of measurement that labs use to report your results can vary from lab to lab. It is similar to the way, for example, your doctor chooses to record your weight during an examination. He may decide to note your weight in pounds or in kilograms. In this same way, labs may choose to use different units of measurement for your test results. Regardless of the units that the lab uses, your results will be interpreted in relation to the reference ranges supplied by the laboratory.

Reference intervals (or reference ranges): These are the ranges in which normal values are expected to fall. The ranges that appear on your report are established and supplied by the laboratory that performed your test. They are made available to the doctor who requested the test(s) and to other health care providers to aid in the interpretation of the results.

Interpretation of results: In certain circumstances, the lab may note on the report what certain test results may indicate.

Condition of specimen: Any pertinent information regarding the condition of specimens that do not meet the laboratory's criteria for acceptability will be noted. This type of information may include a variety of situations in which the specimen was not the best possible sample needed for testing. For example, if the specimen was not collected or stored in optimal conditions or if it was visually apparent that a blood sample was hemolyzed or lipemic, it will be noted on the report. In some cases, the condition of the specimen may preclude analysis (the test is not run and results are not generated) or may generate additional comments directing the use of caution in interpreting results.

Deviations from test preparation procedures: Some tests have specific procedures to follow before a sample is collected or a test is performed. If such procedures are not followed for some reason, it may be noted on the report. For example, if a patient forgets to fast before having a glucose test performed, the report may reflect this fact.

Medications, health supplements, and so forth taken by the patient: Some tests results are affected by medications, vitamins, and other health supplements, so laboratories may obtain this information from the test request form and transcribe it onto the lab report.

Reference Ranges and What They Mean

"Your test was out of the normal range," your doctor says to you, handing you a sheet of paper with a set of test results, numbers on a page. Your heart starts to race in fear that you are really sick. But what does this statement mean, out of the normal range? Is it cause for concern? The brief answer is that a result out of the normal or reference range is a signal that further investigation is needed.

The term normal range is not used very much today because it is considered to be misleading. If a patient's results are outside the range for that test, it does not automatically mean that the result is abnormal. Therefore, today reference range or reference values are considered the more appropriate terms. The term reference value is increasing in use and is often used interchangeably with reference range. For simplicity, the term reference range is used in this article.

Tests results—all medical data—can only be understood once all the pieces are together. Take one of the simplest medical indicators of all—your heart rate. You can take your resting heart rate right now by putting your fingers on your pulse and counting for a minute. Most people know that the average heart rate is about 70 beats per minute. How do you know what a normal heart rate is? We know this on the basis of taking the pulse rate of millions of people over time.

You probably also know that if you are a regular runner or are otherwise in good physical condition, your pulse rate could be considerably lower—so a pulse rate of 55 could also be normal. Say you walk up a hill—your heart rate is now 120 beats a minute. That would be high for a resting heart rate but normal for the rate during this kind of activity.

Your heart rate, like any medical observation, must be considered in context. Without the proper context, any observation or test result is meaningless. To understand what is normal for you, your doctor must know what is normal for most other people of your age and what you were doing at the time—or just before—the test or observation was conducted.

The interpretation of any clinical laboratory test must consider this important concept when comparing the patient's results to the test's reference range.

Common Misconceptions

There are two main misconceptions about test results and reference ranges:

Myth: "An abnormal test result is a sign of a real problem."

Truth: A test result outside the reference range may or may not indicate a problem—the only sure signal it sends is that your doctor should investigate it further. You can have an abnormal value and have nothing wrong—but your doctor should try to determine the cause.

It's possible that your result falls in that 5% of healthy people who fall outside the statistical reference range. In addition, there are many things that could throw off a test without indicating a major problem: High blood sugar could be diet-related rather than caused by diabetes. A lipid result could be high because you did not fast before the test. High liver enzymes can be the temporary result of a recent drinking binge rather than a sign of cirrhosis. New drugs come on the market constantly, faster than laboratories can evaluate whether they might interfere with test results. It is not uncommon for many of these drugs to interfere with certain laboratory tests, resulting in falsely high or low values.

Most likely, your doctor will want to rerun the test. Some abnormal results may disappear on their own, especially if they are on the border of the reference range. Your doctor will also seek explanations for an abnormal result. A key point your doctor will address is, how far out of the reference range is the result? If these investigations point to a problem, then your doctor will address it. But there are very few medical questions that can be answered by a single test.

Myth: "If all my test results are normal, I have nothing to worry about."

Truth: It is certainly a good sign, but it is only one set of tests, not a guarantee. There is a large overlap among results from healthy people and those with diseases, so there is still a small chance that there is an undetected problem. Just as some healthy people's results fall outside the reference range, lab test results in some people with disease fall within the reference range.

If you are trying to follow a healthy lifestyle, take it as a good sign, and keep it up. But if you are engaging in high-risk behavior, such as drug and alcohol abuse or a poor diet, it only means so far so good, and the potential consequences have not caught up with you yet. A good test result is not a license for an unhealthy lifestyle.

If you had abnormal results previously, normal results certainly provide good news. But your doctor may want to conduct follow-up tests some months later to make sure you are still on track and to document any trends.

Chapter 10

Point-of-Care Rapid Diagnostic Tests

PATH Toward New Point-of-Care Diagnostics

Imagine you come down with a fever and the nearest hospital is hours away. The local doctor makes an educated guess as to what you have based on your symptoms. If he is wrong, you may receive the wrong treatment while the illness continues ravaging your body, possibly until it is too late.

Bringing Diagnostics to the Patient

The approach, known as point-of-care (POC) diagnostics, is used in the United States for relatively few specific applications, such as blood glucose tests for diabetics, home pregnancy tests, and strep throat tests at the doctor's office, as well as tests for sexually transmitted diseases administered in health clinics and during home visits to disadvantaged communities. Future applications of POC technology might take the form of an inexpensive lab-in-a-box that could be stored long-term for immediate use in the event of a natural disaster, such as flooding or earthquake. Another possible application is a home test kit that tracks

This chapter includes excerpts from "PATH Toward New Point-of-Care Diagnostics for Low-Resource Settings: September 30, 2010," National Institute of Biomedical Imaging and Bioengineering (NIBIB), September 20, 2010; an excerpt from "Rapid Diagnostic Tests for Influenza," Centers for Disease Control and Prevention (CDC), September 22, 2010; and excerpts from "Rapid Lead Screening Test," U.S. Food and Drug Administration (FDA), March 26, 2009.

your biomarker signature and flags the doctor if there is a worrisome trend, such as indications of early-stage cancer or heart disease.

Transforming Health Care Delivery in Developing Countries

In the United States, most diagnostics are performed in large, factory-like centralized laboratories. The picture is quite different in developing countries, where there are scant resources to set up and maintain laboratories and keep samples refrigerated during transportation. In situations like this, "POC methodology has the opportunity to transform health care in developing countries, enabling them to build lean, efficient systems based on decentralized healthcare delivery rather than emulating the sometimes wasteful systems of the developed world," says Bernhard Weigl, PhD, MSc, Group Leader, Diagnostic Development Teams, Program for Appropriate Technology in Health (PATH) and Director, NIBIB Center for POC Diagnostics for Global Health.

Although the greatest demand for POC diagnostics for low-resource settings still lies in the infectious disease arena (human immunodeficiency virus [HIV], tuberculosis, malaria), there is an emerging need for chronic disease (for example, diabetes) testing. "POC could be the main way people diagnose diseases in developing countries. Implementing POC diagnostics everywhere would eliminate the need for centralized laboratory testing. In countries where central labs were never built in the first place, they may never actually be needed," indicates Weigl.

Rapid Diagnostic Tests for Influenza

The availability and use of commercial influenza rapid diagnostic tests by laboratories and clinics have substantially increased in recent years.

- Influenza rapid diagnostic tests are screening tests for influenza virus infection.

- They can provide results within 15 minutes.

- More than ten rapid influenza tests have been approved by the U.S. Food and Drug Administration (FDA).

- Rapid tests differ in some important respects:

    - Some can identify influenza A and B viruses and distinguish between them.

- Some can identify influenza A and B viruses but cannot distinguish between them.

- Some tests are waived from requirements under the Clinical Laboratory Improvement Amendments of 1988 (CLIA).

- Most tests can be used with a variety of specimen types, but the accuracy of the tests can vary based on the type of specimen collected (for example throat swab versus nasal swab).

- FDA approval is based upon specific specimen types.

- The rapid tests vary in terms of sensitivity and specificity when compared with viral culture or reverse transcription-polymerase chain reaction (RT-PCR). Product insert information and research publications indicate that: sensitivities are approximately 50%–70%; and specificities are approximately 90%–95%.

- Specimens to be used with rapid tests generally should be collected as close as is possible to the start of symptoms and usually no more than 4–5 days later in adults. In very young children, influenza viruses can be shed for longer periods; therefore, in some instances, testing for a few days after this period may still be useful.

Accuracy Depends Upon Prevalence

The positive and negative predictive values vary considerably depending upon the prevalence of influenza in the community.

- False-positive (and true-negative) influenza test results are more likely to occur when disease prevalence is low, which is generally at the beginning and end of the influenza season.

- False-negative (and true-positive) influenza test results are more likely to occur when disease prevalence is high, which is typically at the height of the influenza season.

Selecting Tests

Many factors should be considered when selecting a test, including the following:

- Tests with high sensitivity and specificity will provide better positive and negative predictive values.

- Types of specimens that provide the most accurate results.

When Rapid Diagnostic Tests Are Beneficial

Testing during an outbreak of acute respiratory disease can determine if influenza is the cause. During influenza season, testing of selected patients presenting with respiratory illnesses compatible with influenza can help establish whether influenza is present in a specific patient population and help health care providers determine how to use their clinical judgment for diagnosing and treating respiratory illness. (Testing need not be done for all patients.)

Rapid Lead Screening Test

There is now a test that provides immediate results on lead levels in children and adults that can be used at thousands of places nationwide, including health clinics, mobile healthcare units, and doctors' offices. Broader availability and easier access to this test means lead exposure can be detected and treated earlier before the damaging effects of lead poisoning occur.

U.S. Department of Health and Human Services (HHS) is allowing the LeadCare II Blood Lead Test System, made by ESA Biosciences (Chelmsford, MA), to be used at more than 115,000 certified point-of-care settings because the company proved to the U.S. Food and Drug Administration that the test is simple, accurate, and poses very little risk of harm to a patient.

The Centers for Disease Control and Prevention (CDC) has found that more than 300,000 children under age six each year have blood levels that exceed 10 micrograms/deciliter (μg/dL), the threshold used to indicate lead poisoning. The American Academy of Pediatrics (AAP) estimates one out of four homes with children under age six has lead contamination. The CDC and AAP recommend screening children at ages one and two who live in high-risk homes.

Symptoms of lead poisoning include headaches, stomach cramps, fatigue, memory loss, high blood pressure, and seizures. Lead poisoning in children has been linked to learning disabilities and developmental delays.

The LeadCare II Blood Test System measures lead in blood samples using a finger stick or taking a blood sample from a person's vein, and gives results in as little as three minutes. The rapid result means a second sample for further testing can be obtained quickly if needed, reducing the need for a follow-up visit.

Chapter 11

Common Blood Tests

Blood tests help doctors check for certain diseases and conditions. They also help check the function of your organs and show how well treatments are working. Specifically, blood tests can help doctors evaluate how well organs are working, diagnose diseases and conditions, screen for risk factors for heart disease, and check whether medicines are working.

Blood tests are very common. When you have routine checkups, your doctor may recommend blood tests to see how your body is working. Many blood tests do not require any special preparations. For some, you may need to fast (not eat any food) for 8–12 hours before the test. Your doctor will let you know how to prepare for blood tests.

During a blood test, a small amount of blood is taken from your body. It is usually drawn from a vein in your arm using a needle. A finger prick also may be used. The procedure usually is quick and easy, although it may cause some short-term discomfort. Most people don't have serious reactions to having blood drawn.

Lab workers draw the blood and analyze it. They use either whole blood to count blood cells, or they separate the blood cells from the fluid that contains them. This fluid is called plasma or serum. The fluid is used to measure different substances in the blood. The results can help detect health problems in early stages, when treatments or lifestyle changes may work best.

Excerpted from "Common Blood Tests," National Heart, Lung, and Blood Institute (NHLBI), January 2010. Table 11.3 is excerpted from "Your Kidney Test Results," National Kidney Disease Education Program (NKDEP), April 2010.

Types of Blood Tests

Complete Blood Count (CBC)

The CBC is one of the most common blood tests. It is often done as part of a routine checkup. The CBC can help detect blood diseases and disorders, such as anemia, infections, clotting problems, blood cancers, and immune system disorders. This test measures many different parts of your blood.

Red blood cells carry oxygen from your lungs to the rest of your body. Abnormal red blood cell levels may be a sign of anemia, dehydration (too little fluid in the body), bleeding, or another disorder.

White blood cells are part of your immune system, which fights infections and diseases. Abnormal white blood cell levels may be a sign of infection, blood cancer, or an immune system disorder. A CBC measures the overall number of white blood cells in your blood. A CBC with differential looks at the amounts of different types of white blood cells in your blood.

Platelets are blood cell fragments that help your blood clot. They stick together to seal cuts or breaks on blood vessel walls and stop bleeding. Abnormal platelet levels may be a sign of a bleeding disorder (not enough clotting) or a thrombotic disorder (too much clotting).

Hemoglobin is an iron-rich protein in red blood cells that carries oxygen. Abnormal hemoglobin levels may be a sign of anemia, sickle cell anemia, thalassemia, or other blood disorders. If you have diabetes, excess glucose in your blood can attach to hemoglobin and raise the level of hemoglobin A1c.

Hematocrit is a measure of how much space red blood cells take up in your blood. A high hematocrit level might mean you're dehydrated. A low hematocrit level might mean you have anemia. Abnormal hematocrit levels also may be a sign of a blood or bone marrow disorder.

Mean corpuscular volume (MCV) is a measure of the average size of your red blood cells. Abnormal MCV levels may be a sign of anemia or thalassemia.

Blood Chemistry Tests/Basic Metabolic Panel

The basic metabolic panel (BMP) is a group of tests that measures different chemicals in the blood. These tests usually are done on the fluid (plasma) part of blood. The tests can give doctors information about your muscles (including the heart), bones, and organs, such as the kidneys and liver. The BMP includes blood glucose, calcium, and electrolyte tests, as well as blood tests that measure kidney function. Some of these tests require you to fast (not eat any food) before the test, and others don't. Your doctor will tell you how to prepare for the test(s) you are having.

Blood glucose: Glucose is a type of sugar that the body uses for energy. Abnormal glucose levels in your blood may be a sign of diabetes. For some blood glucose tests, you have to fast before your blood is drawn. Other blood glucose tests are done after a meal or at any time with no preparation.

Calcium is an important mineral in the body. Abnormal calcium levels in the blood may be a sign of kidney problems, bone disease, thyroid disease, cancer, malnutrition, or another disorder.

Electrolytes are minerals that help maintain fluid levels and acid-base balance in the body. They include sodium, potassium, bicarbonate, and chloride. Abnormal electrolyte levels may be a sign of dehydration, kidney disease, liver disease, heart failure, high blood pressure, or other disorders.

Kidney function blood tests measure levels of blood urea nitrogen (BUN) and creatinine. Both of these are waste products that the kidneys filter out of the body. Abnormal BUN and creatinine levels may be signs of a kidney disease or disorder.

Blood Enzyme Tests

Enzymes are chemicals that help control chemical reactions in your body. There are many blood enzyme tests. This section focuses on blood enzyme tests used to check for heart attack. These include troponin and creatine kinase (CK) tests.

Troponin is a muscle protein that helps your muscles contract. When muscle or heart cells are injured, troponin leaks out, and its levels in your blood rise. For example, blood levels of troponin rise when you have a heart attack. For this reason, doctors often order troponin tests when patients have chest pain or other heart attack signs and symptoms.

Creatine kinase: A blood product called CK-MB is released when the heart muscle is damaged. High levels of CK-MB in the blood can mean that you've had a heart attack.

95

What to Expect with Blood Tests

Before Blood Tests

Many blood tests don't require any special preparation and take only a few minutes. Other blood tests require fasting (not eating any food) for 8–12 hours before the test. Your doctor will tell you how to prepare for your blood test(s).

What to Expect during Blood Tests

Blood usually is drawn from a vein in your arm or other part of your body using a needle. It also can be drawn using a finger prick.

The person who draws your blood might tie a band around the upper part of your arm or ask you to make a fist. Doing this can make the veins in your arm stick out more, which makes it easier to insert the needle. The needle that goes into your vein is attached to a small test tube. The person who draws your blood removes the tube when it's full, and the tube seals on its own. The needle is then removed from your vein. If you're getting a few blood tests, more than one test tube may be attached to the needle before it's withdrawn.

Some people get nervous about blood tests because they're afraid of needles. Others may not want to see blood leaving their bodies. If you are nervous or scared, it can help to look away or talk to someone to distract yourself. You might feel a slight sting when the needle goes in or comes out. Drawing blood usually takes less than three minutes.

After Blood Tests

Once the needle is withdrawn, you'll be asked to apply gentle pressure with a piece of gauze or bandage to the place where the needle was inserted. This helps stop bleeding. It also helps prevent swelling and bruising. Most of the time, you can remove the pressure after a minute or two. You may want to keep a bandage on for a few hours.

Usually, you do not need to do anything else after a blood test. Results can take anywhere from a few minutes to a few weeks to come back. Your doctor should get the results. It is important that you follow up with your doctor to discuss your test results.

What Are the Risks of Blood Tests?

The main risks of blood tests are discomfort and bruising at the site where the needle goes in. These complications usually are minor and go away shortly after the tests are done.

What Do Blood Tests Show?

Blood tests show whether the levels of different substances in your blood fall within a normal range. For many blood substances, the normal range is the range of levels seen in 95% of healthy people in a certain group. For many tests, normal ranges are different depending on your age, gender, race, and other factors.

Many factors can cause your blood test levels to fall outside the normal range. Abnormal levels may be a sign of a disorder or disease. Other factors—such as diet, menstrual cycle, how much physical activity you do, how much alcohol you drink, and the medicines you take (both prescription and over-the-counter)—also can cause abnormal levels. Your doctor should discuss any unusual or abnormal blood test results with you. These results may or may not suggest a health problem.

Blood tests alone cannot be used to diagnose many diseases or medical problems. However, blood tests can help you and your doctor learn more about your health. Blood tests also can help find potential problems early, when treatments or lifestyle changes may work best.

Result Ranges for Common Blood Tests

This section presents the result ranges for complete blood counts and blood glucose. Information about lipoprotein panel tests (cholesterol levels) is available in Chapter 6.3. Note: All values in this section are for adults only.

Table 11.1. Normal Range Results for Complete Blood Count Tests

Test	Normal Range Results*
Red blood cell (varies with altitude)	Male: 5 to 6 million cells/mcL
	Female: 4 to 5 million cells/mcL
White blood cell	4,500 to 10,000 cells/mcL
Platelets	140,000 to 450,000 cells/mcL
Hemoglobin (varies with altitude)	Male: 14 to 17 gm/dL
	Female: 12 to 15 gm/dL
Hematocrit (varies with altitude)	Male: 41% to 50%
	Female: 36% to 44%
Mean corpuscular volume	80 to 95 femtoliter

* Cells/mcL = cells per microliter; gm/dL = grams per deciliter

Complete Blood Count

Table 11.1 shows some normal ranges for different parts of the complete blood count (CBC). Some of the normal ranges are different for men and women. Other factors, such as age and race, also may affect normal ranges. Your doctor should discuss your results with you. He or she will advise you further if your results are outside the normal range for your group.

Blood Glucose

Table 11.2 shows the ranges for blood glucose levels after 8–12 hours of fasting (not eating). It shows the normal range and the abnormal ranges that are a sign of prediabetes or diabetes.

Table 11.2. Fasting Blood Glucose Levels and Normal and Abnormal Ranges

Plasma Glucose Results (mg/dL)*	Diagnosis
99 and below	Normal
100 to 125	Prediabetes
126 and above	Diabetes†

* mg/dL = milligrams per deciliter.
† The test is repeated on another day to confirm the results.

Table 11.3. Other Blood Test Normal Range Results

Test	Normal Range Results	Why It Is Important
Serum albumin	3.4 to 5.0*	Albumin is a protein that helps measure how well you are eating.
Bicarbonate	More than 22	Measures the acid level in your blood.
Blood urea nitrogen (BUN)	Less than 20	Checks how much urea, a waste product, is in your blood.
Potassium	3.5 to 5.0*	Affects how your nerves and muscles work. High or low levels can be dangerous.
Calcium	8.5 to 10.2*	Keeps your bones strong and heart rhythm steady.
Phosphorus	2.7 to 4.6*	Important for strong bones and healthy blood vessels. High levels may cause soft bones, hard blood vessels and itchy skin.
Parathyroid Hormone (PTH)	Less than 65	Controls the calcium and phosphorus levels in blood. Needed to keep bones and blood vessels healthy.
Vitamin D	More than 30	Important for bones and heart health.
A1C	Less than 7	Measures average blood sugar levels over 2–3 months.

* Normal ranges may vary.

Chapter 12

Biopsies

Chapter Contents

Section 12.1

Types of Biopsy Procedures

"Abstracting a Cancer Case: The Biopsy Report," SEER Training Module, National Cancer Institute (NCI), accessed March 27, 2011 from http://train ing.seer.cancer.gov/abstracting/procedures/pathological/histologic/biopsy. Reviewed in April 2011 by David A. Cooke, MD, FACP.

The term biopsy (Bx) refers to the removal and examination, gross and microscopic, of tissue or cells from the living body for the purpose of diagnosis. A variety of techniques exist for performing a biopsy of which the most common ones are the following:

- Aspiration biopsy or bone marrow aspiration: Biopsy of material (fluid, cells or tissue) obtained by suction through a needle attached to a syringe.

- Bone marrow biopsy: Examination of a piece of bone marrow by needle aspiration; can also be done as an open biopsy using a trephine (removing a circular disc of bone).

- Curettage: Removal of growths or other material by scraping with a curette.

- Excisional biopsy (total): The removal of a growth in its entirety by having a therapeutic as well as diagnostic purpose.

- Incisional biopsy: Incomplete removal of a growth for the purpose of diagnostic study.

- Needle biopsy: Same as aspiration biopsy.

- Percutaneous biopsy: A needle biopsy with the needle going through the skin.

- Punch biopsy: Biopsy of material obtained from the body tissue by a punch technique.

- Sponge (gel foam) biopsy: Removal of materials (cells, particles of tissue, and tissue juices) by rubbing a sponge over a lesion or over a mucous membrane for examination.

- Surface biopsy: Scraping of cells from surface epithelium, especially from the cervix, for microscopic examination.

- Surgical biopsy: Removal of tissue from the body by surgical excision for examination.

- Total biopsy: See excisional biopsy.

Note: Any biopsy can be processed quickly by a frozen section technique or by routine fixation (permanent section) by H and E (hematoxylin and eosin) stain which usually takes 48 hours to prepare.

Section 12.2

Breast Biopsy

Excerpted from "Consumer Guide: Having a Breast Biopsy:
A Guide for Women and Their Families," Agency for Healthcare Research and Quality (AHRQ), April 14, 2010.

A biopsy is the only test that can tell for sure if a suspicious area is cancer. During a breast biopsy, the doctor removes a small amount of tissue from the breast. There are two main kinds of breast biopsies. One is called surgical biopsy. The other is called core-needle biopsy.

The kind of breast biopsy a doctor recommends may depend on what the suspicious area looks like. It also might depend on the size and where it is located in the breast. After the biopsy, the tissue is sent to a doctor who will look at the tissue under a microscope. This doctor, called a pathologist, looks for tissue changes. The pathology report tells if there is cancer or not. It takes about a week to get the report. It may help to talk to your family and friends. You also might want someone to come to your appointment with you.

Surgical Biopsy

A surgical biopsy is usually done using local anesthesia. Local anesthesia means that the breast will be numbed. You will have an intravenous (IV) and may have medicine to make you drowsy. The surgeon makes a 1–2-inch cut on the breast and removes part or all of the suspicious tissue. Some of the tissue around it also may be taken out.

Core-Needle Biopsy

A core-needle biopsy is done using local anesthesia. The doctor inserts a hollow needle into the breast and removes a small amount of suspicious tissue. The doctor may place a tiny marker inside the breast. It marks the spot where the biopsy was done. Radiologists or surgeons usually do core-needle biopsies using special imaging equipment.

Ultrasound-guided core-needle biopsy uses ultrasound to guide the needle to the suspicious area. You will lie on your back or side for this procedure. The doctor will hold the ultrasound device against your breast to guide the needle.

Stereotactic-guided core-needle biopsy uses x-ray equipment and a computer to guide the needle. Usually for this kind of biopsy, you lie on your stomach on a special table. The table will have an opening for your breast. Your breast will be compressed like it is for a mammogram.

Freehand core-needle biopsy does not use ultrasound or x-ray equipment. It is used less often and only for lumps that can be felt through the skin.

It is not unusual to feel anxious about having a biopsy. Ask your doctor or nurse what to expect.

Accuracy

Out of every 100 women who have breast cancer:

- Surgical biopsies will find 98 to 99 of those breast cancers.
- Ultrasound or stereotactic-guided biopsies will find 97 to 99 of those breast cancers.
- Freehand biopsies will find about 86 of those breast cancers.

Side Effects

Side effects are rare with any kind of core-needle biopsy. Less than one out of 100 women who have a core-needle biopsy have a problem like severe bruising, bleeding, or infection.

Side effects happen more often with surgical biopsy. Up to ten out of 100 women who have surgical biopsy get severe bruising. About five out of 100 women who have surgical biopsy get an infection.

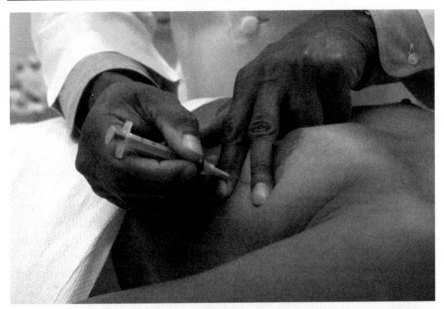

Figure 12.1. *Needle Breast Biopsy (Source: National Cancer Institute (NCI) Visuals Online, "Diagnosis: Biopsy: Needle: Breast Cancer," 1980.)*

Women who have a surgical biopsy sometimes need prescription pain medicine to control pain after the procedure. Women who have a core-needle biopsy rarely need prescription pain medicine.

Biopsy Results

If no cancer is found, the biopsy result is called benign. Benign means it is not cancer. Some benign results need follow-up or treatment. Talk to your doctor or nurse about what they recommend.

If cancer is found, the report will tell you the kind of cancer. It will help you and your doctor talk about the next steps. Usually, you will be referred to a breast cancer specialist. You may need more imaging tests or surgery. Take time to think. Most women with breast cancer have time to consider their options. Ask your doctor if you don't understand your test results and ask for a copy of the pathology report for your records.

Section 12.3

Kidney Biopsy

Excerpted from "Kidney Biopsy," National Institute of
Diabetes and Digestive and Kidney Diseases (NIDDK), July 2008.

A biopsy is a diagnostic test that involves collecting small pieces of tissue, usually through a needle, for examination with a microscope. A kidney biopsy can help in forming a diagnosis and in choosing the best course of treatment. A kidney biopsy may be recommended for any of the following conditions: hematuria, which is blood in the urine; proteinuria, which is excessive protein in the urine; or impaired kidney function, which causes excessive waste products in the blood.

A pathologist will look at the kidney tissue samples to check for unusual deposits, scarring, or infecting organisms that would explain a person's condition. The doctor may find a condition that can be treated and cured. If a person has progressive kidney failure, the biopsy may show how quickly the disease is advancing. A biopsy can also help explain why a transplanted kidney is not working properly. Patients should talk with their doctors about what information might be learned from the biopsy and the risks involved so the patients can help make a decision about whether a biopsy is worthwhile.

What are the preparations for a kidney biopsy?

Patients must sign a consent form saying they understand the risks involved in this procedure. The risks are slight, but patients should discuss these risks in detail with their doctors before signing the form.

Doctors should be aware of all the medicines a patient takes and any drug allergies that patient might have. The patient should avoid aspirin and other blood-thinning medicines for 1–2 weeks before the procedure. Some doctors advise their patients to avoid food and fluids before the test, while others tell patients to eat a light meal. Shortly before the biopsy, blood and urine samples are taken to make sure the patient does not have a condition that would make doing a biopsy risky.

What are the procedures for a kidney biopsy?

Kidney biopsies are usually done in a hospital. The patient is fully awake with light sedation. A local anesthetic is given before the needle is inserted.

Patients lie on their stomachs to position the kidneys near the surface of their backs. Patients who have a transplanted kidney lie on their backs. The doctor marks the entry site, cleans the area, and injects a local painkiller. For a biopsy using a needle inserted through the skin, the doctor uses a locating needle and x-ray or ultrasound equipment to find the kidney and then a collecting needle to gather the tissue. Patients are asked to hold their breath as the doctor uses a spring-loaded instrument to insert the biopsy needle and collect the tissue, usually for about 30 seconds or a little longer for each insertion. The spring-loaded instrument makes a sharp clicking noise that can be startling to patients. The doctor may need to insert the needle three or four times to collect the needed samples.

The entire procedure usually takes about an hour, including time to locate the kidney, clean the biopsy site, inject the local painkiller, and collect the tissue samples.

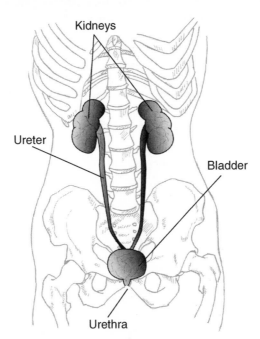

Figure 12.2. *Kidneys filter wastes and extra fluid from the blood and direct them to the bladder as urine.*

What happens after a kidney biopsy?

After the test, patients lie on their backs in the hospital for a few hours. Patients who have a transplanted kidney lie on their stomachs. During this time, the staff will monitor blood pressure and pulse and take blood samples to assess for blood loss. On rare occasions when bleeding does not stop on its own, a transfusion may be necessary to replace lost blood. Most patients leave the hospital the same day. Patients may notice some blood in their urine for 24 hours after the test.

A rare complication is infection from the biopsy. Patients should tell their doctors or nurses if they have any of these problems: bloody urine more than 24 hours after the test, inability to urinate, fever, worsening pain in the biopsy site, faintness, or dizziness.

How are kidney biopsy results reported?

After the biopsy, the doctor will inspect the tissue samples in the laboratory using one or more microscopes, perhaps using dyes to identify different substances that may be settled in the tissue. Electron microscopes may be used to see small details. Getting the complete biopsy results usually takes a few days. In urgent cases, a preliminary report may be given within a few hours.

Section 12.4

Liver Biopsy

Excerpted from "Liver Biopsy," National Institute of
Diabetes and Digestive and Kidney Diseases (NIDDK), May 2009.

A liver biopsy is a procedure to remove a small piece of the liver so it can be examined with a microscope for signs of damage or disease. The three main types of liver biopsy are percutaneous, transvenous, and laparoscopic. A liver biopsy is performed when a liver problem is difficult to diagnose with blood tests or imaging techniques, such as ultrasound and x-ray. More often, a liver biopsy is performed to estimate the degree of liver damage—a process called staging. Staging helps guide treatment.

How does a person prepare for a liver biopsy?

At least one week before a scheduled liver biopsy, patients should inform their doctor of all medications they are taking. Patients may be asked to temporarily stop taking medications that affect blood clotting or interact with sedatives, which are sometimes given during a liver biopsy.

Medications that may be restricted before and after a liver biopsy include:

- nonsteroidal anti-inflammatory drugs, such as aspirin, ibuprofen, and naproxen;

- blood thinners;

- high blood pressure medication;

- diabetes medications;

- antidepressants;

- antibiotics;

- asthma medications; and

- dietary supplements.

Prior to liver biopsy, blood will be drawn to determine its ability to clot. People with severe liver disease often have blood clotting problems that can increase the risk of bleeding after the procedure. A medicine given just before a liver biopsy, called clotting factor concentrates, reduces the risk of bleeding in patients with blood clotting abnormalities.

Patients who will be sedated should not eat or drink for eight hours before the liver biopsy and should arrange a ride home, as driving is prohibited for 12 hours after the procedure. Mild sedation is sometimes used during liver biopsy to help patients stay relaxed. Unlike general anesthesia where patients are unconscious, patients can communicate while sedated but then often have no memory of the procedure. Sedatives are often given through an intravenous (IV) tube placed in a vein. The IV can also be used to give pain medication, if necessary, after the procedure.

How is a liver biopsy performed?

All three main types of liver biopsy remove liver tissue with a needle; however, each takes a different approach to needle insertion. A liver biopsy may be performed at a hospital or outpatient center.

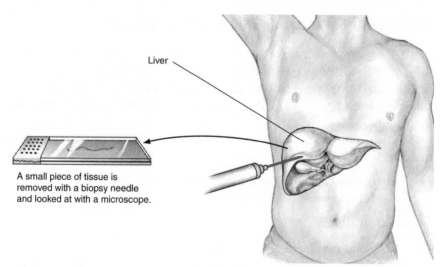

Liver

A small piece of tissue is removed with a biopsy needle and looked at with a microscope.

Figure 12.3. *Percutaneous Liver Biopsy*

Percutaneous Liver Biopsy

The most commonly used technique for collecting a liver sample is percutaneous liver biopsy. For this method, a hollow needle is inserted through the abdomen into the liver to remove a small piece of tissue.

To help find the liver and avoid sticking other organs with the biopsy needle, doctors often use ultrasound, computerized tomography (CT), or other imaging techniques.

During the procedure, patients lie on their back on a table with their right hand resting above their head. A local anesthetic is applied to the area where the biopsy needle will be inserted. If needed, an IV tube is used to give sedatives and pain medication. The doctor makes a small incision in the abdomen, either toward the bottom of the rib cage or just below it, and inserts the biopsy needle. Patients will be asked to exhale and hold their breath while the needle is inserted and a liver sample is quickly withdrawn. Several samples may be collected, requiring multiple needle insertions.

After the biopsy, patients must lie on their right side for up to two hours to reduce the risk of bleeding. Patients are then monitored an additional 2–4 hours after the biopsy before being sent home.

Transvenous Liver Biopsy

Transvenous liver biopsy is used when a person's blood clots slowly or when excess fluid is present in the abdomen, a condition called ascites. During the procedure, patients lie on their back on an x-ray table and a local anesthetic is applied to one side of the neck. If needed, an IV tube is used to give sedatives and pain medication.

A small incision is made in the neck and a specially designed hollow tube called a sheath is inserted into the jugular vein. The doctor threads the sheath down the jugular vein, along the side of the heart, and into one of the hepatic veins, which are located in the liver. To see the veins, the doctor injects liquid contrast material into the sheath. The contrast material lights up when x-rayed, highlighting the blood vessels and showing the location of the sheath. The doctor threads a biopsy needle through the sheath and into the liver and a liver sample is quickly withdrawn. Several samples may be collected, requiring multiple needle insertions. The sheath is carefully withdrawn and the incision is closed with a bandage. Patients are monitored for 4–6 hours for signs of bleeding.

Laparoscopic Liver Biopsy

Doctors use laparoscopic liver biopsy to obtain a tissue sample from a specific area or from multiple areas of the liver or when the risk of spreading cancer or infection exists. Laparoscopic surgery is a technique that avoids making a large incision by instead making one or a few small incisions. The doctor works with special tools—including a small, lighted video camera—passed through the incisions. A doctor may take a liver sample during laparoscopic surgery performed for other reasons, including liver surgery.

During laparoscopy, patients lie on their back on an operating table. An IV is inserted in a vein to give sedatives and pain medication. A small incision is made in the abdomen, usually just below the rib cage. A plastic, tube-like instrument, called a cannula, is inserted in the incision and the abdomen is inflated with gas. Inflation allows the doctor space to work inside the abdominal cavity. A biopsy needle is inserted through the cannula and into the abdomen. The needle is inserted into the liver and a tissue sample is quickly withdrawn. Several samples may be collected, requiring multiple needle insertions. Any excessive bleeding because of the surgery is easily spotted with the camera and treated using an electric probe.

After liver samples are collected, the cannula is removed and the incision is closed with dissolvable stitches. Patients will need to remain at the hospital or outpatient center for a few hours while the sedatives wear off.

How soon do results come back from a liver biopsy?

Results from a liver biopsy take a few days to come back. The liver sample goes to a pathology laboratory where the tissue is stained. Staining highlights important details within the liver tissue and helps the pathologist—a doctor who specializes in diagnosing disease—identify signs of liver disease. The pathologist looks at the tissue with a microscope and sends a report to the patient's doctor.

How long does it take to recover from a liver biopsy?

Most patients fully recover from a liver biopsy in 1–2 days. Patients should avoid intense activity, exercise, or heavy lifting during this time. Soreness around the incision site may persist for about a week. Acetaminophen (Tylenol) or other pain medications that do not interfere with blood clotting may help. Patients should check with their doctor before taking any pain medications.

What are the risks of liver biopsy?

Pain at the biopsy site is the most frequent risk of percutaneous liver biopsy, occurring in about 20% of patients. The risk of excessive bleeding, called hemorrhage, is about one in 500 to one in 1,000. Risk of death is about one in 10,000 to one in 12,000. If hemorrhage occurs, a procedure called embolization, assisted by an x-ray procedure used to visualize blood vessels called angiography, can be used to stop the bleeding. In some cases, a blood transfusion is necessary. Surgery can also be used to stop a hemorrhage. Other risks include puncture of other internal organs, infection, and spread of cancer cells, called cancer seeding. Transvenous liver biopsy carries an additional risk of adverse reaction to the contrast material.

Section 12.5

Lung Needle Biopsy

"Lung Needle Biopsy," © 2011 A.D.A.M., Inc. Reprinted with permission.

A lung needle biopsy is a method to remove a piece of lung tissue for examination. If it is done through the wall of your chest, it is called a transthoracic lung biopsy.

How the Test Is Performed

A chest x-ray or chest computed tomography (CT) scan may be used to find the exact spot for the biopsy. If the biopsy is done using a CT scan, you may be lying down during the exam.

A needle biopsy of the lung may also be performed during bronchoscopy or mediastinoscopy. You sit with your arms resting forward on a table. You should try to keep still and not cough during the biopsy. The doctor will ask you to hold your breath. The skin is scrubbed and a local pain-killing medicine (anesthetic) is injected.

The physician will make a small (about 1/8ᵗʰ inch) cut in the skin, and will insert the biopsy needle into the abnormal tissue, tumor, or lung tissue. A small piece of tissue is removed with the needle and sent to a laboratory for examination.

When the biopsy is done, pressure is placed over the site. Once bleeding has stopped, a bandage is applied. A chest x-ray is taken immediately after the biopsy. The procedure usually takes 30–60 minutes. Laboratory analysis usually takes a few days.

How to Prepare for the Test

You should not eat for 6–12 hours before the test. Your health care provider will likely tell you to avoid aspirin, nonsteroidal anti-inflammatory drugs (NSAIDs) such as ibuprofen, or blood thinners such as warfarin for a period of time before the procedure. Always check with your health care provider before changing or stopping any medications.

Before a needle biopsy of the lung, a chest x-ray or chest CT scan may be performed. Sometimes, you will be given a mild sedative before the biopsy to relax you. You must sign a consent form. It is important to remain as still as possible for the biopsy and avoid coughing.

How the Test Will Feel

You will receive an injection of anesthetic before the biopsy. This injection will sting for a moment. You will feel pressure and a brief, sharp pain when the needle touches the lung.

Why the Test Is Performed

A lung needle biopsy is performed when there is an abnormal condition near the surface of the lung, in the lung itself, or on the chest wall. Most often, it is done to rule out cancer. The biopsy is usually performed after abnormalities appear on chest x-ray or CT scan.

Normal Results

In a normal test, the tissues are normal and there is no growth of bacteria, viruses, or fungi if a culture is performed.

What Abnormal Results Mean

Bacterial, viral, or fungal lung infection; cancerous cells (lung cancer, mesothelioma); or pneumonia. The test may also be performed for metastatic cancer to the lung or pneumonia with lung abscess.

Risks

In a very small percentage of lung needle biopsies, a collapsed lung (also called a pneumothorax) occurs. A chest x-ray will be done after the needle biopsy to check for this. The risk is higher if you have certain lung diseases such as emphysema. However, if the pneumothorax is large, a chest tube may need to be inserted to expand your lung. In rare cases, pneumothorax can be life threatening if air escapes from the lung, gets trapped in the chest, and presses on the rest of your lungs or heart.

Whenever a biopsy is done, there is a risk of excessive bleeding (hemorrhage). Some bleeding is common, and a health care provider will monitor the amount of bleeding. Rarely, major and life-threatening bleeding may occur.

A needle biopsy should not be performed if other tests show that you have the following:

- Blood coagulation disorder of any type
- Bullae (enlarged alveoli that occur with emphysema)
- Cor pulmonale
- Cysts of the lung
- Pulmonary hypertension
- Severe hypoxia (low oxygen)

Considerations

Signs of a collapsed lung include blueness of the skin, chest pain, rapid heart rate (rapid pulse), and shortness of breath. If any of these occur, report them to your health care provider immediately.

Alternative Names

Transthoracic needle aspiration; percutaneous needle aspiration

Section 12.6

Muscle Biopsy

"Simply Stated...Muscle Biopsies," reprinted by permission of the Muscular Dystrophy Association of the United States (www.mda.org), © 2000. Reviewed in April 2011 by David A. Cooke, MD, FACP.

A muscle biopsy is a surgical procedure in which one or more small pieces of muscle tissue are removed for further microscopic or biochemical examination. The procedure, often used in the diagnosis of a neuromuscular disorder, is considered minor surgery and is usually performed under local anesthetic.

A doctor is likely to call for a muscle biopsy after looking at preliminary blood tests, performing an electromyogram (EMG) and physical examination, and determining that the patient's symptoms indicate an underlying neuromuscular disorder. The muscle biopsy can help distinguish between muscular and neurological problems and can help pinpoint the exact neuromuscular disorder present.

Not everyone suspected of having a neuromuscular disease requires a muscle biopsy. In some cases, diagnosis can be made by symptoms and a deoxyribonucleic acid (DNA) test based on a blood sample.

Open or Needle Biopsy

There are two types of muscle biopsy. The open biopsy involves the removal of one or more small pieces of muscle tissue with sharp scissors.

The neuromuscular specialist selects a muscle, usually the biceps, triceps, deltoid or quadriceps muscle, that should yield the most information about the disease. Usually moderately affected muscles are chosen; the weakest muscles may already be too degraded for analysis. The procedure involves a 2- to 3-inch incision, which is then closed with stitches and may feel sore for a few days.

In a needle biopsy, used since the 1960s, a pea-sized muscle sample is collected with a large bore needle. Although this is less invasive than the open biopsy, the doctor loses the ability to examine the muscle visually first, and the specimen collected is smaller.

Analyzing the Sample

When the muscle samples are sent to a laboratory for analysis, the technicians cut them into many thin sections for examination. Using different tests on different sections, they look at the tissue's overall appearance, chemical activities in the tissue, and the presence or absence of critical proteins. The information these tests provide helps determine exactly what disease and what form of it the person has.

Histology tests (histo means tissue) employ chemical stains to see the muscle's overall appearance and the structure of the muscle cells. This analysis can yield information about muscle degeneration and regeneration, fiber type abnormalities, mitochondrial abnormalities, scar tissue, inflammation, and other clues to specific disorders.

Histochemistry uses stains to detect chemical activities in the cells, including the actions of specific enzymes and metabolic processes. A lab that performs only histology may miss important metabolic abnormalities.

Immunohistochemistry uses antibodies to detect the presence or absence of proteins. This analysis can show whether the cells are missing dystrophin (indicating Duchenne or Becker muscular dystrophy [MD]), sarcoglycans (limb-girdle MD), merosin (congenital MD), or other proteins whose absence causes specific muscular dystrophies. Specific antibodies can also be used to identify the nature of inflammatory cells found in the muscle.

The lab may also use electron microscopy to get very high magnification views of the cellular structure, which can confirm structural abnormalities, like the presence of nemaline rods.

Finally, a DNA analysis can be performed on a muscle sample to detect a genetic mutation. Although a blood sample is usually adequate for a DNA test, a muscle sample may be needed to test for mitochondrial DNA mutations.

Multiple Biopsies

Yadollah Harati, a neurologist and director of the Muscle and Nerve Pathology Laboratory at Baylor College of Medicine in Houston, usually takes as many as five separate muscle samples from different regions of the muscle incision. Several are analyzed and at least one is frozen for future use. Harati believes no biopsy should be done unless the amount of tissue removed is adequate for a complete study.

Having at least three muscle samples gives the lab an adequate amount of tissue to work with. In some disorders, particularly "patchy" disorders like the inflammatory myopathies, signs of the disease may not be present in all regions of the muscles, so more samples give a better chance of accuracy.

It's important that the tissue samples be frozen promptly and properly after the biopsy and be stored carefully. If they're not handled and stored correctly, the results may be inaccurate.

Your doctor may occasionally recommend a new biopsy even though you've had one in the past, especially if you've been given a tentative diagnosis or now suspect your diagnosis was incorrect. With many new muscle-protein antibodies now available for testing biopsy samples, as well as new understanding of mitochondrial disorders and new DNA tests, a new biopsy may be desirable.

According to Harati, tissue that was frozen promptly after removal and maintained carefully is useful for many years. In autoimmune diseases, tissue changes over time in your body may necessitate a new biopsy for the most accurate diagnosis.

Getting Results

The analysis of a muscle biopsy sample is a very tedious and labor-intensive process in which many sections of the muscle must be cut, many different types of procedures performed, and the results carefully analyzed. Harati's lab usually performs a few basic histology tests immediately after the biopsy and then, based on these results, determines what further tests should be made. His lab typically makes an initial report on the day of the biopsy and a full report in two to three weeks.

Section 12.7

Sentinel Lymph Node Biopsy

Excerpted from "Sentinel Lymph Node Biopsy," National Cancer Institute (NCI), April 2005. Reviewed in April 2011 by David A. Cooke, MD, FACP.

A lymph node is part of the body's lymphatic system. In the lymphatic system, a network of lymph vessels carries clear fluid called lymph. Lymph vessels lead to lymph nodes, which are small, round organs that trap cancer cells, bacteria, or other harmful substances that may be in the lymph. Groups of lymph nodes are found in the neck, underarms, chest, abdomen, and groin.

The sentinel lymph node is the first lymph node to which cancer is likely to spread from the primary tumor. Cancer cells may appear in the sentinel node before spreading to other lymph nodes. In some cases, there can be more than one sentinel lymph node.

What is sentinel lymph node (SLN) biopsy?

SLN biopsy is a procedure in which the sentinel lymph node is removed and examined under a microscope to determine whether cancer cells are present. SLN biopsy is based on the idea that cancer cells spread (metastasize) in an orderly way from the primary tumor to the sentinel lymph node(s), then to other nearby lymph nodes.

A negative SLN biopsy result suggests that cancer has not spread to the lymph nodes. A positive result indicates that cancer is present in the SLN and may be present in other lymph nodes in the same area (regional lymph nodes). This information may help the doctor determine the stage of cancer (extent of the disease within the body) and develop an appropriate treatment plan.

What happens during the SLN biopsy procedure?

In SLN biopsy, one or a few lymph nodes (the sentinel node or nodes) are removed. To identify the sentinel lymph node(s), the surgeon injects a radioactive substance, blue dye, or both near the tumor. The surgeon then uses a scanner to find the sentinel lymph nodes(s) containing the radioactive substance or looks for the lymph node(s) stained with dye.

Once the SLN is located, the surgeon makes a small incision (about ½ inch) in the skin overlying the SLN and removes the lymph node(s).

The sentinel node(s) is/are checked for the presence of cancer cells by a pathologist (a doctor who identifies diseases by studying cells and tissue under a microscope). If cancer is found, the surgeon will usually remove more lymph nodes during the biopsy procedure or during a follow-up surgical procedure. SLN biopsy may be done on an outpatient basis or require a short stay in the hospital.

What are the possible benefits of SLN biopsy?

To understand the possible benefits of SLN biopsy, it helps to know about standard lymph node removal. Standard lymph node removal involves surgery to remove most of the lymph nodes in the area of the tumor (regional lymph nodes). For example, breast cancer surgery may include removing most of the axillary lymph nodes, the group of lymph nodes under the arm. This is called axillary lymph node dissection (ALND).

If SLN biopsy is done and the sentinel node does not contain cancer cells, the rest of the regional lymph nodes may not need to be removed. Because fewer lymph nodes are removed, there may be fewer side effects. When multiple regional lymph nodes are removed, the patient may experience side effects such as lymphedema (swelling caused by excess fluid build-up), numbness, a persistent burning sensation, infection, and difficulty moving the affected body area.

What are the side effects and disadvantages of SLN biopsy?

Side effects of SLN biopsy can include pain or bruising at the biopsy site and the rare possibility of an allergic reaction to the blue dye used to find the sentinel node. Patients may find that their urine is discolored, or that their skin has been stained the same color as the dye. These problems are temporary.

Although some surgeons consider SLN biopsy to be the standard of care for some cancers, its role and benefit are yet to be determined. We do not know whether SLN biopsy improves a patient's survival or reduces the chance that the cancer will recur (come back).

Section 12.8

Skin Lesion Biopsy

A skin lesion biopsy is the removal of a piece of skin to diagnose or rule out an illness.

How the Test Is Performed

There are several ways to do a skin biopsy. Most procedures can be easily done in outpatient medical offices or your doctor's office. Which procedure you have depends on several factors, including the location, size, and type of lesion. You will receive some type of numbing medicine (anesthetic) before any type of skin biopsy.

Types of skin biopsies include the following:

- Shave biopsy

- Punch biopsy

- Excisional biopsy

The shave biopsy is the least invasive of all three techniques. Your doctor will remove the outermost layers of skin. You will not need stitches.

Punch biopsies are most often used for deeper skin lesions. Your doctor removes a small round piece of skin (usually the size of a pencil eraser) using a sharp, hollow instrument. If a large sample is taken, the area may be closed with stitches.

An excisional biopsy is done to remove the entire lesion. A numbing medicine is injected into the area. Then the entire lump, spot, or sore is removed, going as deep as necessary to get the entire area. The area is closed with stitches. Pressure is applied to the area to stop any bleeding. If a large area is biopsied, a skin graft or flap of normal skin may be used to replace the skin that was removed.

How to Prepare for the Test

Tell your health care provider:

- About the medications you are taking (including vitamins and supplements, herbal remedies, and over-the-counter preparations)
- If you have any allergies
- If you have bleeding problems
- If you are pregnant

Why the Test Is Performed

Your doctor may order a skin biopsy if you have signs or symptoms of skin cancer, benign growths, chronic bacterial and fungal skin infections, or other skin conditions.

Normal Results

Normal value ranges may vary slightly among different laboratories. Talk to your doctor about the meaning of your specific test results.

What Abnormal Results Mean

The test may reveal skin cancers or noncancerous (benign) conditions. Bacteria and fungi can be identified. The test may also reveal some inflammatory diseases of the skin. Once the diagnosis is confirmed with the biopsy, a treatment plan is usually started.

Risks

Risks may include infection or scars (keloids). You will bleed slightly during the procedure. Tell your doctor if you have a history of bleeding problems.

Considerations

Fluid-filled lesions may be examined by skin lesion aspiration instead of skin lesion biopsy.

Section 12.9

Thyroid Fine Needle Aspiration

"Fine Needle Aspiration of the Thyroid,"
© 2011 A.D.A.M., Inc. Reprinted with permission.

A fine needle aspiration of the thyroid gland is a procedure to remove thyroid cells for examination. The thyroid is located in front of the trachea (windpipe) at the top of the neck.

How the Test Is Performed

This test may be done in the health care provider's office or in a hospital. Usually numbing medicine (anesthesia) is not needed because the needle is very thin. You will lie on your back with a pillow under your shoulders and your neck extended. The biopsy site is cleaned. A thin needle is inserted into the thyroid, and a sample of thyroid cells and fluid are removed. The needle is then taken out. Pressure will be applied to the biopsy site to stop any bleeding. The site will be covered with a bandage.

How to Prepare for the Test

Tell your health care provider if you have drug allergies, bleeding problems, or are pregnant. You should also make sure your health care provider has a current list of all medications you take, including herbal remedies and over-the-counter drugs.

Why the Test Is Performed

This is a test to diagnose thyroid disease or thyroid cancer. It is often used to get information on thyroid lumps that can either be felt by the doctor or seen by ultrasound.

Normal Results

The thyroid tissue is normal in structure and the cells appear non-cancerous under a microscope.

Abnormal Results May Mean

Diffuse thyroid disease such as goiter or thyroiditis, noncancerous tumors, or thyroid cancer.

Risks

The main risk is bleeding into or around the thyroid gland. If bleeding is severe, the windpipe (trachea) may be compressed. This complication is rare.

Chapter 13

Bone Marrow Tests

What are bone marrow tests?

Bone marrow tests are used to check whether your bone marrow is healthy. These tests also show whether your bone marrow is making normal amounts of blood cells. Bone marrow is the sponge-like tissue inside the bones. It contains stem cells that develop into the three types of blood cells that the body needs:

- Red blood cells carry oxygen through the body.
- White blood cells fight infection.
- Platelets (PLATE-lets) stop bleeding.

Another type of stem cell, called an embryonic stem cell, can develop into any type of cell in the body. These cells are not found in bone marrow.

Overview: Doctors use bone marrow tests to diagnose blood and bone marrow diseases and conditions, including the following:

- Conditions in which a person produces too few or too many of certain types of blood cells
- Problems with the structure of red blood cells

Excerpted from "Bone Marrow Tests," National Heart, Lung, and Blood Institute (NHLBI), August 2009.

- Bone marrow disorders, such as myelofibrosis

- Some cancers, such as leukemia

Bone marrow tests also help doctors figure out how severe a cancer is and how much it has spread in the body. The tests also are used to diagnose fevers and infections. The two bone marrow tests are aspiration and biopsy.

Bone marrow aspiration usually is done first. For this test, your doctor removes a small amount of fluid bone marrow through a needle. He or she may have some idea of what the problem is, and the sample gives him or her useful information about the cells in the marrow.

A bone marrow biopsy is a follow-up test. It is done when an aspiration does not give needed information. Or, it is done if your doctor wants to examine the bone marrow structure itself. For a bone marrow biopsy, your doctor removes a small amount of bone marrow tissue through a larger needle.

Who needs bone marrow tests?

Your doctor may recommend bone marrow tests if he or she thinks you have a blood or bone marrow disease or condition. These diseases and conditions include the following:

Myelodysplastic syndrome: This is a group of diseases in which your bone marrow does not make enough normal blood cells.

Neutropenia: This is a condition in which you have a lower than normal number of white blood cells in your blood.

Anemia: This is a condition in which you have a lower than normal number of red blood cells, or your red blood cells do not have enough of an iron-rich protein that carries oxygen from the lungs to the rest of the body. Bone marrow tests also are used to diagnose aplastic anemia. This is a rare and serious condition in which bone marrow stops making enough new blood cells.

Myelofibrosis: This is a serious bone marrow disorder that disrupts normal production of blood cells and leads to severe anemia.

Thrombocytopenia: This group of conditions occurs when your body does not make enough platelets and your blood does not clot as it should.

Essential thrombocythemia: This is a disease in which your bone marrow makes too many blood cells, especially platelets.

Leukemia: This is a cancer of the white blood cells. Types of leukemia include acute and chronic leukemias and multiple myeloma.

Your doctor also may recommend bone marrow tests if you have other types of cancer. These may include breast cancer that has spread to the bone or Hodgkin and non-Hodgkin lymphomas (cancers of a particular type of white blood cell).

Bone marrow tests help show what stage the cancer is in. That is, the tests help doctors know how serious the cancer is and how much it has spread in the body. Bone marrow tests also can show what's causing a fever. The tests may be used for people who have diseases in which their immune systems aren't working properly. The tests also are used for patients who may have uncommon bacterial infections.

What can a person expect during bone marrow tests?

Bone marrow aspiration and biopsy take about 20 minutes each. Before the tests, a doctor or nurse will explain the testing process. Your breathing, heart rate, and any pain will be closely checked during the test.

Bone marrow tests generally are done on the pelvic bone. Part of this bone is accessible in most people on the lower back. If your doctor uses that part of the pelvic bone, you will lie on your stomach for the test. Aspiration may be done on the breastbone.

The area on your body where your doctor will insert the needle is cleaned and draped with a cloth. Your doctor will see only the site where the needle is inserted. He or she will numb the skin at the site and then make a small incision (cut). This makes it easier to insert the needle into the bone. Stitches may be needed to close the cut after the test.

For bone marrow aspiration, your doctor will insert the needle into the marrow and remove a small amount of fluid bone marrow. You may feel a brief, sharp pain. The fluid that is removed from the bone marrow will be taken to a lab and studied under a microscope.

If your doctor decides to do a bone marrow biopsy, it will be done after the aspiration. For the biopsy, your doctor will use a needle to remove a small amount of the bone marrow tissue. Thin sections of this tissue will be studied under a microscope. During both tests, it's important for you to remain still and as relaxed as possible.

What can a person expect after bone marrow tests?

After the bone marrow tests, a nurse will hold a bandage on the site where the needle was inserted until the bleeding stops. Then he or she will put a smaller bandage on the site. Most people can go home the same day.

After 24 hours, you can take off the bandage. Call your doctor if you develop a fever, have a lot of pain, or see redness, swelling, or discharge at the site. These are signs of infection. Expect mild discomfort for about a week. Your doctor may tell you to take an over-the-counter pain medicine.

What do bone marrow tests show?

Bone marrow tests show whether your bone marrow is making enough healthy blood cells. If it is not, the results can tell your doctor which cells are unhealthy and why. Bone marrow tests are an important tool. They are used to diagnose a variety of blood and bone marrow disorders, including anemia and certain kinds of cancer. Bone marrow tests also are used to find out how serious a cancer is and how much it has spread to other areas of the body. The tests also help doctors determine the cause of fevers and infections.

Chapter 14

Lumbar Puncture
(Spinal Tap)

Note: This information explains lumbar puncture procedures done on children with specific information for parents; however, the information is applicable for adults undergoing the procedure.

What It Is

A lumbar puncture (also called a spinal tap) is a common medical test that involves taking a small sample of cerebrospinal fluid (CSF) for examination. CSF is a clear, colorless liquid that delivers nutrients and "cushions" the brain and spinal cord, or central nervous system. In a lumbar puncture, a needle is carefully inserted into the lower spine to collect the CSF sample.

Why It's Done

Medical personnel perform lumbar punctures and test the cerebrospinal fluid to detect or rule out suspected diseases or conditions. CSF testing looks for signs of possible infection by analyzing the white blood cell count, glucose levels, protein, and bacteria or abnormal cells that can help identify specific diseases in the central nervous system.

"Lumbar Puncture (Spinal Tap)," September 2008, reprinted with permission from www.kidshealth.org. Copyright © 2008 The Nemours Foundation. This information was provided by KidsHealth, one of the largest resources online for medically reviewed health information written for parents, kids, and teens. For more articles like this one, visit www.KidsHealth.org, or www.TeensHealth.org.

Most lumbar punctures are done to test for meningitis, but they also can determine if there is bleeding in the brain, detect certain conditions affecting the nervous system such as Guillain Barré syndrome and multiple sclerosis, and administer chemotherapy medications.

Preparation

After the procedure is explained to you, you'll be asked to sign an informed consent form—this states that you understand the procedure and its risks and give your permission for it to be performed.

The doctor doing the lumbar puncture will know your child's medical history but might ask additional questions, such as whether your child is allergic to any medicines.

You might be able to stay in the room with your child during the procedure, or you can step outside to a waiting area.

The Procedure

A lumbar puncture takes about 30 minutes. The doctor carefully inserts a thin needle between the bones of the lower spine (below the spinal cord) to withdraw the fluid sample.

The patient will be positioned with the back curved out so the spaces between the vertebrae are as wide as possible. This allows the doctor to easily find the spaces between the lower lumbar bones (where the needle will be inserted). Older children may be asked to either sit on an exam table while leaning over with their head on a pillow or lie on their side. Infants and younger children are usually positioned on their sides with their knees under their chin.

A small puncture through the skin on the lower back is made and liquid anesthetic medicine is injected into the tissues beneath the skin to prevent pain. In many cases, before the injected anesthesia medication is given, a numbing cream is applied to the skin to minimize discomfort.

The spinal needle is thin and the length varies according to the size of the patient. It has a hollow core, and inside the hollow core is a "stylet," another type of thin needle that acts kind of like a plug. When the spinal needle is inserted into the lower lumbar area, the stylet is carefully removed, which allows the cerebrospinal fluid to drip out into the collection tubes.

After the CSF sample is collected (this usually takes about five minutes), the needle is withdrawn and a small bandage is placed on the site. Collected samples are sent to a lab for analysis and testing.

What to Expect

While some notice a brief pinch and some discomfort, most people don't consider a lumbar puncture to be painful. Depending on the doctor's recommendations, your child might have to lie on his or her back for a few hours after the procedure. Your child might feel tired and have a mild backache the day after the procedure.

Getting the Results

Some results from a lumbar puncture are available within 30 to 60 minutes. However, to look for specific bacteria growing in the sample, a bacterial culture is sent to the lab and these results are usually available in 48 hours. If it's determined there might be an infection, the doctor will start antibiotic treatment while waiting for the results of the culture.

Risks

A lumbar puncture is considered a safe procedure with minimal risks. Most of the time, there are no complications. In some instances, a patient may get a headache (it's recommended that patients lie down for a few hours after the test and drink plenty of fluids to help prevent headaches). And in rare cases, infection or bleeding can occur.

Helping Your Child

You can help prepare your child for a lumbar puncture by explaining that while the test might be uncomfortable, it shouldn't be painful and won't take long. Also explain the importance of lying still during the test, and let your child know that a nurse might hold him or her in place. After the procedure, make sure your child rests and follow any other instructions the doctor gives you.

If You Have Questions

It's important to understand any procedure your child undergoes. If you have questions or concerns about the lumbar puncture procedure, be sure to speak with your doctor.

Chapter 15

Stool Tests

Chapter Contents

Section 15.1

Stool Culture

This section includes information from "Stool Culture," © 2011 American Association for Clinical Chemistry. Reprinted with permission. For additional information about clinical lab testing, visit the Lab Tests Online website at www.labtestsonline.org.

The Test Sample

What is being tested? The stool culture is a test that allows the detection and identification of pathogenic bacteria in the stool. In the laboratory, the test is initiated by applying a small amount of a fresh fecal sample to a variety of nutrient media. These thin layers of gelatin-like material in sterile, covered plastic dishes allow the growth of potential pathogens and discourage the growth of normal bacteria. Once inoculated with stool, the media are incubated and checked daily for bacterial growth. Bacteria that are present in the stool grow as colonies that look like dots on the surface of the gel. The physical characteristics of the colonies—their shape, color, and some of their chemical properties are unique to each type of bacteria and allow them to be differentiated.

The bacteria in the stool are representative of the bacteria that are present in the gastrointestinal tract. Bacteria and fungi called normal flora inhabit everyone's gastrointestinal tract. They play an important role in the digestion of food, and they form a protective barrier against the growth of pathogenic bacteria. The balance of the normal flora may be upset by the administration of broad-spectrum antibiotics, which inhibit the growth of normal flora and allow bacteria resistant to the antibiotic to survive.

Pathogenic bacteria enter the body when someone eats food or drinks water that has been contaminated. This may include raw or undercooked eggs, poultry or beef, unpasteurized milk, and contaminated water from lakes, streams, and (occasionally) from community water supplies. People who travel outside the U.S., especially to developing nations, may face a greater risk of being exposed to disease-causing bacteria. Some of these bacteria may be true pathogens while others are strains of gastrointestinal bacteria that are normal flora for the local inhabitants but cause gastrointestinal distress to the tourist. Visitors may become infected by eating or drinking anything that has been contaminated with the bacteria, even things as simple as tap water, ice cubes in a drink, a fresh salad, or food from a vendor's stall.

The most common symptoms of a pathogenic bacterial infection are prolonged diarrhea, bloody diarrhea, mucus in the stool, abdominal pain, and nausea. If diarrhea lasts more than a few days, it may lead to dehydration and electrolyte imbalance—dangerous conditions, especially in children and the elderly. Dehydration can cause symptoms such as dry skin, fatigue, light-headedness, and fever. Severely affected patients may require hospitalization to replace lost fluids and electrolytes. Hemolytic uremic syndrome (the destruction of red blood cells and kidney failure) is a serious complication that may occasionally arise from an infection with a toxin-producing bacteria, *Escherichia coli*. It is most frequently seen in children and the elderly.

The most common pathogenic bacteria seen in the stool and their most frequently encountered sources include the following:

- **Salmonella,** often found in raw eggs (even intact disinfected eggs), raw poultry, and in reptiles. Pets, such as lizards and turtles, may carry salmonella in their intestines without being ill themselves. Some humans may become carriers of salmonella. Salmonella may be transmitted person-to-person.

- **Shigella,** from fecally contaminated food and water, and from infected-person to person when careful sanitation is not observed. For instance, it can be a challenge to prevent the spread of shigella within a family and in a daycare or nursing home setting since very few organisms may cause disease.

- **Campylobacter,** from raw or undercooked poultry. It is the most common cause of bacterial diarrhea in the U.S. It may become especially serious if it spreads to the bloodstream, and it occasionally causes long-term complications such as arthritis and Guillain-Barré syndrome.

- ***Escherichia coli 0157:H7*** and other toxin-producing *E. coli* (most strains of *E. coli* are considered normal flora). Found in raw or undercooked hamburger/beef, spinach, or unpasteurized cider. Causes bloody diarrhea and may lead to hemolytic uremic syndrome.

Other bacteria that may cause diarrhea include: *Staphylococcus aureus*, *Clostridium difficile*, *Yersinia enterocolitica*, and *Vibrio cholerae* and other Vibrio species.

How is the sample collected for testing? A fresh stool sample is collected in a sterile container. The stool sample should not be contaminated with urine or water. Once it has been collected, the stool should be taken to the laboratory within about an hour after collection or should be transferred into a vial containing a preservative and taken to the lab as soon as possible. The vial should be labeled with the patient's name and the date and time of the stool collection.

Special measures will need to be taken with diaper-wearing infants, both to prevent urine contamination of the sample and to prevent the samples from touching the inside surface of disposable diapers. The diapers often contain a bacteriostatic agent that will inhibit the growth of the bacteria in the sample and interfere with the results of the stool culture.

Is any test preparation needed to ensure the quality of the sample? No test preparation is needed.

The Test

How is it used? A stool culture is used, often along with other tests such as an ova and parasites (O and P) test that detects parasites in the stool and/or a *Clostridium difficile* toxin test, to help determine the cause of your prolonged diarrhea.

When is it ordered? Stool cultures may be ordered when you have had diarrhea for several days and when you have blood and/or mucus in your loose stools. This is especially true when you have eaten food or drunk fluids that you or your doctor suspect may have been contaminated with a pathogenic bacteria, such as undercooked meat or raw eggs, or the same food that has made others ill. Recent travel outside the United States may also suggest possible food contamination. When your doctor suspects that you may have a parasitic infection, he may also order an O and P test. When your diarrhea begins during or after antibiotic treatment, then your doctor may order a *Clostridium difficile* toxin test along with a stool culture.

If you have had a previous pathogenic bacterial infection of your gastrointestinal tract and have been treated for it or gotten better on your own, your doctor may order one or more stool cultures to verify that the pathogenic bacteria are no longer detectable. This can be important because in some cases people can become carriers of the bacteria. Carriers are not ill themselves, but they can infect other people.

What does the test result mean? Results are frequently reported out with the name of the pathogenic bacteria and whether it was isolated (found in your stool sample) or not isolated (that bacteria was not found). Negative results usually reflect the fact that the stool culture was checked for pathogens at several intervals and none were found (not isolated). A report may say something like: "No campylobacter isolated," "No salmonella or shigella isolated," and so forth. If the culture is negative for the major pathogens, then it is likely that your diarrhea is due to another cause. It is also possible that the pathogenic bacteria are present in the gastrointestinal tract but were not found in this particular stool sample. If your doctor suspects this is the case and your symptoms continue, he may order another stool culture.

If your stool culture is positive for pathogenic bacteria, then that is the most likely cause of your prolonged diarrhea. The stool culture report may state "*Salmonella enteritidis* isolated" (which means that you have an infection caused by this particular pathogenic bacterium). Most diarrheal disease is caused by a single pathogen, but it is possible to have an infection with more than one.

Is there anything else I should know? Severe pathogenic bacterial infections of the gastrointestinal tract and those causing complications may be treated with antibiotics, but many uncomplicated cases are best untreated with antibiotics. Patients with competent immune systems will usually get better on their own within a week or so. Patients are instructed in how to prevent the spread of the infection and are treated and monitored for symptoms such as dehydration.

Pathogenic bacterial infections are monitored on a community level. Other than travel-related cases, health officials want to try to determine where your infection came from so that they can address any potential public health concerns. For instance if your salmonella or shigella infection is due to eating food from a particular restaurant, the health department will want to investigate whether or not other people have also become ill from their food. They will visit the restaurant to determine the source of the infection and take steps to ensure that the spread of the infection is stopped.

Section 15.2

Colorectal Cancer Stool Tests

This section is excerpted from "Screen for Life National Colorectal
Cancer Action Campaign: Screening Tests At-a-Glance," Centers for
Disease Control and Prevention (CDC), February 2009.

The U.S. Preventive Services Task Force (USPSTF) recommends
colorectal cancer screening for men and women aged 50–75 using high-
sensitivity fecal occult blood testing (FOBT), sigmoidoscopy, or colonoscopy. The decision to be screened after age 75 should be made on an
individual basis. If you are older than 75, ask your doctor if you should be
screened. The benefits and potential harms of the recommended screening methods vary. Discuss with your doctor which test is best for you.
Getting screened could save your life.

**High-sensitivity fecal occult blood test (FOBT), or fecal im-
munochemical test (FIT):** There are two types of FOBT: one uses the
chemical guaiac to detect blood; the other—a fecal immunochemical test
(FIT) uses antibodies to detect blood in the stool. Ask your doctor for a
high-sensitivity FOBT or FIT. The one-time FOBT done by the doctor in the
doctor's office is not appropriate as a screening test for colorectal cancer.

Your doctor may recommend that you follow a special diet before
taking the FOBT. You receive a test kit from your health care provider.
At home, you use a stick or brush to obtain a small amount of stool.
You may be asked to do this for several bowel movements in a row. You
return the test to the doctor or a lab, where stool samples are checked
for blood. This test should be done every year. (If anything unusual is
found, your doctor will recommend a follow-up colonoscopy.)

Flexible sigmoidoscopy: Your doctor will tell you what foods you
can and cannot eat before the test. The evening before the test, you use
a strong laxative and/or enema to clean out the colon. During the test,
the doctor puts a short, thin, flexible, lighted tube into the rectum. This
tube allows the doctor to check for polyps or cancer inside the rectum
and lower third of the colon. This test should be done every five years.
When it is done in combination with the high-sensitivity FOBT, the
FOBT should be done every three years.

Colonoscopy: May be used as a follow-up test if anything unusual is found during one of the other screening tests. Before this test, your doctor will tell you what foods you can and cannot eat. You use a strong laxative to clean out the colon. Some doctors recommend that you also use an enema. Make sure you arrange for a ride home, as you will not be allowed to drive. You will receive medication during this test, to make you more comfortable.

This test is similar to flexible sigmoidoscopy, except the doctor uses a longer, thin, flexible, lighted tube to check for polyps or cancer inside the rectum and the entire colon. During the test, the doctor can find and remove most polyps and some cancers. This test should be done every ten years. If polyps or cancers are found during the test, you will need more frequent colonoscopies in the future.

Double contrast barium enema: The American Cancer Society recommends this test every five years. Before this test, you follow a special diet and use a strong laxative or enema to clean out the colon. During the test, you receive an enema with a liquid called barium that flows from a tube into the colon, followed by an air enema. The barium and air create an outline around your colon, allowing the doctor to see the outline of your colon on an x-ray.

Virtual colonoscopy: American Cancer Society recommends this every five years. You prepare for this test as you would for a colonoscopy. Before the test, you follow a special diet and use a strong laxative to clean out the colon. Virtual colonoscopy uses x-rays and computers to produce images of the entire colon. The images are displayed on the computer screen.

Some groups say more studies are needed to measure this test's effectiveness and to better understand its benefits and potential harms. Many insurance plans do not yet cover this test for screening.

Stool deoxyribonucleic acid (DNA) test: Recommended by the American Cancer Society. For this test you collect an entire bowel movement and send it to a lab to be checked for cancer cells. This test costs more than the other FOBT or stool tests. If something is found, you will need a colonoscopy. It is not yet known how often this test should be done. Most insurance plans do not cover this test.

Section 15.3

Detecting Parasite Antigens

Excerpted from "Diagnostic Procedures: Stool Specimens,
Detection of Parasite Antigens," Centers for Disease Control and
Prevention (CDC), July 20, 2009.

The diagnosis of human intestinal protozoa depends on microscopic detection of the various parasite stages in feces, duodenal fluid, or small intestine biopsy specimens. Since fecal examination is very labor-intensive and requires a skilled microscopist, antigen detection tests have been developed as alternatives using direct fluorescent antibody (DFA), enzyme immunoassay (EIA), and rapid, dipstick-like tests. Antigen detection methods can be performed quickly and do not require an experienced and skilled morphologist. Much work has been accomplished on the development of antigen detection tests, resulting in commercially available reagents for the intestinal parasites Cryptosporidium spp., *Entamoeba histolytica, Giardia intestinalis (lamblia)*, and *Trichomonas vaginalis.* In addition, antigen detection tests using blood or serum are available for Plasmodium and *Wuchereria bancrofti.*

Specimens for antigen detection: Fresh or preserved stool samples are the appropriate specimen for antigen detection testing with most kits, but refer to the recommended collection procedures included with each specific kit.

Amebiasis

Enzyme immunoassay (EIA) kits are commercially available for detection of fecal antigens for the diagnosis of intestinal amebiasis. Organisms of both the pathogenic *E. histolytica* and the nonpathogenic *Entamoeba dispar* strains are morphologically identical. These assays use monoclonal antibodies that detect the galactose-inhibitable adherence protein in the pathogenic *E. histolytica.* The primary drawback of these assays is the requirement for fresh, unpreserved stool specimens. Several EIA kits for antigen detection of the *E. histolytica / E. dispar* group are available in the U.S., but only the TechLab kit is specific for *E. histolytica.*

Cryptosporidiosis

Immunodetection of antigens on the surface of organisms in stool specimens, using monoclonal antibody-based direct immunofluorescence assay (DFA) assays, is the current test of choice for diagnosis of cryptosporidiosis and provides increased sensitivity over modified acid-fast staining techniques. There are commercial products (DFA, indirect immunofluorescence assay [IFA], EIA, and rapid tests) available in the United States for the diagnosis of cryptosporidiosis. Several kits are combined tests for Cryptosporidium, Giardia, and *E. histolytica*. Factors such as ease of use, technical skill and time, single versus batch testing, and test cost must be considered when determining the test of choice for individual laboratories. The most sensitive (99%) and specific (100%) method is reported to be the DFA test, which identifies oocysts in concentrated or unconcentrated fecal samples by using a fluorescein isothiocyanate (FITC)-labeled monoclonal antibody. A combined DFA test for the simultaneous detection of Cryptosporidium oocysts and Giardia cysts is available.

Some commercial EIA tests are available in the microplate format for the detection of Cryptosporidium antigens in fresh or frozen stool samples and also in stool specimens preserved in formalin, or sodium acetate-acetic acid-formalin (SAF) fixed stool specimens. Concentrated or polyvinyl alcohol-treated (PVA) samples are unsuitable for testing with available antigen detection EIA kits. The kits are reportedly superior to microscopy, especially acid-fast staining, and show good correlation with the DFA test. Kit sensitivities and specificities reportedly range from 93% to 100% when used in a clinical setting. Laboratories which use these EIA kits need to be aware of potential problems with false-positive results and take steps to monitor kit performance.

Rapid immunochromatographic assays are available for the combined antigen detection of either Cryptosporidium and Giardia or Cryptosporidium, Giardia, and *E. histolytica*. These offer the advantage of short test time and multiple results in one reaction device. Initial evaluations indicate comparable sensitivity and specificity to previously available tests.

The Meridian Merifluor DFA Kit for Cryptosporidium/Giardia, modified acid-fast stain for Cryptosporidium spp., or Wheatley's trichrome stain for Giardia spp. are used at the Centers for Disease Control and Prevention (CDC) for routine identification of these parasites. These techniques can be used to confirm suspicious or discrepant diagnostic results.

Giardiasis

Detection of antigens on the surface of organisms in stool specimens is the current test of choice for diagnosis of giardiasis and provides increased sensitivity over more common microscopy techniques. Commercial products (DFA, EIAs, and rapid tests) are available in the United States for the immunodiagnosis of giardiasis. DFA assays may be purchased that employ FITC-labeled monoclonal antibody for detection of Giardia cysts alone or in a combined kit for the simultaneous detection of Giardia cysts and Cryptosporidium oocysts. The sensitivity and specificity of these kits were both 100% compared to those of microscopy. They may be used for quantitation of cysts and oocysts, and thus may be useful for epidemiologic and control studies.

Some commercial EIA tests are available in the microplate format for the detection of Giardia antigen in fresh or frozen stool samples and also in stool specimens preserved in formalin, migration-inhibitory factor (MIF), or sodium acetate-acetic acid-formalin (SAF) fixatives. EIA kit sensitivity rates were recently reported as ranging from 94%–100% while specificity rates were all 100%.

Rapid immunochromatographic assays are available for the combined antigen detection of either Cryptosporidium and Giardia or Cryptosporidium, Giardia, and *E. histolytica*. These offer the advantage of short test time and multiple results in one reaction device. Initial evaluations indicate comparable sensitivity and specificity to previously available tests.

The Meridian Merifluor DFA Kit for Cryptosporidium/Giardia, modified acid-fast stain for Cryptosporidium spp., or Wheatley's trichrome stain for Giardia spp. are used at CDC for routine identification of these parasites. These techniques can be used to confirm suspicious or discrepant diagnostic results.

Trichomoniasis

Trichomoniasis, an infection caused by *Trichomonas vaginalis*, is a common sexually transmitted disease. Diagnosis is made by detection of trophozoites in vaginal secretions or urethral specimens by wet mount microscopic examination, DFA staining of specimens, or culture. Sensitivity of the assays was reported as 60% for wet mounts and 86% for DFA when compared to cultures. A kit which employs FITC- or enzyme-labeled monoclonal antibodies for use in a DFA or EIA procedure is available for detection of whole parasites in fluids. A latex agglutination test for antigen detection in vaginal swab specimens is available; the manufacturer's evaluation indicated good sensitivity and specificity.

Chapter 16

Throat Culture

What It Is

A throat culture or strep test is performed by using a throat swab to detect the presence of group A streptococcus bacteria, the most common cause of strep throat. Group A streptococcus bacteria also can cause other infections, including pneumonia, tonsillitis, and meningitis.

A sample swabbed from the back of the throat is put on a special plate (culture) that enables bacteria to grow. The specific type of infection is determined using chemical tests. If bacteria don't grow, the culture is negative and the person doesn't have a strep throat infection.

Strep throat is a bacterial infection that affects the back of the throat and the tonsils, which become irritated and swell, causing a sore throat that's especially bothersome when swallowing. White or yellow spots or a coating on the throat and tonsils also might be present, and the lymph nodes in the neck may swell.

Strep throat is most common among school-age children. The infection may cause headaches, stomachaches, nausea, vomiting, and listlessness. Strep throat infections don't usually include cold symptoms such as sneezing, coughing, or a runny or stuffy nose.

"Strep Test: Throat Culture," February 2009, reprinted with permission from www.kidshealth.org. Copyright © 2009 The Nemours Foundation. This information was provided by KidsHealth, one of the largest resources online for medically reviewed health information written for parents, kids, and teens. For more articles like this one, visit www.KidsHealth.org, or www.TeensHealth.org.

While symptoms of strep throat usually go away within a few days without direct treatment, doctors will prescribe antibiotics to help prevent related complications such as rheumatic fever.

Why It's Done

The throat culture test can help determine the cause of a sore throat. Often, a sore throat is caused by a virus, but a throat culture will determine if it's definitely caused by strep bacteria so doctors can provide proper treatment.

Preparation

Encourage your child to stay still during the procedure. Be sure to tell the doctor if your child has taken any antibiotics recently, and try to have your child avoid antiseptic mouthwash before the test as this could affect test results.

The Procedure

A health professional will ask your child to tilt his or her head back and open his or her mouth as wide as possible. If the back of the throat cannot be seen clearly, the tongue will be pressed down with a flat stick (tongue depressor) to provide a better view. A clean cotton swab will be rubbed over the back of the throat, over the tonsils, and over any red or sore areas to collect a sample.

You may wish to hold your child on your lap during the procedure to prevent movement that could make it difficult for the health professional to obtain an adequate sample.

What to Expect

Your child may have some gagging when the cotton swab touches the back of the throat. If your child's throat is sore, the swabbing may cause brief discomfort.

Getting the Results

Throat culture test results are generally ready in two days.

Risks

Throat swabbing can be uncomfortable, but no risks are associated with a throat culture test.

Helping Your Child

Explaining the test in terms your child can understand might help ease any fear. During the test, encourage your child to relax and stay still so the health professional can adequately swab the throat and tonsils.

If You Have Questions

If you have questions about the throat culture strep test, speak with your doctor.

Chapter 17

Toxicology Screen

A toxicology screen refers to various tests to determine the type and approximate amount of legal and illegal drugs a person has taken.

How the Test Is Performed

Toxicology screening is most often done using a blood or urine sample. However, it may be done soon after swallowing the medication, using stomach contents that are obtained through gastric lavage or after vomiting. In some circumstances, you may need to provide the urine sample in the presence of the nurse or technician to verify that the urine sample came from you and was not tampered with.

How to Prepare for the Test

No special preparation is needed. If able, tell your health care provider what drugs (including over-the-counter medications) you have taken, including when and how much.

This test is sometimes part of an investigation for drug use or abuse. Special consents, handling and labeling of specimens, or other special procedures may be required.

Excerpted from "Toxicology Screen," © 2011 A.D.A.M., Inc. Reprinted with permission.

How the Test Will Feel

Blood test: When the needle is inserted to draw blood, some people feel moderate pain, while others feel only a prick or stinging sensation. Afterward, there may be some throbbing.

Urine test: A urine test involves normal urination. There is no discomfort.

Why the Test Is Performed

This test is often done in emergency medical situations. It can be used to evaluate possible accidental or intentional overdose or poisoning. It may help determine the cause of acute drug toxicity, to monitor drug dependency, and to determine the presence of substances in the body for medical or legal purposes.

Additional reasons the test may be performed:

- Alcoholism
- Alcohol withdrawal state
- Altered mental state
- Analgesic nephropathy
- Complicated alcohol abstinence (delirium tremens)
- Delirium
- Dementia
- Drug abuse monitoring
- Fetal alcohol syndrome
- Intentional overdose
- Seizures
- Stroke secondary to cocaine
- Unconscious patient

If the test is used as a drug screen, it must be done during a certain time period after the drug has been taken or while forms of the drug can still be detected in the body. Examples are below:

- Alcohol: 3–10 hours
- Amphetamines: 24–48 hours

- Barbiturates: up to six weeks
- Benzodiazepines: up to six weeks with high level use
- Cocaine: 2–4 days; up to 10–22 days with heavy use
- Codeine: 1–2 days
- Heroin: 1–2 days
- Hydromorphone: 1–2 days
- Methadone: 2–3 days
- Morphine: 1–2 days
- Phencyclidine (PCP): 1–8 days
- Propoxyphene: 6–48 hours
- Tetrahydrocannabinol (THC): 6–11 weeks with heavy use

Normal Results

Normal value ranges for over-the-counter or prescription medications may vary slightly among different laboratories. Talk to your doctor about the meaning of your specific test results. A negative value usually means that alcohol, prescription medications that have not been prescribed, and illegal drugs have not been detected.

A blood toxicology screen can determine the presence and level (amount) of a drug in your body. Urine sample results are usually reported as positive (substance is found) or negative (no substance is found).

What Abnormal Results Mean

Elevated levels of alcohol or prescription drugs can be a sign of intentional or accidental intoxication or overdose. The presence of illegal drugs or drugs not prescribed for the person indicates illicit drug use.

Considerations

Commonly found substances on a toxicology screen include the following:

- Alcohol (ethanol)—"drinking" alcohol
- Amphetamines
- Antidepressants

- Barbiturates and hypnotics
- Benzodiazepines
- Cocaine
- Marijuana
- Narcotics
- Non-narcotic pain medicines including acetaminophen and anti-inflammatory drugs
- Phencyclidine (PCP)
- Phenothiazines (antipsychotic or tranquilizing medications)
- Prescription medications, any type

Chapter 18

Urine Tests

Note: Urine tests for adults are similar as described in this chapter.

Doctors order urine tests for kids to make sure that the kidneys and certain other organs are functioning properly, or when they suspect that a child might have an infection in the kidneys, bladder, or other parts of the urinary tract.

The kidneys make urine as they filter wastes from the bloodstream while leaving substances in the blood that the body needs, like protein and glucose. So when urine contains glucose, too much protein, or has other irregularities, it's usually a sign of a health problem.

Urinalysis

A urinalysis is usually ordered when a doctor suspects that a child has a urinary tract infection or a health problem that can cause an abnormality in the urine. This test can measure:

- the number and variety of red and white blood cells;

- the presence of bacteria or other organisms;

- the presence of substances, such as glucose, that usually shouldn't be found in the urine;

- the pH, which shows how acidic or basic the urine is;
- the concentration of the urine.

Sometimes, when the urine contains white blood cells or protein, or the test results seem abnormal for another reason, it's because of how or when the urine was collected. For example, a dehydrated child may have a few white blood cells or a small amount of protein in the urine. But that may not necessarily mean that there's an infection or a health problem. Once the child is rehydrated, these "abnormal" results may disappear. Depending on the amount of protein or white blood cells in the urine, the doctor may repeat the urine test at another time, just to make sure that everything is back to normal.

How a Urinalysis Is Done

In most cases, urine is collected in a clean container, then a plastic stick that has patches of chemicals on it (the dipstick) is placed in the urine. The patches change color to indicate things like the presence of white blood cells or glucose.

The doctor or laboratory technologist also usually examines the urine under a microscope to check for other substances that indicate different conditions.

If a urinalysis shows white blood cells and bacteria—which may mean that there's an infection in the kidneys or the bladder—the doctor may decide to send the urine to a lab for a urine culture to identify bacteria that may be causing the infection.

Getting a urine sample: It can be difficult to get urine samples from kids to analyze for a possible infection. That's because the skin around the urinary opening normally is home to some of the same bacteria that cause infections in the urinary tract. If these bacteria contaminate the urine, the doctors may not be able to use the sample to tell if there is an infection or not.

To avoid this, the skin surrounding the urinary opening has to be cleaned and rinsed immediately before the urine is collected. In this "clean-catch" method, the patient (or parent) cleans the skin around the urinary opening. The child then urinates, stops momentarily (if the child is old enough to cooperate), then urinates again into the collection container. Catching the urine in "midstream" is the goal.

In some cases, like when the child is not yet toilet trained, the doctor will insert a catheter (a narrow, soft tube) through the urinary tract opening into the bladder to get the urine sample.

If you have any questions about urine tests, talk with your doctor.

Part Three

Imaging Tests

Chapter 19

Risks of Medical Imaging

Chapter Contents

Section 19.1

Increasing Use of Radiation-Emitting Procedures

Excerpted from "The Downside of Diagnostic Imaging,"
National Cancer Institute (NCI), January 26, 2010.

Modern diagnostic imaging has revolutionized medicine. In a matter of seconds, a computed tomography (CT) machine can produce extremely detailed images of any part of the body. Nuclear medicine tests, such as positron emission tomography (PET) or the technetium-based stress tests used widely in cardiovascular medicine, let doctors observe the inner workings of cells and tissues.

CT and nuclear medicine tests do have a downside, however: they deliver doses of ionizing radiation from 50 to over 500 times that of a standard x-ray, such as a chest x-ray or mammogram. Scientists have raised concerns that such large doses of radiation plus the widespread and increasing use these diagnostic procedures may, in a small but significant way, pose a cancer risk in the general population. Data from several studies released in the second half of 2009 have helped to quantify this risk and the pace at which it is growing.

Unacceptable on the Job, But Not in the Clinic?

In the United States, people exposed to radiation at their jobs are monitored and limited to an effective dose of 100 millisieverts (mSv) every five years (an average of 20 mSv per year, with a maximum of 50 mSv in any single year). The concept of effective dose and the mSv measurement estimate the potential future risk of cancer from radiation exposure. However, the available evidence indicates that most patients exposed to radiation from diagnostic imaging are not subject to similar monitoring or exposure limits. In a study published in the *New England Journal of Medicine* in August 2009, researchers led by Dr. Reza Fazel of the Emory University School of Medicine examined the medical records of 952,420 people in four states from 2005 through 2007 to estimate the number of people who might receive radiation doses from diagnostic imaging at a level that would cause concern in an occupational health setting.

Between 1980 and 2006, the annual per-capita effective radiation dose in the United States nearly doubled. Almost all of this increased dose came from exposure through medical imaging, which increased by about 600%.

In that three-year period, their patient sample underwent more than three million imaging procedures delivering radiation exposure. Almost 194 per 1,000 people each year received moderate radiation doses (between 3–20 mSv). Almost 19 per 1,000 received high doses (between 20 and 50 mSv), and almost two per 1,000 received very high doses (over 50 mSv) each year. Using this data, the authors estimated that about four million Americans each year receive radiation doses higher than 20 mSv from medical imaging.

Worldwide Exposure

These data are particularly concerning, experts say, given the recent and continuing increase in the use of imaging procedures using ionizing radiation in the United States and worldwide. A report published November 2009 in *Radiology* using data from the U.S. National Council on Radiation Protection and Measurements and the United Nations Scientific Committee on the Effects of Atomic Radiation concluded that, worldwide, the annual effective radiation dose per capita from medical imaging has doubled in the past 10–15 years. The increase in the United States was much greater than anywhere else in the world.

The authors, led by Dr. Fred A. Mettler of the New Mexico Veterans Administration Health Care System reported that in the United States this dose increased by about six-fold between 1980 and 2006. Over the past 56 years, the estimated number of annual radiologic and nuclear medicine procedures increased by about 15-fold.

"The use of CT in particular has gone up dramatically, and we've drastically lowered the threshold for using it," said Dr. Rebecca Smith-Bindman, a visiting research scientist with National Cancer Institute's (NCI) Radiation Epidemiology Branch (REB). "There's a general belief that if you get a CT scan, you must be reasonably sick and must really need it. This is no longer true, and we are increasingly using CT scans in patients who are not that sick. There's been drift not only in how often we use it but in how we use it."

"We've only talked about the benefits of CT for the past 20 years, without considering any potential harm" she continued. "I'm hoping the medical community can start a dialogue about when it should be used.

CT is a fabulous test, but we have to use it prudently, and only when there is clear evidence of benefit that outweighs its potential harm."

Considering Benefit, Reducing Harm

The failure to optimize and standardize diagnostic protocols and techniques was highlighted in a study led by Dr. Smith-Bindman, published in the December 2009 *Archives of Internal Medicine.* She and her colleagues gathered data on radiation dose from CT scanning at four hospitals, all of which used equipment from the same manufacturer. Even with this homogeneity in CT equipment, the researchers observed a mean 13-fold variation between the lowest and highest radiation doses seen in each type of CT study measured, both within and across the four institutions. This variation is due to different institutions and individual physicians choosing different technical parameters on the machines when running similar types of CT scans done for similar indications, explained the authors.

"There are no standards set for what's an acceptable radiation dose for different types of scans, and no group is monitoring the radiation doses patients receive," said Dr. Smith-Bindman. "Thus, the variation in dose is high and unacceptable. With available technology we could lower the doses by 30% to 50% immediately, but there's currently no mandate to do this."

The Coming Storm?

In addition to measuring variability in dose, Dr. Smith-Bindman and her colleagues used data from the National Research Council to estimate the number of excess cancers expected to develop from exposure to high-dose diagnostic imaging. Their results suggested that one in 270 women and one in 600 men undergoing CT heart scans (a potentially high-dose procedure) at the age of 40 will develop cancer related to that CT scan. Lower-dose imaging procedures carried lower risks, but increased risks nonetheless. When these tests were performed in younger patients, the risks were higher.

Dr. Amy Berrington de González, of REB, and her colleagues used National Research Council data to estimate the number of excess cancers expected to be caused by CT scans performed in the United States in 2007. Their research estimated that approximately 29,000 future cancers could be related to CT scans performed in the United States in that year alone, with women being at higher risk than men. About 35% of these cancers were projected to be related to scans performed in patients 35–54 years old, and 15% related to scans performed in children younger than 18.

The medical community has proposed many ways to reduce radiation exposure from diagnostic medicine without negatively impacting the quality of patient care:

- Reduce the number of CT exams by using other technologies (such as ultrasound or magnetic resonance imaging [MRI]) in cases where they would provide equal diagnostic quality.

- Limit the use of CT in healthy patients who would obtain little benefit (such as whole-body CT screening).

- Limit the use of repeat CT surveillance of patients in whom a diagnosis has already been made, when repeat scanning would lead to little change in their treatment.

- Tailor the radiation dose carefully to a patient's individual size. This point is particularly important for children.

- Educate both doctors and patients about radiation exposure from diagnostic imaging. In a recent survey, nearly all physicians polled significantly underestimated radiation doses from a CT scan.

- Track and collect information on radiation exposure for individual patients through a system such as the International Atomic Energy Agency's proposed Smart Card digital record system.

- Improve communication between doctors as a patient moves through the diagnostic process to avoid unnecessary imaging and repeated imaging in different departments or hospitals.

- Optimize and standardize diagnostic protocols and techniques to limit exposure from any individual procedure.

Section 19.2

Doses from Medical Radiation Sources

Excerpted from "Radiation Exposure from Medical Exams
and Procedures," © 2010 The Health Physics Society
(http://hps.org). Reprinted with permission.

Ionizing radiation is used daily in hospitals and clinics to perform diagnostic imaging exams and medical interventions. For the purposes of this document, the word radiation refers to ionizing radiation; the most common forms of radiation in medicine are x-rays and gamma rays.

Exams and procedures that use radiation are necessary for accurate diagnosis of disease and injury. They provide important information about your health to your doctor and help ensure that you receive appropriate care.

Physicians can also use radiation to make some procedures, such as heart valve replacement, less time-consuming and invasive. Physicians and technologists performing these procedures are trained to use the minimum amount of radiation necessary for the procedure. Benefits from medical procedures greatly outweigh the potential small risk of harm from the amount of radiation used.

A recent report from the National Council on Radiation Protection and Measurements (NCRP) states that exposure to the U.S. population from medical procedures has increased since the 1980s (NCRP 2009). These findings can be attributed to the growth in the use of medical imaging procedures, especially from increased use of computed tomography (CT) and nuclear medicine. The NCRP, the American College of Radiology, the World Health Organization, and others are working to improve the referral process for procedures involving CT and nuclear medicine so that they are based on objective, medically relevant criteria.

Which types of diagnostic imaging procedures use radiation?

- In x-ray procedures, x-rays pass through the body to form pictures on a computer or television monitor, which are viewed by a radiologist. If you have an x-ray, it will be performed with a standard x-ray machine or with a more sophisticated x-ray machine called a CT machine.

- During interventional procedures, fluoroscopy is used by cardiologists, gastroenterologists, pain specialists, and radiologists to perform procedures inside the body.

- In nuclear medicine procedures, a small amount of radioactive material is inhaled, injected, or swallowed by the patient. If you have a nuclear medicine procedure, a special camera will be used to detect energy given off by the radioactive material in your body and form a picture of your organs and their level of function on a computer monitor. A nuclear medicine physician views these pictures. The radioactive material typically disappears from your body within a few hours or days.

Do benefits from medical examinations using radiation outweigh the risks from the radiation?

Your doctor will order an x-ray for you when it is needed for accurate diagnosis of your condition. There is no conclusive evidence of radiation causing harm at the levels patients receive from diagnostic x-ray exams. Although high doses of radiation are linked to an increased risk of cancer, the effects of low doses of radiation used in diagnostic imaging are either nonexistent or too small to observe. The benefits of diagnostic medical exams are vital to good patient care.

What are typical doses from medical procedures involving radiation?

Radiation dose can be estimated for some common diagnostic x-ray, fluoroscopic, and nuclear medicine procedures. It is important to note that these are only typical values. Radiation doses differ for each person because of differences in x-ray machines and their settings, the amount of radioactive material given in a nuclear medicine procedure, and the patient's metabolism.

Many diagnostic exposures are less than or similar to the exposure we receive from natural background radiation. For comparison, in the United States each person receives about 3.0 millisievert (mSv) (300 millirem [mrem]) of radiation exposure from background sources every year. The effective dose listed is a comparable whole-body dose from the exam. The effective dose is given in mSv (an international unit of radiation measurement) and mrem (the traditional unit used in the United States).

159

How can I obtain an estimate of my radiation dose from medical exams?

Ask your doctor to refer you to a medical health physicist or diagnostic medical physicist for information on medical radiation exposure and an estimate of exposure. You can also get an estimate of typical doses for procedures online at http://www.doseinfo-radar.com/RADARDoseRiskCalc.html.

Do magnetic resonance imaging (MRI) and ultrasound use radiation?

No. MRI and ultrasound procedures do not use ionizing radiation. If you have either of these types of studies, you are not exposed to radiation.

Glossary

dose: A general term used to refer either to the amount of energy absorbed by a material exposed to radiation (absorbed dose) or to the potential biological effect in tissue exposed to radiation (equivalent dose).

Sv or sievert: The International System of Units (SI) unit for dose equivalent equal to one joule/kilogram. The sievert has replaced the rem; one sievert is equal to 100 rem. One millisievert is equal to 100 millirem.

References

Health Physics Society. People exposed to more radiation from medical exams. Available at http://hps.org/media/documents/NCRP_Report-People_Exposed_to_More_Radiation_from_Medical_Exams_9Mar.pdf. Accessed 8 February 2010.

Mettler FA Jr, Huda W, Yoshizumi TT, Mahesh M. Effective doses in radiology and diagnostic nuclear medicine: A catalog. *Radiology 248(1)*:254–263; 2008. Available at: http://radiology.rsna.org/content/248/1/254.long. Accessed 8 February 2010.

National Council on Radiation Protection and Measurements. Ionizing radiation exposure of the population of the United States. Washington, DC: National Council on Radiation Protection and Measurements; *NCRP Report No. 160*; 2009. Summary of the report available at: http://www.ncrponline.org/Press_Rel/Rept_160_Press_Release.pdf. Accessed 8 February 2010.

Section 19.3

Radiation Exposure and Pregnancy

"Radiation Exposure and Pregnancy," © 2010 The Health Physics Society (http://hps.org). Reprinted with permission.

Everyone is exposed to radiation every day. People are continuously exposed to low-level radiation found in food, soils, building materials, and the air and from outer space. All of this radiation originates from naturally occurring sources. For example, bananas contain naturally occurring radioactive potassium-40 and air contains radon, a radioactive gas. Your average natural background radiation dose is about 3.0 mSv (300 mrem) each year (millisieverts and millirem are units of radiation dose, much like a gram or an ounce is a unit of weight).

In addition to natural background radiation, you may be exposed to radiation from medical x-rays and medical radiation tests or treatments. If you think, or there is a possibility, that you may be pregnant and need a medical x-ray or radiation procedure, the information below will help answer your question: "Does a medical procedure involving radiation increase my baby's health risks?"

What are the health risks from medical x-rays or radionuclide medical tests performed during pregnancy?

There is a lot of reliable information about the effects of radiation exposure during pregnancy. Potential radiation effects vary depending on the fetal stage of development and the magnitude of the doses. Our best knowledge indicates that there is a threshold below which negative effects are not observed.

According to the American College of Radiology, routine x-rays of a mother's abdomen, back, hips, and pelvis are not likely to pose a serious risk to the child (ACR/RSNA 2010). However, certain procedures (such as a computerized tomography [CT scan] or a lower gastrointestinal [GI] fluoroscope exam) to the mother's stomach or hips may give higher doses. If you are administered a radioactive drug (nuclear medicine), radioactivity in your urine or intestines could give a moderate dose to the fetus, and some compounds can cross the placenta as well. If you are a candidate for a therapeutic use of radiation from either machine-produced radiation or a nuclear medicine treatment, this may be delayed until after pregnancy, or if urgent, special precautions should be taken to protect the fetus.

Very high radiation doses (for example, in survivors of the Japanese atomic bombings who were pregnant) resulted in some fetal abnormalities and neurological effects, but in diagnostic uses of radiation the doses are below these thresholds. Some have discussed possible risks of cancer appearing later from children irradiated in utero, but the chance of these effects occurring are very small and, if they exist at all, they are well below the natural occurrence rates for these cancers and even farther below the other normal risks of all pregnancies. Every pregnancy carries about a 3% risk for birth defects (American College of Obstetricians and Gynecologists [ACOG] 2009) and a 15% risk of miscarriage (ACOG 2002).

Most diagnostic x-ray or radionuclide medical procedures do not result in a radiation dose that can be associated with any significant increase in risk. If you have a test or treatment that might give your fetus a higher dose, a medical physicist or health physicist in consultation with your doctor can evaluate the possible radiation dose and risk. A medical physicist or health physicist may be contacted through your hospital's radiology or radiation safety department.

What if I find out I'm pregnant after being exposed to radiation?

If you discover you are pregnant after you have had a test or treatment that causes you concern, you should consult with the doctor who ordered the test. You and your doctor should contact a medical physicist or health physicist, who will estimate the radiation dose to your fetus. The calculated radiation dose and developmental stage of your fetus will help the medical physicist or health physicist determine the potential health risks. This information should be shared with your doctor.

Most standard radiological tests and treatments produce radiation doses below 50 mSv (5,000 millirem). The National Council on Radiation Protection and Measurements and the American College of Obstetricians and Gynecologists both agree that the potential health risks to your fetus are not increased from most standard medical tests with a radiation dose below 50 mSv. Potential health risks, however, may increase for a few medical tests or combinations of tests that result in radiation doses that exceed 50 mSv, depending on the dose and on the stage of pregnancy.

Does it matter how far along in the pregnancy I am?

The sensitivity of a developing fetus to radiation can vary with the stage of development, the magnitude of the dose, and the length of time of the total exposure (minutes, hours, days, or weeks). The most radiosensitive period appears to be between eight and 15 weeks after conception. The medical physicist or health physicist will consider all these factors in determining the risks to your fetus.

I am not pregnant now, but will an x-ray or a radionuclide medical test cause my future children to have birth defects?

There is no evidence that your future children will be at a greater risk for birth defects from x-rays or radionuclide medical tests that you receive before becoming pregnant. This conclusion is based on extensive studies of women exposed to atomic-bomb radiation at Hiroshima and Nagasaki and those pregnant women who received x-ray studies, radionuclide medical tests, and other medical radiation procedures. Since the discovery of x-rays over a century ago, the number of women exposed to medical radiation has increased dramatically while the rate of birth defects and miscarriages has not changed.

What else do I need to know?

As a precaution, if during your pregnancy you are considering having an abdominal/pelvic x-ray or a radionuclide medical test, consult your doctor. The doctor, in consultation with the medical physicist or health physicist, will help you determine if any increased risk is significant. If there is a considerable risk, your doctor can determine if the procedures can be delayed until after birth or whether another medical procedure, such as an ultrasound or magnetic resonance imaging (MRI), could be used instead.

If you are pregnant and abdominal x-rays or radionuclide medical procedures are scheduled without consultation with your doctor, inform the person performing the exam that you are pregnant. As a precaution, you should inform a person performing any type of x-ray or radiation procedure that you are pregnant.

What if I am breast feeding and I need a nuclear medicine exam?

A woman who is a breast feeding mother may have to stop breast feeding for a period of time after receiving a radiopharmaceutical for a nuclear medicine exam. The nuclear medicine staff will provide information to women regarding cessation. In the case of x-rays and computed tomography (CT) scans, the breast milk is not affected by the exam so the woman can continue to breast-feed.

Glossary

dose: A general term used to refer either to the amount of energy absorbed by a material exposed to radiation (absorbed dose) or to the potential biological effect in tissue exposed to radiation (equivalent dose).

Sv or sievert: The International System of Units (SI) unit for dose equivalent equal to one joule/kilogram. The sievert has replaced the rem; one sievert is equal to 100 rem. One millisievert is equal to 100 millirem.

References

American College of Obstetricians and Gynecologists. *Reducing your risk of birth defects.* August 2009. Available at: http://www.acog.org/publications/patient_education/bp146.cfm. Accessed 24 June 2010.

American College of Radiology/Radiological Society of North America. *Pregnancy and x-rays.* RadiologyInfo.org. March 2010. Available at: http://www.radiologyinfo.org/en/safety/index.cfm?pg=sfty_xray#part6. Accessed 6 May 2010.

American College of Obstetricians and Gynecologists. *Early pregnancy loss: Miscarriage and molar pregnancy.* May 2002. Available at: http://www.acog.org/publications/patient_education/bp090.cfm. Accessed 24 June 2010.

Section 19.4

Radiology and Children

Excerpted from "Radiology and Children: Extra Care Required,"
U.S. Food and Drug Administration (FDA), June 23, 2008.

Children may be more sensitive to radiation received from medical imaging scans than adults. One factor to consider is that children have more rapidly dividing cells that can be exposed to the low-level radiation. Also, they have a longer expected lifetime for the effects of radiation exposure to manifest as cancer. That is why it is important that with children, the lowest radiation dose necessary is used for providing an image from which an accurate diagnosis can be made.

Image Gently, a national initiative of the Alliance for Radiation Safety in Pediatric Imaging aims to educate parents and health care professionals about the specific precautions required for children undergoing radiological imaging. The campaign's introductory focus is on child-safety awareness in regard to computed tomography (CT) scans.

CT scans are taken in large machines containing a round hole and tunnel chamber. Patients lie on a table that slides into the chamber, where an x-ray camera rotates around them and snaps pictures offering health care professionals three-dimensional views of internal organs, bone, soft tissue, and blood vessels. CT has helped improve the diagnosis and care for conditions such as cancer, heart disease, brain disorders, and cardiovascular illnesses. But the technology does expose patients to higher doses of radiation than most other radiological exams.

CT: Tips for Parents

The Image Gently campaign advises parents to do the following:

- **Talk with your child's physician.** He or she will know or can find out if the imaging center to which they refer uses appropriate pediatric CT scanning techniques, and if a non-radiation imaging test might be as useful for your child's situation.

- **Be your child's advocate.** Learn about ways health care professionals can lower and limit radiation dose in the CT imaging of children without compromising diagnostic quality. Ask questions.

- **Be sure that the imaging facility is using appropriate reduced radiation techniques.** You may not know unless you ask, and it is reasonable and within your rights to do so.

- **Check credentials.** Ask whether the facility has American College of Radiology accreditation, whether the CT technologists have the proper credentials, and if the person interpreting the studies is a board-certified radiologist or pediatric radiologist.

Section 19.5

Reducing Radiation from Medical X-Rays

Excerpted from "Reducing Radiation from Medical X-Rays," U.S. Food and Drug Administration (FDA), February 2009.

X-rays are used for much more than identifying injuries from accidents. They are used to screen for, diagnose, and treat various medical conditions. X-rays can be used on just about any part of the body—from the head down to the toes—to identify health problems ranging from a broken bone to pneumonia, heart disease, intestinal blockages, and kidney stones. And x-rays cannot only find cancerous tumors, but can often destroy them. Along with their tremendous value, medical x-rays have a drawback: they expose people to radiation.

Steps for Consumers

Consumers have an important role in reducing radiation risks from medical x-rays. FDA recommends these steps:

Ask your health care professional how an X-ray will help. How will it help find out what's wrong or determine your treatment? Ask if there are other procedures that might be lower risk but still allow a good assessment or treatment for your medical situation.

Don't refuse an x-ray. If your health care professional explains why it is medically needed, then don't refuse an x-ray. The risk of not having a needed x-ray is greater than the small risk from radiation.

Don't insist on an x-ray. If your health care professional explains there is no need for an x-ray, then don't demand one.

Tell the x-ray technologist in advance if you are, or might be, pregnant.

Ask if a protective shield can be used. If you or your children are getting an x-ray, ask whether a lead apron or other shield should be used.

Table 19.1. Radiation Dose of Common Medical Exams Compared to Natural Source of Radiation

For this procedure:	Your effective radiation dose is:	Comparable to natural background radiation for:
Abdominal region:		
Computed tomography (CT)-Abdomen	10 mSv	3 years
Computed tomography (CT)-Body	10 mSv	3 years
Radiography–Lower GI tract	4 mSv	16 months
Radiography–Upper GI tract	2 mSv	8 months
Bone:		
Radiography–Extremity	0.001 mSv	Less than 1 day
Chest:		
Computed tomography (CT)-Chest	8 mSv	3 years
Radiography–Chest	0.1 mSv	10 days
Women's imaging:		
Mammography	0.7 mSv	3 months

Copyright © 2009 RadiologyInfo.org; Courtesy: American College of Radiology and Radiological Society of North America.

Ask your dentist if he/she uses the faster (E or F) speed film for x-rays. It costs about the same as the conventional D speed film and offers similar benefits with a lower radiation dose. Using digital imaging detectors instead of film further reduces radiation dose.

Know your x-ray history. When an x-ray is taken, fill out the card with the date and type of exam, referring physician, and facility and address where the images are kept. Show the card to your health care professionals to avoid unnecessary duplication of x-rays of the same body part. Keep a record card for everyone in your family.

Medical X-rays: How Much Radiation Are You Getting?

Table 19.1 shows the radiation dose of some common medical x-ray exams compared to the radiation people are exposed to from natural sources in the environment. For example, the radiation exposure from one chest x-ray equals the amount of radiation a person is exposed to from their natural surroundings in ten days.

The unit of measurement for an effective radiation dose is the millisievert (mSv). The average person in the United States receives a dose of about three mSv per year from naturally occurring radiation.

Three types of x-ray procedures are listed:

- Computed tomography (CT) generates a three-dimensional image of part of the body.

- Radiography generates a two-dimensional image.

- Mammography is radiography of the breast.

Chapter 20

Radiography

Chapter Contents

Section 20.1

Medical X-Rays

Excerpted from "Medical X-Rays," U.S. Food and
Drug Administration (FDA), March 21, 2011.

X-rays refer to radiation, waves, or particles that travel through the air like light or radio signals. X-ray energy is high enough that some radiation passes through objects (such as internal organs, body tissues, and clothing) and onto x-ray detectors (such as film or a detector linked to a computer monitor). In general, objects that are more dense (such as bones and calcium deposits) absorb more of the radiation from the x-rays and do not allow as much to pass through them. These objects leave a different image on the detector than less dense objects. Specially trained or experienced physicians can read these images to diagnose medical conditions or injuries.

Procedures

Medical x-rays are used in many types of examinations and procedures. Some examples include:

- x-ray radiography (to find orthopedic damage, tumors, pneumonias, foreign objects, and so forth);

- mammography (to image the internal structures of breasts);

- CT (computed tomography) (to produce cross-sectional images of the body);

- fluoroscopy (to dynamically visualize the body for example to see where to remove plaque from coronary arteries or where to place stents to keep those arteries open);

- radiation therapy in cancer treatment.

Risks/Benefits

Medical x-rays have increased the ability to detect disease or injury early enough for a medical problem to be managed, treated, or cured.

When applied and performed appropriately, these procedures can improve health and may even save a person's life.

X-ray energy also has a small potential to harm living tissue. The most significant risks are a small increase in the possibility that a person exposed to x-rays will develop cancer later in life; and, cataracts and skin burns only at very high levels of radiation exposure and in only very few procedures. The risk of developing cancer from radiation exposure is generally small, and it depends on at least three factors—the amount of radiation dose, the age at exposure, and the sex of the person exposed with women at a somewhat higher lifetime risk than men.

Note: Chapter 19 provides specific information about reducing your radiation risks from medical x-ray procedures.

Section 20.2

Chest X-Ray

Excerpted from "Chest X-Ray," National Heart,
Lung, and Blood Institute (NHLBI), August 2010.

A chest x-ray is a painless, noninvasive test that creates pictures of the structures inside your chest, such as your heart, lungs, and blood vessels. Noninvasive means that no surgery is done and no instruments are inserted into your body. This test is done to find the cause of symptoms such as shortness of breath, chest pain, chronic cough (a cough that lasts a long time), and fever.

A chest x-ray takes pictures of the inside of your chest. The different tissues in your chest absorb different amounts of radiation. Your ribs and spine are bony and absorb radiation well. They normally appear light on a chest x-ray. Your lungs, which are filled with air, normally appear dark. A disease in the chest that changes how radiation is absorbed also will appear on a chest x-ray.

Chest x-rays help doctors diagnose conditions such as pneumonia, heart failure, lung cancer, lung tissue scarring, and sarcoidosis. Doctors also may use chest x-rays to see how well treatments for certain conditions are working. Also, doctors often use chest x-rays before surgery to look at the structures in the chest. Chest x-rays are the most common x-ray test used to diagnose health problems.

Chest x-rays have few risks. The amount of radiation used in a chest x-ray is very small. A lead apron may be used to protect certain parts of your body from the radiation. The test gives out a radiation dose similar to the amount of radiation you're naturally exposed to over ten days.

What to Expect before a Chest X-Ray

You don't have to do anything special to prepare for a chest x-ray. However, you may want to wear a shirt that is easy to take off. Before the test, you'll be asked to undress from the waist up and wear a gown. You also may want to avoid wearing jewelry and other metal objects. You'll be asked to take off any jewelry, eyeglasses, and metal objects that might interfere with the x-ray picture. Let the x-ray technician (a person specially trained to do x-ray tests) know if you have any body piercings on your chest.

Let your doctor know if you're pregnant or may be pregnant. In general, women should avoid all x-ray tests during pregnancy. Sometimes, though, having an x-ray is important to the health of the mother and fetus. If an x-ray is needed, the technician will take extra steps to protect the fetus from radiation.

What to Expect during a Chest X-Ray

Chest x-rays are done at doctors' offices, clinics, hospitals, and other health care facilities. The location depends on the situation. An x-ray technician oversees the test. This person is specially trained to do x-ray tests. The entire test usually takes about 15 minutes.

Depending on your doctor's request, you'll stand, sit, or lie for the chest x-ray. The technician will help position you correctly. He or she may cover you with a heavy lead apron to protect certain parts of your body from the radiation.

The x-ray equipment usually consists of two parts. One part, a box-like machine, holds the x-ray film or a special plate that records the picture digitally. You'll sit or stand next to this machine. The second part is the x-ray tube, which is located about six feet away. Before the pictures are taken, the technician will walk behind a wall or into the next room to turn on the x-ray machine. This helps reduce his or her exposure to the radiation.

Usually, two views of the chest are taken. The first is a view from the back. The second is a view from the side. For a view from the back, you'll sit or stand so that your chest rests against the image plate. The x-ray tube will be behind you. For the side view, you'll turn to your side and raise your arms above your head. If you need to lie down for the test, you'll lie on a table that contains the x-ray film or plate. The x-ray tube will be over the table.

You'll need to hold very still while the pictures are taken. The technician may ask you to hold your breath for a few seconds. These steps help prevent a blurry picture. Although the test is painless, you may feel some discomfort from the coolness of the exam room and the x-ray plate. If you have arthritis or injuries to the chest wall, shoulders, or arms, you may feel discomfort holding a position during the test. The technician may be able to help you find a more comfortable position.

When the test is done, you'll need to wait while the technician checks the quality of the x-ray pictures. He or she needs to make sure that the pictures are good enough for the doctor to use.

What to Expect after a Chest X-Ray

A radiologist will analyze, or "read," your x-ray images. This doctor is specially trained to supervise x-ray tests and look at the x-ray pictures. The radiologist will send a report to your doctor (who requested the x-ray test). Your doctor will discuss the results with you.

In an emergency, you'll get the x-ray results right away. Otherwise, it may take 24 hours or more. Talk with your doctor about when you should expect the results.

What Does a Chest X-Ray Show?

Chest x-rays show the structures in and around the chest. The test is used to look for and track conditions of the heart, lungs, bones, and chest cavity. For example, chest x-ray pictures may show signs of pneumonia, heart failure, lung cancer, lung tissue scarring, or sarcoidosis.

Chest x-rays do have limits. They only show conditions that change the size of tissues in the chest or how the tissues absorb radiation. Also, chest x-rays create two-dimensional pictures. This means that denser structures, like bone or the heart, may hide some signs of disease. Very small areas of cancer and blood clots in the lungs usually don't show up on chest x-rays. For these reasons, your doctor may recommend other tests to confirm a diagnosis.

Section 20.3

Dental X-Rays

Excerpted from "Radiation-Emitting Products: The Selection of Patients
for Dental Radiographic Examinations," American Dental Association
and the U.S. Food and Drug Administration (FDA), May 6, 2009.

Radiographs and other imaging modalities are used to diagnose and
monitor oral diseases, as well as to monitor dentofacial development
and the progress or prognosis of therapy. Radiographic examinations
can be performed using digital imaging or conventional film. The available evidence suggests that either is a suitable diagnostic method.
Digital imaging may offer reduced radiation exposure and the advantage of image analysis that may enhance sensitivity and reduce error
introduced by subjective analysis. In addition, new imaging technology
offers the possibility of three-dimensional visualization of skeletal and
other structures.

Dental radiographs are recommended in the following situations:

1. Intraoral radiography is useful for the evaluation of dentoal-
   veolar trauma. If the area of interest extends beyond the den-
   toalveolar complex, extra-oral imaging may be indicated.

2. Care should be taken to examine all radiographs for any evidence of caries, bone loss from periodontal disease, developmental anomalies and occult disease.

3. Radiographic screening for the purpose of detecting disease
   before clinical examination should not be performed. A thorough clinical examination, consideration of the patient history,
   review of any prior radiographs, caries risk assessment, and
   consideration of both the dental and the general health needs
   of the patient should precede radiographic examination.

In the practice of dentistry, patients often seek care on a routine
basis in part because dental disease may develop in the absence of
clinical symptoms. Since attempts to identify specific criteria that will
accurately predict a high probability of finding interproximal carious
lesions have not been successful for individuals, it was necessary to

recommend time-based schedules for making radiographs intended primarily for the detection of dental caries. Professional judgment should be used to determine the optimum time for radiographic examination within the suggested interval.

Once a decision to obtain radiographs is made, it is the dentist's responsibility to follow the ALARA principle (as low as reasonably achievable) to minimize the patient's exposure to radiation. Examples of good radiologic practice include:

- use of the fastest image receptor compatible with the diagnostic task;

- collimation of the beam to the size of the receptor whenever feasible;

- proper film exposure and processing techniques; and

- use of leaded aprons and thyroid collars.

The amount of scattered radiation striking the patient's abdomen during a properly conducted radiographic examination is negligible. However, there is some evidence that radiation exposure to the thyroid during pregnancy is associated with low birth weight. Protective thyroid collars substantially reduce radiation exposure to the thyroid during dental radiographic procedures. Because every precaution should be taken to minimize radiation exposure, protective thyroid collars and aprons should be used whenever possible. This practice is strongly recommended for children, women of childbearing age, and pregnant women.

Clinical situations for which radiographs may be indicated include, but are not limited to, the following:

1. Previous periodontal or endodontic treatment

2. History of pain or trauma

3. Familial history of dental anomalies

4. Postoperative evaluation of healing

5. Remineralization monitoring

6. Presence of implants or evaluation for implant placement

Positive clinical signs/symptoms that indicate need for radiographs include these:

1. Clinical evidence of periodontal disease

2. Large or deep restorations

3. Deep carious lesions

4. Malposed or clinically impacted teeth

5. Swelling

6. Evidence of dental/facial trauma

7. Mobility of teeth

8. Sinus tract (fistula)

9. Clinically suspected sinus pathology

10. Growth abnormalities

11. Oral involvement in known or suspected systemic disease

12. Positive neurologic findings in the head and neck

13. Evidence of foreign objects

14. Pain and/or dysfunction of the temporomandibular joint

15. Facial asymmetry

16. Abutment teeth for fixed or removable partial prosthesis

17. Unexplained bleeding

18. Unexplained sensitivity of teeth

19. Unusual eruption, spacing or migration of teeth

20. Unusual tooth morphology, calcification or color

21. Unexplained absence of teeth

22. Clinical erosion

Section 20.4

Dual-Energy X-Ray Absorptiometry (DXA) Test for Bone Density

Excerpted from "Bone Mass Measurement: What the Numbers Mean,"
National Institute of Health (NIH)–Osteoporosis and Related Bone
Diseases National Resource Center, May 2009.

A bone mineral density (BMD) test is the best way to determine your bone health. The test can identify osteoporosis, determine your risk for fractures (broken bones), and measure your response to osteoporosis treatment. The most widely recognized BMD test is called a dual-energy x-ray absorptiometry, or DXA test. It is painless—a bit like having an x-ray. The test can measure bone density at your hip and spine.

A DXA test measures your bone mineral density and compares it to that of an established norm or standard to give you a score. Although no bone density test is 100% accurate, the DXA test is the single most important predictor of whether a person will have a fracture in the future.

T-Score

Most commonly, your DXA test results are compared to the ideal or peak bone mineral density of a healthy 30-year-old adult, and you are given a T-score. A score of 0 means your BMD is equal to the norm for a healthy young adult. Differences between your BMD and that of the healthy young adult norm are measured in units called standard deviations (SDs). The more standard deviations below 0, indicated as negative numbers, the lower your BMD and the higher your risk of fracture.

A T-score between +1 and -1 is considered normal or healthy. A T-score between -1 and -2.5 indicates that you have low bone mass, although not low enough to be diagnosed with osteoporosis. A T-score of -2.5 or lower indicates that you have osteoporosis. The greater the negative number, the more severe the osteoporosis.

Z-Score

Sometimes your bone mineral density is compared to that of a typical individual whose age is matched to yours. This comparison gives you a Z-score. Because a low BMD level is common among older adults, comparisons with the BMD of a typical individual whose age is matched to yours can be misleading. Therefore, the diagnosis of osteoporosis or low bone mass is based on your T-score. However, a Z-score can be useful for determining whether an underlying disease or condition is causing bone loss.

Low Bone Mass Versus Osteoporosis

The information provided by a BMD test can help your doctor decide which prevention or treatment options are right for you. If you have low bone mass that is not low enough to be diagnosed as osteoporosis, this is sometimes referred to as osteopenia. Low bone mass can be caused by many factors such as heredity, the development of less-than-optimal peak bone mass in your youth, a medical condition or medication to treat such a condition that negatively affects bone, and abnormally accelerated bone loss. Although not everyone who has low bone mass will develop osteoporosis, everyone with low bone mass is at higher risk for the disease and the resulting fractures.

As a person with low bone mass, you can take steps to help slow down your bone loss and prevent osteoporosis in your future. Your doctor will want you to develop—or keep—healthy habits such as eating foods rich in calcium and vitamin D and doing weight-bearing exercise such as walking, jogging, or dancing. In some cases, your doctor may recommend medication to prevent osteoporosis.

Osteoporosis: If you are diagnosed with osteoporosis, these healthy habits will help, but your doctor will probably also recommend that you take medication. Several effective medications are available to slow—or even reverse—bone loss. If you do take medication to treat osteoporosis, your doctor can advise you concerning the need for future BMD tests to check your progress.

Who Should Get a Bone Density Test?

The U.S. Preventive Services Task Force recommends that women age 65 and older be screened routinely for osteoporosis. The task force also recommends that routine screening begin at age 60 for women who are at increased risk for osteoporotic fractures.

In addition, a panel convened by the National Institutes of Health in 2000 recommended that bone density testing be considered in people taking glucocorticoid medications for two months or more and in those with conditions that place them at high risk for an osteoporosis-related fracture. However, the panel did not find enough scientific evidence upon which to base universal recommendations about when all women and men should obtain a BMD test. Instead, an individualized approach is recommended.

Chapter 21

Contrast Radiography

Chapter Contents

Section 21.1

Angiography

Angiography is an x-ray examination of the blood vessels after they have been filled with a contrast agent (a type of fluid that makes the vessels visible on an x-ray image). Angiography is performed when your physician suspects blockages in your arteries or veins that may interfere with the normal flow of blood through the body. It also is used to detect aneurysms, to image malformation in a blood vessel, to detect stroke or bleeding in the brain, and to find irregularities that can affect the heart or other organs. Some people reserve the term angiography to refer to an x-ray examination of the arteries, while preferring the term venography to refer to an x-ray examination of the veins. The procedure is similar for both.

Patient Preparation

A few days before your angiography examination, a number of blood tests will be performed, and you will be asked about the medications you take, whether prescription or over-the-counter. You also will be asked if you have any allergies. It is important to list all allergies to food and medicine, as well as hay fever or asthma. Existing allergies may indicate a possible reaction to the contrast agent that will be used during the examination. If you are a woman of childbearing age, you also will be asked if there is any possibility that you are pregnant, because a fetus is sensitive to radiation. Before you leave, you will receive detailed instructions about how to prepare for your procedure. Follow these instructions carefully.

When you arrive for your angiogram, a radiologic technologist will explain the procedure to you and answer any questions you might have. A radiologic technologist is a skilled medical professional who has received specialized education in the areas of radiation protection, patient care, radiation exposure, and radiographic positioning and procedures. Before the exam begins, you will be asked to remove all clothing and jewelry and put on a hospital gown.

During the Examination

The radiologic technologist will position you on the exam table. A radiologist, a physician who specializes in the diagnostic interpretation of medical images, will administer a local anesthetic and then make a small incision in your skin so that a thin catheter can be inserted into an artery or vein. The catheter is a flexible, hollow tube about the size of a strand of spaghetti. It usually is inserted into an artery in your groin, although in some cases your arm or another site will be selected for the catheter.

The radiologist will ease the catheter into the artery or vein and gently guide it to the area under investigation. The radiologist will be able to watch the movement of the catheter on a fluoroscope, which is an x-ray unit combined with a television monitor.

When the catheter reaches the area under study, the contrast agent is injected through the catheter. By watching the fluoroscope screen, the radiologist will be able to see the outline of your blood vessels and identify any blockages or other irregularities.

Angiography procedures can range in time from less than an hour to three hours or more. It is important that you relax, follow breathing instructions, and remain as still as possible during the examination. The radiologic technologist and radiologist will stay in the room with you throughout the procedure. If you experience any difficulty, let them know.

Angiography also can be performed using magnetic resonance instead of x-rays to produce images of the blood vessels; this procedure is known as magnetic resonance angiography (MRA) or magnetic resonance venography (MRV).

Therapeutic Uses of Angiography

In addition to imaging the blood vessels, angiography can be used to help repair them. During a procedure known as balloon angioplasty, angiography is used to guide a balloon through the catheter to a blocked or narrowed area of an artery. The balloon is inflated, compressing plaque against the walls of the artery and widening it. Then the balloon is deflated and the catheter is removed. In cases where the artery cannot be stretched by balloon angioplasty, a surgical stent can be inserted into the vessel to help keep it open. Stents are small, metal mesh tubes.

Post-Examination Information

After the angiography examination is complete, you will be moved to a room where you can rest and recover. Depending upon your overall health and medical condition, you may be released after just a few hours, or you may be admitted to the hospital for observation and recovery.

Before you go home, you will be given instructions explaining how to care for the site where the catheter was inserted. Your physician also may recommend that you restrict your activities at home or rest in bed, possibly with your head elevated. Follow the physician's instructions carefully.

Any contrast agent that remains in your system will be excreted by your kidneys. You may be advised to drink lots of water to help flush the contrast from your system. The amount of contrast is very small, and it has no odor or color. You will not notice any discoloration of your urine. In addition, the radiation that you are exposed to during this examination, like the radiation produced during any other x-ray procedure, passes through you immediately.

Your angiograms will be reviewed by the radiologist or a cardiologist, and your personal physician will receive a report of the findings. Your physician then will advise you of the results and discuss what further procedures, if any, are needed.

Section 21.2

Cystogram

A cystogram is an x-ray examination of the urinary bladder, which
is located in the lower pelvic area. A cystogram can show the bladder's
position and shape, and the exam often is used to diagnose a condition
called reflux. Reflux occurs when urine in the bladder moves back up
the ureters, the tubes that transport urine from the kidneys to the
bladder. This condition can cause repeated urinary tract infections. A
cystogram may be performed after a patient has experienced a pelvic
injury to ensure that the bladder has not torn. Cystograms also are
used to detect polyps or tumors in the bladder.

Preparation

Before your examination, a radiographer will explain the procedure
to you and answer any questions you might have. A radiographer, also
known as a radiologic technologist, is a skilled medical professional
who has specialized education in the areas of radiation protection,
patient care, and radiographic positioning and procedures.

If you are a woman of childbearing age, the radiographer will ask
the date of your last menstrual period and if there is any possibility
you are pregnant. Next, the radiographer will ask if you have any allergies. It is important to list all allergies to food and medicine, as well
as to let the radiographer know if you have a history of hay fever or
asthma. Some allergies may indicate a possible reaction to the contrast
agent that will be used during the examination.

You will be asked to put on a hospital gown, and then the radiographer will direct you to the restroom and ask you to completely empty
your bladder.

During the Examination

You will be positioned on your back on the x-ray table, with your
knees flexed. Your pubic area will be washed, and then the radiographer

or a radiology nurse will gently insert a small, flexible catheter into your urethra, the duct from which you urinate. Skin tape may be used to hold the catheter to your inner thigh.

Next, a radiologist (a physician who specializes in the diagnostic interpretation of medical images) or a urologist (a physician who specializes in conditions of the urinary system) will slowly fill your bladder with a contrast agent. The contrast agent is a substance that helps make organs easier to see on radiographs and is administered through the catheter. You will feel pressure and fullness in your bladder and will have an urge to urinate.

After your bladder is full, the physician will take radiographs using fluoroscopy. A fluoroscope is an x-ray unit attached to a television screen. You will be asked to lie on your side or to turn slightly from side to side while the physician watches your bladder on the TV screen. The radiographer also may take a few additional x-ray images.

Following this portion of the exam, the catheter will be removed, and you will be allowed to use the restroom. In addition to being sticky, the contrast agent that you expel is clear and odorless, so it will not be visible to you. After you return to the x-ray room, an additional x-ray image will be taken. This final radiograph will show whether any contrast agent stays in your bladder following urination. Any remaining contrast will be expelled the next time you urinate.

Voiding Cystourethrogram

Voiding cystourethrograms follow the same routine as cystograms with one difference. Toward the end of the examination, when the urinary catheter is removed, you will be asked to urinate into a special urinal. Radiographs will be taken while you urinate. These images will show the size and shape of the bladder when it is under stress caused by urination.

Post-Examination Information

Your radiographs will be reviewed by the radiologist, and your personal physician will receive a report of the findings. Your physician then will advise you of the results and discuss what further procedures, if any, are needed.

Section 21.3

Upper Gastrointestinal (GI) Series

Excerpted from "Upper GI Series," National Institute of Diabetes and Digestive and Kidney Diseases (NIDDK), December 2009.

An upper gastrointestinal (GI) series uses x-rays to help diagnose problems of the upper GI tract, which includes the esophagus, stomach, and duodenum. The duodenum is the first part of the small intestine.

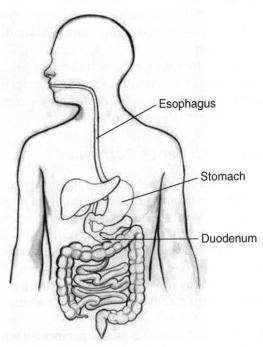

Figure 21.1. *Upper GI Tract*

An upper GI series can help detect ulcers, abnormal growths, scars or strictures—narrowings of the GI tract, hiatal hernia, diverticula (bulges in the wall of the esophagus or intestine), and esophageal varices (enlarged veins in the esophagus).

An upper GI series can be used to help determine the cause of:

- abdominal pain,

- nausea,

- vomiting,

- swallowing difficulties,

- gastroesophageal reflux—a condition in which food and digestive juices rise from the stomach into the esophagus, and

- unexplained weight loss.

How to Prepare for an Upper GI Series

The upper GI tract must be empty prior to an upper GI series. Generally, no eating or drinking is allowed for eight hours before the procedure. Smoking and chewing gum are also prohibited during this time. Patients should tell their doctor about all health conditions they have—especially allergies to medications or foods—and about all medications they are taking.

Women should let their doctor know if they are pregnant. Developing fetuses are particularly sensitive to x-rays. Special precautions can be taken to minimize exposure, or the doctor may suggest an alternate procedure such as upper GI endoscopy.

How Is an Upper GI Series Performed?

An upper GI series is conducted by a radiology technologist or a radiologist—a doctor who specializes in x-ray imaging—at a hospital or outpatient center. While sitting or standing in front of an x-ray machine, the patient drinks barium liquid, which is often white and has a chalky consistency and taste. The barium liquid coats the lining of the upper GI tract and makes signs of disease show up more clearly on x-rays. X-ray video, called fluoroscopy, is used to view the barium liquid moving through the esophagus, stomach, and duodenum.

Additional x-rays and fluoroscopy are performed while the patient lies on an x-ray table. To fully coat the upper GI tract with barium liquid, the technologist or radiologist may press on the abdomen or ask the patient to change position. Patients hold still in various positions, allowing the technologist or radiologist to take x-rays of the upper GI tract at different angles. If a technologist conducts the upper GI series, a radiologist will later examine the images to look for problems.

What Is a Double Contrast Study?

The double contrast study gets its name from the combination of air and liquid barium working together to create a more detailed view of the stomach lining. The patient swallows gas-forming crystals, which are activated when they mix with the barium liquid. The gas expands the barium-coated stomach, exposing finer details of the stomach lining, and additional x-rays are taken.

Recovery from an Upper GI Series

Patients may experience bloating and nausea for a short time after an upper GI series. Not eating before the test and the test itself may cause one to feel tired. For several days afterward, barium liquid in the GI tract causes stools to be white or light colored. Unless otherwise directed, patients may immediately resume their normal diet once they leave the hospital or outpatient center.

What Are the Risks Associated with an Upper GI Series?

Mild constipation from the barium liquid is the most common complication of an upper GI series. Rarely, barium liquid causes bowel obstruction, a life-threatening condition that blocks the intestines. Drinking plenty of liquids after an upper GI series flushes out the barium and helps reduce the risks of constipation and bowel obstruction.

Although infrequent, barium can cause an allergic reaction, which is treated with antihistamines. Some barium liquids contain flavorings, which may also cause an allergic reaction.

The risk of radiation-related damage to cells or tissues from an upper GI series is low. People who have recently undergone other x-ray tests should talk with their doctor about potential risks.

Patients who experience any of the following rare symptoms should contact their doctor immediately:

- Severe abdominal pain
- Failure to have a bowel movement within two days after the procedure
- Inability to pass gas
- Fever

Section 21.4

Lower GI Series (Barium Enema)

Excerpted from "Lower GI Series," National Institute of Diabetes
and Digestive and Kidney Diseases (NIDDK), December 2009.

A lower gastrointestinal (GI) series uses x-rays to help diagnose
problems of the large intestine, which includes the colon and rectum.
A lower GI series is sometimes called a barium enema because the
large intestine is filled with barium liquid. The barium liquid coats
the lining of the large intestine and makes signs of disease show up
more clearly on x-rays.

A lower GI series can detect problems of the large intestine, including:

- polyps;
- diverticula—bulges in the intestinal wall;
- cancerous growths;
- ulcers;
- fistulae—abnormal openings in the intestinal wall that lead to
  the abdominal cavity, other organs, or the skin's surface;
- inflammation.

A lower GI series can be used to help determine the cause of:

- chronic diarrhea,
- rectal bleeding,
- abdominal pain,
- changes in bowel habits, and
- unexplained weight loss.

How to Prepare for a Lower GI Series

To prepare for a lower GI series, patients must empty all solids from
the GI tract during a bowel prep, which is usually done at home. The

doctor provides written bowel prep instructions. Generally, patients follow a clear liquid diet for 1–3 days before the procedure. Acceptable liquids include fat-free bouillon or broth, strained fruit juice, water, plain coffee, plain tea, sports drinks (such as Gatorade), and gelatin.

A laxative or enema is usually used the evening before a lower GI series. A laxative is medicine that loosens stool and increases bowel movements. Laxatives are usually swallowed as a pill or as a powder dissolved in water. An enema involves flushing a liquid solution into the anus using a special squirt bottle. Enemas are sometimes repeated the morning of the test.

Sometimes, especially when only the rectum or end of the colon is being evaluated, emptying all solids from the entire GI tract beforehand is not necessary. Instead, the patient undergoes one or more enemas the day of the procedure to remove solids from just the large intestine.

Before starting the bowel prep, patients should tell their doctor about all health issues and medications. Women who may be pregnant should discuss getting an alternate test, such as colonoscopy, or taking precautions to minimize radiation exposure to their unborn child.

How Is a Lower GI Series Performed?

A lower GI series is conducted by a radiology technologist or a radiologist—a doctor who specializes in x-ray imaging—at a hospital or outpatient center. While the patient lies on an x-ray table, a lubricated tube is inserted into the anus and the large intestine is filled with barium liquid. Patients may experience some discomfort and will feel the urge to have a bowel movement. Leakage of barium liquid is prevented by an inflated balloon on the end of the tube. To evenly coat the inside of the large intestine with barium liquid, patients are asked to change positions several times.

X-ray pictures and possibly x-ray video are taken while patients hold still in various positions, allowing the technologist or radiologist to see the large intestine at different angles. If a technologist conducts the lower GI series, a radiologist will later examine the images to look for problems.

When the imaging is complete, the balloon on the tube is deflated and most of the barium liquid drains through the tube. The patient expels the remaining barium liquid into a bed pan or nearby toilet. An enema may be used to flush out the remaining barium liquid. The entire procedure takes 30 to 60 minutes—longer if it includes a double contrast study.

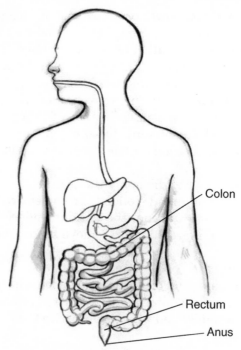

Figure 21.2. Lower GI series uses x-rays to help diagnose problems of the large intestine, which includes the colon and rectum.

What Is a Double Contrast Study?

The double contrast study gets its name from the combination of air and barium liquid working together to create a more detailed view of the intestinal lining on x-rays. If performed, a double contrast study takes place after the patient has expelled most of the barium liquid. What remains clings to the intestinal wall. The large intestine is inflated with air, expanding the barium-coated large intestine, and additional x-rays are taken.

Recovery from a Lower GI Series

For an hour or so after the procedure, most patients experience bloating. Not eating before the test and the test itself may cause one to feel tired. Repeated bowel movements and enemas during the bowel prep may cause anal soreness. And for several days, traces of barium liquid in the large intestine cause stools to be white or light colored. Unless otherwise directed, patients may immediately resume their normal diet.

What Are the Risks Associated with a Lower GI Series?

Mild constipation from the barium enema is the most common complication of a lower GI series. Rarely, a barium enema causes bowel obstruction, a life-threatening condition that blocks the intestines. Drinking plenty of liquids after a lower GI series flushes out the barium and reduces the risks of constipation and bowel obstruction.

A 1%–4% risk of acute kidney injury exists from sodium phosphate—a commonly used laxative for lower GI series bowel preps. Laxatives can also lead to temporary but potentially serious imbalances in electrolytes—salts and minerals in the body—possibly causing sluggishness, confusion, muscle cramps, and seizures. People with—or those at risk for—kidney disease should discuss options for minimizing bowel prep-related risks with their doctor.

Rarely, barium liquid causes an allergic reaction, which is treated with antihistamines. Leakage of barium liquid into the abdomen through a tear in the lining of the large intestine is a rare but serious complication that usually requires emergency surgery to repair. The risk of radiation-related damage to cells or tissues from a lower GI series is low. People who have recently undergone other x-ray tests should talk with their doctor about potential risks.

Patients who experience any of the following rare symptoms after a lower GI series should contact their doctor immediately:

- Severe abdominal pain

- Rectal bleeding

- Failure to have a bowel movement within two days after the procedure

- Inability to pass gas

- Fever

Section 21.5

Lung Ventilation/Perfusion Scan

Excerpted from "Lung Ventilation/Perfusion Scan," National
Heart, Lung, and Blood Institute (NHLBI), May 2008.

A lung ventilation/perfusion scan, or VQ scan, is a test that measures air and blood flow in your lungs. This test most often is used
to help diagnose or rule out a pulmonary embolism, or PE. A PE is a
blood clot that travels to the lungs and blocks blood flow. This results in
low blood oxygen levels, damage to the lungs, or even death. The scan
also can detect poor blood flow in the lungs' blood vessels and provide
pictures that help doctors prepare for some types of lung surgery.

A VQ scan involves two types of scans: ventilation and perfusion.
The ventilation scan shows where air flows in your lungs. The perfusion
scan shows where blood flows in your lungs. Both scans use radioisotopes (a low-risk radioactive substance).

VQ scans involve little pain or risk for most people. During the
perfusion scan, you may feel some discomfort when the radioisotopes
are injected. You also may have a bruise at the injection site after the
test. The amount of radiation in the radioisotopes used for both tests is
very small. The amount of radiation in the gas and injection together
are about the same as the amount a person is naturally exposed to in
one year. Very rarely the radioisotopes used in VQ scans can cause an
allergic reaction. Hives or a rash may result. Medicines can relieve
this reaction.

Who Needs a Lung Ventilation/Perfusion Scan?

People who have signs or symptoms of a pulmonary embolism (PE)
may need lung ventilation/perfusion (VQ) scans. A PE occurs when a
blood clot travels to the lungs and blocks blood flow. Signs and symptoms of PE include chest pain, trouble breathing, rapid breathing,
coughing, coughing up blood, and a rapid heart rate. Some clots travel
to the lungs from veins deep in the legs. This can cause pain and
swelling in the affected limb(s). Doctors use VQ scans to help find out
whether a PE is causing these signs and symptoms. A VQ scan alone,

however, will not confirm whether you have PE. Your doctor also will consider other factors when making a diagnosis. Doctors also use VQ scans to detect poor blood flow in the lungs' blood vessels and to examine the lungs before some types of surgery.

What to Expect during a Lung Ventilation/Perfusion Scan

A lung ventilation/perfusion (VQ) scan is done at a radiology clinic. You will lie on a table for about one hour and have two types of scans: ventilation and perfusion. The ventilation scan shows where air flows in your lungs. The perfusion scan shows where blood flows in your lungs. You must lie very still for the tests, or the pictures may blur. If you're having trouble staying still, your doctor may give you medicine to help you relax.

Both scans use radioisotopes (a low-risk radioactive substance). This substance releases energy inside your body. Special scanners outside of your body use the energy to create images of air and blood flow to your lungs. The radioisotopes used in VQ scans can cause an allergic reaction, including itching and hives. If this happens, your doctor will give you medicine to relieve the symptoms.

Ventilation: For this scan, you lie on an open table that moves under the arm of the scanner. You wear a breathing mask over your nose and mouth and inhale a small amount of radioisotope gas mixed with oxygen. As you breathe, the scanner takes pictures that show air going into your lungs. You'll need to hold your breath for a few seconds at the start of each picture. The scan is painless, and each picture takes only a few minutes. However, wearing the mask can make some people feel anxious. If this happens, your doctor may give you medicine to help you relax.

Perfusion: For this scan, a member of the health care team will inject a small amount of radioisotope into a vein in your arm. The scanner then takes pictures of blood flow through your lungs. The scan itself does not hurt, but you may feel some discomfort when the radioisotopes are injected.

What to Expect after a Lung Ventilation/Perfusion Scan

Most people can return to their normal routines right after a lung ventilation/perfusion (VQ) scan. If you got medicine to help you relax during the scan, your doctor will tell you when you can return to your normal routine. The medicine may make you tired, so you will need someone to drive you home. You may have a bruise on your arm where the radioisotopes were injected. You will need to drink plenty of fluids to flush the radioisotopes out of your body. Your doctor can advise you about how much fluid to drink.

If you are breast feeding, ask your doctor how long you should wait after the test before you breast feed. The radioisotopes used for VQ scans can be passed to your baby through your breast milk. You may want to prepare for the scan by pumping and saving milk for 24 to 48 hours in advance. You can bottle feed your baby in the hours after the VQ scan.

What does a Lung Ventilation/Perfusion Scan Show?

A lung ventilation/perfusion (VQ) scan shows how well air and blood are flowing through your lungs. Normal results will show full air and blood flow to all parts of your lungs.

If air flow is normal but blood flow is not, you may have a pulmonary embolism (PE). PE occurs when a blood clot travels to the lungs and blocks blood flow.

The results of the scan will show whether you're at high, medium, or low risk for PE. However, a VQ scan alone will not confirm whether you have PE. A scan showing low blood flow in spots may reflect other lung problems, such as lung damage from COPD (chronic obstructive pulmonary disease). Your doctor will use the VQ scan results along with results from a physical exam, chest x-ray, and other tests to make a diagnosis.

What Are the Risks of a Lung Ventilation/Perfusion Scan?

Lung ventilation/perfusion (VQ) scans involve little risk for most people. The radioisotopes used for both tests expose you to a small amount of radiation. The amount of radiation in the gas and injection together are about the same as the amount a person is naturally exposed to in one year. Although rare, the radioisotopes may cause an allergic reaction.

Section 21.6

Myelography

Myelography is an x-ray examination of the structures within your spinal column. The examination can show conditions such as spinal tumors, spinal cord swelling, and herniated (slipped) disks.

Patient Preparation

Before the exam, a radiographer will explain the procedure and answer any questions you might have. A radiographer, also known as a radiologic technologist, is a skilled medical professional who has received specialized education in radiation protection, patient care, and radiographic positioning and procedures.

If you are a woman of childbearing age, the radiographer will ask if you could be pregnant. It is important that you tell the radiographer the date of your last menstrual period and whether there is a chance you may be pregnant. It is also important to tell the radiographer if you have any allergies to food or medicine, or a history of hay fever or asthma. Allergies may indicate a possible reaction to the contrast agent that is used during the exam.

During the Examination

Before your spine can be imaged, a contrast agent is injected into the space around your spinal cord. A contrast agent is a substance that makes it easier to see parts of your body that are not normally visible on a radiograph. A physician first injects a local anesthetic to numb the area before inserting a spinal needle. This will sting slightly.

You will be positioned in one of the following ways:

- Lying on your side with knees pulled up to the chest and chest curled forward.

- Lying face down on the table with large pillows under your stomach.

- Sitting on the edge of the table, leaning forward and grasping your ankles.

Each of these positions opens the spaces between your vertebrae to allow a needle to be inserted. Once the needle is in place, the physician removes a small amount of fluid from your spinal canal. It will be sent to a laboratory for analysis. The physician then slowly injects the contrast agent through the needle.

While the contrast is administered, a fluoroscope, which combines an x-ray unit with a television screen, is used to take images of your spine. As the contrast agent fills the space around your spinal cord, the radiographer and radiologist watch the screen to observe any problems or defects. The room lights will be dimmed so they can see the images more clearly.

After the contrast is administered, the needle is removed, and the radiographer positions you on the x-ray table, stomach down. A brace will be placed against your shoulders to support you as the table is tipped slowly. You will never be alone in the room, and the radiographer and radiologist will monitor you closely. If you experience any discomfort, tell them immediately.

As the table is tipped gently toward your head or feet, the radiologist will take images of your back. He or she may ask you to turn slightly onto one hip and then the other. You will be asked to hold your breath as the images are taken. Next, the radiographer will place an imaging cassette against the side of your abdomen and take a radiograph of your back.

Post-Examination Information

Once the exam is complete, the radiographer processes your images, determines if they are technically acceptable, and decides whether additional images are needed. Follow-up images may be taken at this time. A radiologist will interpret the final images, and your personal physician will receive a report of the findings.

You may be asked to wait in the radiology department for about an hour so that caregivers can ensure that you recover fully. Before you leave, the radiographer will give you a set of instructions. It is important to follow these instructions to avoid a headache or other side effects.

Section 21.7

Intravenous Pyelogram

"Intravenous Pyelogram," © 2011 A.D.A.M., Inc.
Reprinted with permission.

An intravenous pyelogram (IVP) is a special x-ray examination of the kidneys, bladder, and ureters (the tubes that carry urine from the kidneys to the bladder).

How the Test Is Performed

An IVP is done in a hospital radiology department or a health care provider's office by an x-ray technician. You will need to empty your bladder immediately before the procedure starts. The health care provider will inject an iodine-based contrast (dye) into a vein in your arm. A series of x-ray images are taken at different times to see how the kidneys remove the dye and how it collects in your urine. A compression device (a wide belt containing two balloons that can be inflated) may be used to keep the contrast material in the kidneys. You will need to remain still during the procedure, which may take up to an hour. Before the final image is taken, you will be asked to urinate again, to see how well the bladder has emptied. You can resume your normal diet and medications after the procedure. You should drink plenty of fluids to help remove all the contrast dye from your body.

How to Prepare for the Test

As with all x-ray procedures, tell your health care provider if you:

- are allergic to contrast material,
- are pregnant, or
- have any drug allergies.

Your health care provider will tell you whether you can eat or drink before this test. You may be given a laxative to take the afternoon before the procedure to clear the intestines so your kidneys can be clearly seen. You must sign a consent form. You will be asked to wear a hospital gown and to remove all jewelry.

How the Test Will Feel

You may feel a burning or flushing sensation in your arm and body as the contrast dye is injected. You may also have a metallic taste in your mouth. This is normal and will quickly disappear. Some people develop a headache, nausea, or vomiting after the dye is injected. The belt across the kidneys may feel tight over your belly area.

Why the Test Is Performed

An IVP can be used to evaluate:

- an abdominal injury,
- bladder and kidney infections,
- blood in the urine,
- flank pain (possibly due to kidney stones),
- tumors.

What Abnormal Results Mean

The test may reveal kidney diseases, birth defects of the urinary system, tumors, kidney stones, or damage to the urinary system.

Risks

There is a chance of an allergic reaction to the dye, even if you have received contrast dye in the past without any problem. If you have a known allergy to iodine-based contrast, an alternate test should be performed. Alternatives include retrograde pyelography, magnetic resonance imaging (MRI), or ultrasound.

There is low radiation exposure. X-rays are monitored and regulated to provide the minimum amount of radiation exposure needed to produce the image. Most experts feel that the risk is low compared with the benefits. Pregnant women and children are more sensitive to the risks of radiation.

Considerations

Computed tomography (CT) scans have replaced IVP as the main tool for checking the urinary system. CT takes less time to perform and provides additional views of the abdomen, which can help rule out other possible reasons for the patient's symptoms. Magnetic resonance imaging (MRI) is also used to look at the kidneys, ureters, and bladder.

Chapter 22

Ultrasound (Sonography) Exams

Chapter Contents

Section 22.1

Ultrasound Overview

Excerpted from "Taking a Close Look at Ultrasound,"
U.S. Food and Drug Administration (FDA), March 24, 2008.

Medical ultrasound imagery is a common and vital tool used for monitoring fetal health and internal organs, and for diagnosing many conditions. It should only be used by licensed health care professionals and with a prescription. Obstetricians and other health care professionals use ultrasound—also known as sonography—to diagnose pregnancies, determine fetal age, detect abnormalities, evaluate placenta position, and determine multiple pregnancies. They also use ultrasound to check for fetus size, location, and movement, as well as to keep track of fetal breathing and heartbeat.

Other health care professionals use ultrasound to view the heart, blood vessels, kidneys, liver, and other organs of people of all ages. Using ultrasound, doctors can check patients' thyroid glands, diagnose certain infections and cancers, and find abnormalities in men's prostate glands and scrotums. Carotid ultrasound allows viewing of arteries in the neck for plaque-caused narrowing that can lead to stroke.

The types of ultrasound imaging exams used to diagnose medical conditions include the following:

- Doppler ultrasound, used to visualize flow through a blood vessel

- Bone sonography, which helps doctors diagnose osteoporosis

- Echocardiograms, which offer a view of the heart

A Safe Technology

Ultrasound, which was developed from sonar and radar technology, has earned an excellent safety record since being put into widespread use more than 30 years ago. It generates images that can be captured in real-time and show movement of the body's internal organs. The images can also be presented as still pictures.

Ultrasound uses non-ionizing radiation—energy levels that are not great enough to alter atoms and molecules and permanently damage biological tissues. Hence, it does not present the same type of risks as x-rays or other types of ionizing radiation. The technology uses high-frequency sound waves that reflect off of soft tissues such as muscles and internal organs. The returning waves are read by a receiving device, which transforms them into a visual image.

Usually Painless

The sound waves of ultrasound imaging are transmitted by a hand-held device known as a transducer, which sends a beam of ultrasound into the body and then receives the reflected signal. During most ultrasound exams, a doctor or a qualified technician moves the transducer over the skin covering the area of interest. The area of interest is covered before the procedure with a small amount of warm gel that helps keep air pockets from forming between the transducer and skin. An ultrasound exam is usually a painless procedure.

Some exams, called invasive ultrasounds, are done inside the body. A health care professional attaches a transducer to a probe that is inserted into a natural opening in the body. This type of procedure can cause some discomfort or pain.

A typical ultrasound exam takes from 30 minutes to an hour. How a patient prepares for a procedure depends on the part of the body being examined. There may be no special preparation required. However, a physician may instruct a patient not to eat food or drink liquids prior to the procedure. Some types of exams require the patient to have a full bladder. Patients should ask their doctors for full instructions on how to prepare for an ultrasound exam.

Section 22.2

Abdominal Ultrasound

What It Is

An abdominal ultrasound is a safe and painless test that uses sound
waves to make images of the abdomen (belly). During the examination,
an ultrasound machine sends sound waves into the abdominal area
and images are recorded on a computer. The black-and-white images
show the internal structures of the abdomen, such as the appendix,
intestines, liver, gall bladder, pancreas, spleen, kidneys, and urinary
bladder. A complete ultrasound of the abdomen evaluates all of the
abdominal organs. A limited ultrasound of the abdomen evaluates one
or multiple organs, but not all.

Why It's Done

Doctors order an abdominal ultrasound when they're concerned
about symptoms such as abdominal pain, repeated vomiting, abnormal
liver or kidney function tests, or a swollen belly. Abdominal ultrasound
tests can show the size of the abdominal organs and can help evaluate
injuries to or diseases of the abdominal organs. Specific conditions that
ultrasound can help diagnose include:

- appendicitis (inflammation of the appendix);
- pyloric stenosis (narrowing of the lower part of the stomach, which
  blocks the passage of food from the stomach to the intestines);
- stones in the kidneys or gall bladder;
- abdominal masses such as tumors, cysts, or abscesses;
- abnormal fluid in the abdomen.

Abdominal ultrasounds can be used to guide procedures such as needle biopsies or catheter insertion (to help ensure accurate placement of the needle or the catheter). Abdominal ultrasounds also are used to monitor the growth and development of a baby in the uterus during pregnancy.

Preparation

Usually, you don't have to do anything special to prepare for an abdominal ultrasound, although your doctor may ask that your child not eat or drink anything for several hours before the test. You should tell the technician about any medications your child is taking before the test begins.

Procedure

The abdominal ultrasound usually will be done in the radiology department of a hospital or in a radiology center. Parents usually can accompany their child to provide reassurance and support.

Your child will be asked to change into a cloth gown and lie on a table. The room is usually dark so the images can be seen clearly on the computer screen. A technician (sonographer) trained in ultrasound imaging will spread a clear, warm gel on the skin of the abdomen. This gel helps with the transmission of the sound waves.

The technician will then rub a small wand (transducer) over the gel. The transducer emits high-frequency sound waves and a computer measures how the sound waves bounce back from the body. The computer changes those sound waves into images to be analyzed. Sometimes a doctor will come in at the end of the test to meet your child and take a few more pictures. The procedure usually takes less than 30 minutes.

What to Expect

The abdominal ultrasound is painless. Your child may feel a slight pressure on the belly as the transducer is moved over the body, and the gel may feel wet or cold. You'll need to tell your child to lie still during the procedure so the sound waves can reach the area effectively. The technician may ask your child to lie in different positions or hold his or her breath briefly. Babies might cry in the ultrasound room, especially if they're restrained, but this won't interfere with the procedure.

Getting the Results

A radiologist (a doctor who's specially trained in reading and interpreting x-ray and ultrasound images) will interpret the ultrasound results and then give the information to your doctor, who will review the results with you. If the test results appear abnormal, your doctor may order further tests.

In an emergency, the results of an ultrasound can be available quickly. Otherwise, they're usually ready in 1–2 days. In most cases, results can't be given directly to the patient or family at the time of the test.

Risks

No risks are associated with an abdominal ultrasound. Unlike x-rays, radiation isn't involved with this test.

Helping Your Child

Some younger children may be afraid of the machinery used for the ultrasound. Explaining in simple terms how the abdominal ultrasound will be conducted and why it's being done can help ease any fears.

You can tell your child that the equipment takes pictures of the belly, and encourage him or her to ask the technician questions. Tell your child to try to relax during the procedure, as tense muscles can make it more difficult to get accurate results.

If You Have Questions

If you have questions about the abdominal ultrasound, speak with your doctor. You can also talk to the technician before the exam.

Section 22.3

Carotid Ultrasound

Excerpted from "Carotid Ultrasound,"
National Heart, Lung, and Blood Institute (NHLBI), May 2009.

Carotid ultrasound is a painless and harmless test that uses high-frequency sound waves to create pictures of the insides of the two large arteries in your neck. These arteries, called carotid arteries, supply your brain with oxygen-rich blood. You have one carotid artery on each side of your neck. Carotid ultrasound shows whether a substance called plaque has narrowed your carotid arteries. Plaque is made up of fat, cholesterol, calcium, and other substances found in the blood. Plaque builds up on the insides of your arteries as you age. This condition is called carotid artery disease.

You have two common carotid arteries—one on each side of your neck—that divide into internal and external carotid arteries. Too much plaque in a carotid artery can cause a stroke. The plaque can slow down or block the flow of blood through the artery, allowing a blood clot to form. A piece of the blood clot can break off and get stuck in the artery, blocking blood flow to the brain. This is what causes a stroke.

A standard carotid ultrasound shows the structure of your carotid arteries. Your carotid ultrasound test may include a Doppler ultrasound. Doppler ultrasound is a special test that shows the movement of blood through your blood vessels. Your doctor often will need results from both types of ultrasound to fully assess whether there is a problem with blood flow through your carotid arteries.

Preparation: Carotid ultrasound is a painless test, and typically there is little to do in advance. Your doctor will tell you how to prepare for your carotid ultrasound.

What to Expect with a Carotid Ultrasound

Carotid ultrasound usually is done in a doctor's office or hospital. The test is painless and often does not take more than 30 minutes.

The ultrasound machine includes a computer, a video screen, and a transducer. A transducer is a hand-held device that sends and receives ultrasound waves into and from the body.

You will lie on your back on an exam table for the test. Your technician or doctor will put a gel on your neck where your carotid arteries are located. This gel helps the ultrasound waves reach the arteries better. Your technician or doctor will put the transducer against different spots on your neck and move it back and forth. The transducer gives off ultrasound waves and detects their echoes after they bounce off the artery walls and blood cells. Ultrasound waves cannot be heard by the human ear.

A computer uses the echoes to create and record pictures of the insides of the arteries (usually in black and white) and your blood flowing through them (usually in color; this is the Doppler ultrasound). A video screen displays these live images for your doctor to review.

You usually do not have to take any special steps after a carotid ultrasound. You should be able to return to normal activities right away. Often, your doctor will be able to tell you the results of the carotid ultrasound when it occurs or soon afterward.

Section 22.4

Circulation (Vascular) Ultrasound

This section includes "Why Might I Need a Circulation Ultrasound," and "Circulation Ultrasound," © 2008 American Society of Echocardiography (www.asecho.org). Reprinted with permission.

The vascular (circulatory) system is made up of blood vessels called arteries and veins. Arteries carry oxygenated blood from the heart to the body. Blood is pushed through the arteries by pressure created by the heart's beating. Veins carry deoxygenated blood back to the heart. Veins have valves that prevent blood from flowing backwards. Blood flow is slower than in the arteries. The contractions of surrounding muscles help keep the blood moving forward.

You may benefit from this if you have experienced a stroke or ministroke, blood clot in blood vessel, pain in your legs when walking, or a history of disease of the circulation in your family, although there are many other possible reasons that might lead your doctor to want to evaluate your circulation health.

Sonography is a useful way of evaluating the body's circulatory system. Vascular ultrasound is performed to:

- help monitor the blood flow to organs and tissues throughout the body;

- locate and identify blockages and abnormalities like blood clots, plaque, or emboli and help plan for their effective treatment;

- determine whether a patient is a good candidate for a procedure;

- to plan or evaluate the success of procedures that graft or bypass blood vessels.

Doppler ultrasound images can help the physician to see and evaluate:

- blockages to blood flow (such as clots),

- narrowing of vessels (which may be caused by plaque),

- tumors and congenital malformation.

There are some common problems that can occur with the blood vessels. These problems include high blood pressure, atherosclerosis, aneurysm, embolism, varicose veins, and thrombosis.

- High blood pressure, or hypertension, is a condition in which blood pressure levels are measure above the normal ranges. Blood pressure is the force of the blood in your arteries. Your blood pressure is high if it is 140/90 or higher.

- Atherosclerosis is a disease that affects the arteries. It is caused by fatty deposits that begin within the blood vessel wall and eventually progress to cause narrowing of the blood vessel itself. Severe narrowing can stop blood flow.

- An aneurysm is caused by a weakened area in a blood vessel wall. This causes the wall to balloon outward. As the aneurysm becomes larger, the wall becomes weaker and the blood vessel may break open (rupture).

- An embolism is a blood clot that has traveled to another place in the body. These blood clots most commonly form in the veins of the legs. The clots can lodge in smaller arteries, stopping blood flow.

- Varicose veins occur when the valves in a veins do not work properly. As a result, blood pools in the veins and causes the veins to become swollen and twisted. Most commonly, varicose veins occur in the legs.

- A thrombosis is a blood clot that has formed inside a blood vessel. Most commonly they can occur in the veins of the leg (deep vein thrombosis). They can sometimes form in arteries. These blood clots can break off and travel through the blood (embolism).

What is circulation (vascular) ultrasound?

Circulation (vascular) ultrasound provides your doctor with moving images of your circulatory system (arteries and veins), and takes excellent pictures that will help your doctor to evaluate your circulation's health. A specially trained technician (sonographer) will use a gel to slide a microphone-like device called a transducer over your body. Reflected sound waves will provide images of your veins and arteries. Circulation (vascular) ultrasound uses the same technology that allows doctors to see an unborn baby inside the pregnant mother.

In some cases, a special dye may need to be injected into the vein to help enhance the images so that your doctor can better evaluate the health of your circulatory system. This ultrasound does not involve radiation.

What is peripheral vascular ultrasound?

This procedure uses sound waves to obtain images and measure speed (velocity) of blood flow in carotids (neck), arms, legs, abdominal aorta, and renal (kidney) blood vessels. These images are analyzed to determine whether or not you have blockages in your arteries, blood clots in your veins, or if an abdominal aortic aneurysm is present.

What is carotid ultrasound?

This procedure uses sound waves to obtain color images of the arteries in your neck. The physician evaluates the images to determine to what extent these arteries are blocked and how much blood is flowing to your brain and eyes. There are two carotid arteries, one on each side of your neck. Both sides will be checked during the procedure. This test takes one hour and no preparation is needed.

Section 22.5

Echocardiography (Heart)

Excerpted from "Echocardiography," National Heart, Lung, and Blood Institute (NHLBI), August 2009.

Echocardiography, or echo, is a painless test that uses sound waves to create pictures of your heart. The test gives your doctor information about the size and shape of your heart and how well your heart's chambers and valves are working. Echo also can be done to detect heart problems in infants and children. The test also can identify areas of heart muscle that are not contracting normally due to poor blood flow or injury from a previous heart attack. In addition, a type of echo called Doppler ultrasound shows how well blood flows through the chambers and valves of your heart. Echo can detect possible blood clots inside the heart, fluid buildup in the pericardium (the sac around the heart), and problems with the aorta. The aorta is the main artery that carries oxygen-rich blood from your heart to your body.

Types of Echocardiography

There are several types of echocardiography (echo)—all use sound waves to create pictures of your heart. This is the same technology that allows doctors to see an unborn baby inside a pregnant woman. Unlike x-rays and some other tests, echo doesn't involve radiation.

Transthoracic echocardiography is the most common type of echocardiogram test. It is painless and noninvasive.

Stress echocardiography is done as part of a stress test. Some heart problems, such as coronary heart disease, are easier to diagnose when the heart is working hard and beating fast.

Transesophageal echocardiography: During this test, the transducer is attached to the end of a flexible tube which is guided down your throat and into your esophagus. This allows your doctor to get more detailed pictures of your heart.

Fetal echocardiography is used to look at an unborn baby's heart. A doctor may recommend this test to check a baby for heart problems.

Three-dimensional (3D) echocardiography creates 3D images of the heart and may be used to diagnose heart problems in children. This method also may be used for planning and monitoring heart valve surgery.

What to Expect during Echocardiography

Echocardiography (echo) is painless and usually takes less than an hour to do. For some types of echo, your doctor will need to inject saline or a special dye into one of your veins to make your heart show up more clearly on the test images. This special dye is different from the dye used during angiography (a test used to examine the body's blood vessels).

For most types of echo, you will be asked to remove your clothing from the waist up. Women will be given a gown to wear during the test. You will lay on your back or left side on an exam table or stretcher. Soft, sticky patches called electrodes will be attached to your chest to allow an EKG (electrocardiogram) to be done. An EKG is a test that records the heart's electrical activity.

A doctor or sonographer (a person specially trained to do ultrasounds) will apply gel to your chest. The gel helps the sound waves reach your heart. A wand-like device called a transducer will then be moved around on your chest. The transducer transmits ultrasound waves into your chest. Echoes from the sound waves will be converted into pictures of your heart on a computer screen. During the test, the lights in the room will be dimmed so the computer screen is easier to see. The sonographer will make several recordings of the pictures to show various locations in your heart. The recordings will be put on a computer disc or videotape for the cardiologist (heart specialist) to review.

During the test, you may be asked to change positions or hold your breath for a short time so that the sonographer can get good pictures of your heart. At times, the sonographer may apply a bit of pressure to your chest with the transducer. This pressure can be a little uncomfortable, but it helps get the best picture of your heart. You should let the sonographer know if you feel too uncomfortable. This process is similar for fetal echo. However, in that test the transducer is placed over the pregnant woman's belly at the location of the baby's heart.

Stress echocardiography is a transthoracic echo combined with either an exercise or pharmacological stress test. For an exercise stress test, you will walk or run on a treadmill or pedal a stationary bike to make your heart work hard and beat fast. For a pharmacological stress test, you will be given medicine to make your heart work hard and beat fast. A technician will take pictures of your heart using echo before you exercise and as soon as you finish.

What You May See and Hear during Echocardiography

As the doctor or sonographer moves the transducer around, different views of your heart can be seen on the screen of the echo machine. The structures of the heart will appear as white objects, while any fluid or blood will appear black on the screen. Doppler ultrasound techniques often are used during echo tests. Doppler ultrasound is a special ultrasound that shows how blood is flowing through the blood vessels. This test allows the sonographer to see blood flowing at different speeds and in different directions. The speeds and directions appear as different colors moving within the black and white images. The human ear is unable to hear the sound waves used in echo. If Doppler ultrasound is used, you may be able to hear whooshing sounds. Your doctor can use these sounds to learn about blood flow through your heart.

What Does Echocardiography Show?

Echocardiography (echo) shows the size, structure, and movement of the various parts of your heart. This includes the valves, the septum (the wall separating the right and left heart chambers), and the walls of the heart chambers. Doppler ultrasound shows the movement of blood through the heart.

Echo can be used to diagnose heart problems, guide or determine next steps for treatment, monitor changes and improvement, and determine the need for more tests.

Section 22.6

Pelvic Ultrasound

Pelvic ultrasound is a diagnostic tool used to provide pictures of the
structures and organs in the lower belly or pelvis.

There are two types of pelvic ultrasound:

- abdominal (transabdominal—through or across the abdomen), and

- vaginal (transvaginal—across or through the vagina; endovaginal—within the vagina) for women.

Who performs the procedure?

The procedure is performed by a sonographer with the assistance
of a radiologist.

Why is the procedure performed?

A pelvic ultrasound can be performed for different reasons dependent upon your gender. A pelvic ultrasound exam for men and women
can help identify kidney stones, tumors, or other disorders in the urinary bladder.

In women, a pelvic or abdominal ultrasound is most often performed
to evaluate the bladder, ovaries, uterus, and fallopian tubes.

Is there any prep for this procedure?

A full bladder helps to visualize the uterus, ovaries, bladder wall
and prostate gland. Drink a minimum of 32 ounces of clear fluid at
least one hour before your appointment. Do not empty your bladder.

What can I expect before the procedure?

Once you arrive, you will have to register at the front desk. Please
have your insurance information ready at this time. After registration,

you will be taken to the ultrasound department where you will be instructed to remove all clothing and jewelry in the area to be examined.

What can I expect during the procedure?

There are different things to expect dependent upon what type of pelvic exam you are having.

- **Transabdominal:** You will be lying on your back while a gel is applied to the area of the body being studied. The sonographer will then press the transducer firmly against the skin and move it back and forth over the area of interest.

- **Transvaginal:** This ultrasound is performed very much like a gynecologic exam, and involves the insertion of the transducer into the vagina after the patient empties her bladder. A protective cover is placed over the transducer, lubricated with a small amount of gel and then inserted into the vagina. Only two to three inches of the transducer end are inserted into the vagina. The images are obtained from different orientations to get the best views of the uterus and ovaries. Transvaginal ultrasound is usually performed with you lying on your back, possibly with your feet in stirrups similar to a gynecologic exam.

How long is this procedure?

This procedure takes approximately 25 minutes.

What can I expect after the procedure?

After an ultrasound exam, you may be asked to dress and wait until the ultrasound images are reviewed. You should be able to resume your normal activities.

Are there any risks to this procedure?

There are no known risks with this procedure.

Are there any alternatives to this procedure?

No alternatives are available for this procedure.

Section 22.7

Transesophageal Echocardiography

Excerpted from "Transesophageal Echocardiography," National Heart, Lung, and Blood Institute (NHLBI), February 2010.

For transesophageal echocardiography (TEE), a transducer at the tip of a flexible tube (probe) is guided down your throat and into your esophagus. From this position, the sound waves have a more direct path to your heart. This allows your doctor to get more detailed pictures of your heart and its blood vessels. TEE may be used to help diagnose coronary heart disease, congenital heart disease, heart attack, aortic aneurysm, heart infection, cardiomyopathy, heart valve disease, injury to the heart, and blood clots.

Doctors may use TEE to help guide the catheter while doing a cardiac catheterization. Also, doctors may use TEE to help them prepare for a patient's surgery and identify possible risks or problems before, during, and after surgery. For example, they may use TEE to look for possible sources of blood clots in the heart or aorta that could cause a stroke during surgery. At the end of surgery, TEE may be used to check the result of a repair. For example, TEE can show whether heart valves are working properly.

What to Expect before Transesophageal Echocardiography

Transesophageal echocardiography (TEE) most often is done in a hospital. You usually will need to fast (not eat or drink) for eight hours prior to the test. If you have dentures or oral prostheses, you'll need to remove them before the test. You may be given medicine to help you relax during TEE. If so, you will have to arrange for a ride home after the test because the medicine can make you sleepy. Talk with your doctor about whether you or your child needs to take any special precautions before having TEE. He or she can tell you whether you need to change how you take your regular medicines on the day of the test or whether you need to take other steps.

217

What to Expect during Transesophageal Echocardiography

During transesophageal echocardiography (TEE), your doctor or your child's doctor will use a probe with a transducer at its tip. The transducer sends sound waves (ultrasound) to the heart. Probes come in various sizes; smaller probes are used for children and newborns. Your doctor will insert the probe into your mouth or nose. He or she will then gently guide it down your throat into your esophagus (the passage leading from your mouth to your stomach). Your esophagus lies directly behind your heart.

During this process, your doctor will take care to protect your teeth and mouth from injury. The back of your mouth will be numbed with a gel or spray so that you don't gag when the probe is put down your throat. You may feel some discomfort as the probe is guided into your esophagus. Your blood pressure, blood oxygen level, and other vital signs will be checked during the test. You may be given oxygen through a tube in your nose. Children always receive some type of medicine to help them relax or sleep if they're having TEE. This helps them remain still so the doctor can safely insert the probe and take good pictures of the heart and blood vessels. TEE takes less than an hour. However, you may be watched for a few hours after the test because of the effects of the medicine used to help you relax.

What to Expect after Transesophageal Echocardiography

After having transesophageal echocardiography (TEE), your or your child's blood pressure, blood oxygen level, and other vital signs will be closely watched. You can likely go home a few hours after having the test. After the TEE, you may have a sore throat for a few hours. You should not eat or drink for 30 to 60 minutes after having TEE. Most people can return to their normal activities within about 24 hours of the test.

What Does Transesophageal Echocardiography Show?

Transesophageal echocardiography (TEE) provides very high-quality moving pictures of your heart and blood vessels. These pictures help doctors detect and treat heart and blood vessel diseases and conditions. TEE creates pictures from inside the esophagus (the passage leading from the mouth to the stomach) or, sometimes, from inside the stomach. Because the esophagus lies directly behind the heart, TEE provides close-up pictures of the heart. This imaging position also offers different views and may provide more detailed pictures than transthoracic echocardiography (TTE), the most common type of echo. (For TTE, the transducer is placed on the chest, outside of the body.)

What Are the Risks of Transesophageal Echocardiography?

Transesophageal echocardiography (TEE) has a very low risk of serious complications in both adults and children. To reduce your risk, your heart rate and other vital signs will be carefully checked during the test.

Some risks are associated with the medicine given to help you relax during TEE. You may have a bad reaction to the medicine, problems breathing, or nausea (feeling sick to your stomach). Usually, these problems go away without treatment. Your throat also might be sore for a few hours after the test. Rarely, the probe used during TEE can cause minor throat injuries.

Section 22.8

Transvaginal Ultrasound

Transvaginal ultrasound is a type of pelvic ultrasound. It is used to look at a woman's reproductive organs, including the uterus, ovaries, cervix, and vagina. Transvaginal means across or through the vagina.

How the Test Is Performed

You will lie down on a table with your knees bent and feet in holders called stirrups. The health care provider will place a probe, called a transducer, into the vagina. The probe is covered with a condom and a gel. The probe sends out sound waves, which reflect off body structures. A computer receives these waves and uses them to create a picture. The doctor can immediately see the picture on a nearby monitor. The health care provider will move the probe within the area to see the pelvic organs. This test can be used during pregnancy.

In some cases, a special transvaginal ultrasound method called saline infusion sonography (SIS), also called sonohysterography or hysterosonography, may be needed to more clearly view the uterus. This test requires saline (sterile salt water) to be placed into the uterus before the ultrasound. The saline helps outline any abnormal masses, so the doctor can get a better idea of their size. SIS is not done on pregnant women.

How to Prepare for the Test

You will be asked to undress, usually from the waist down. A transvaginal ultrasound is done with your bladder empty or partially filled.

How the Test Will Feel

The test is usually painless, although some women may have mild discomfort from the pressure of the probe. Only a small part of the probe is placed into the vagina.

Why the Test Is Performed

Transvaginal ultrasound may be done for the following problems:

- Abnormal findings on a physical exam, such as cysts, fibroid tumors, or other growths
- Abnormal vaginal bleeding and menstrual problems
- Certain types of infertility
- Ectopic pregnancy
- Pelvic pain

Transvaginal ultrasound is also used during pregnancy to:

- evaluate cases of threatened miscarriage,
- listen to the unborn baby's heartbeat,
- look at the placenta,
- look for the cause of bleeding,
- monitor the growth of the embryo or fetus early in the pregnancy,
- see if the cervix is changing or opening up when labor is starting early.

What Abnormal Results Mean

An abnormal result may be due to many conditions. Some problems that may be seen include:

- birth defects;
- cancers of the uterus, ovaries, vagina, and other pelvic structures;
- infection, including pelvic inflammatory disease;
- non-cancerous growths of the uterus and ovaries (such as cysts or fibroids);
- twisting of the ovaries.

Some problems or conditions that may be found specifically in pregnant women include:

- ectopic pregnancy;
- more than one fetus (twins, triplets, and so forth);

- miscarriage;

- placenta previa;

- placental abruption;

- problems with the baby's growth or the fluid level around the baby;

- shortened cervix, which increases the risk for preterm delivery or late miscarriage;

- structural problems in the baby;

- tumors of pregnancy, including gestational trophoblastic disease.

Risks

There are no known harmful effects of transvaginal ultrasound on humans. Unlike traditional x-rays, there is no radiation exposure with this test.

Chapter 23

Computed Tomography (CT)

Chapter Contents

Section 23.1

Introduction to CT

Excerpted from "What Is Computed Tomography?" U.S.
Food and Drug Administration (FDA), June 18, 2009.

Although also based on the variable absorption of x-rays by different tissues, computed tomography (CT) imaging, also known as "CAT scanning" (computerized axial tomography), provides a different form of imaging known as cross-sectional imaging. The origin of the word "tomography" is from the Greek word *tomos* meaning slice or section, and *graphe* meaning drawing. A CT imaging system produces cross-sectional images or slices of anatomy, like the slices in a loaf of bread. The cross-sectional images are used for a variety of diagnostic and therapeutic purposes.

How a CT System Works

First, a motorized table moves the patient through a circular opening in the CT imaging system. As the patient passes through the CT imaging system, a source of x-rays rotates around the inside of the circular opening. A single rotation takes about one second. The x-ray source produces a narrow, fan-shaped beam of x-rays used to irradiate a section of the patient's body. The thickness of the fan beam may be as small as one millimeter or as large as ten millimeters. In typical examinations there are several phases; each made up of 10–50 rotations of the x-ray tube around the patient in coordination with the table moving through the circular opening. The patient may receive an injection of a "contrast material" to facilitate visualization of vascular structure.

Next, detectors on the exit side of the patient record the x-rays exiting the section of the patient's body being irradiated as an x-ray "snapshot" at one position (angle) of the source of x-rays. Many different "snapshots" (angles) are collected during one complete rotation.

Then, the data are sent to a computer to reconstruct all of the individual "snapshots" into a cross-sectional image (slice) of the internal organs and tissues for each complete rotation of the source of x-rays.

Advances in Technology and Clinical Practice

Today most CT systems are capable of spiral (also called helical) scanning as well as scanning in the formerly more conventional "axial" mode. In addition, many CT systems are capable of imaging multiple slices simultaneously. Such advances allow relatively larger volumes of anatomy to be imaged in relatively less time. Another advancement in the technology is electron beam CT, also known as EBCT. Although the principle of creating cross-sectional images is the same as for conventional CT, whether single- or multi-slice, the EBCT scanner does not require any moving parts to generate the individual "snapshots." As a result, the EBCT scanner allows a quicker image acquisition than conventional CT scanners.

Section 23.2

Chest CT Scan

Excerpted from "Chest CT Scan," National Heart, Lung, and Blood Institute (NHLBI), March 2008.

A chest computed tomography scan, or chest CT scan, is a painless, noninvasive test. It creates precise pictures of the structures in your chest, such as your lungs. "Noninvasive" means that no surgery is done and no instruments are inserted into your body.

A chest CT scan is a type of x-ray. However, a CT scan's pictures show more detail than pictures from a standard chest x-ray. Like other x-ray tests, chest CT scans use a form of energy called ionizing radiation. This energy helps create pictures of the inside of your chest.

The chest CT scanning machine takes many pictures, called slices, of the lungs and the inside of the chest. A computer processes these pictures; they can be viewed on a screen or printed on film. The computer also can stack the pictures to create a very detailed, three-dimensional (3D) model of organs. Sometimes, a substance called contrast dye is injected into a vein in your arm for the CT scan. This substance highlights areas in your chest, which helps create clearer images.

Types of Chest CT Scans

High-resolution chest CT scans provide more than one slice in a single rotation of the x-ray tube. Each slice is very thin and provides a lot of details about the organs and other structures in your chest.

Spiral chest CT scan: For this scan, the table moves continuously through the tunnel-like hole as the x-ray tube rotates around you. This allows the x-ray beam to follow a spiral path. The machine's computer can process the many slices into a very detailed, three-dimensional (3D) picture of the lungs and other structures in the chest.

Who Needs a Chest CT Scan?

Your doctor may recommend a chest CT scan if you have symptoms of lung problems, such as chest pain or trouble breathing. The scan can help find the cause of the symptoms. A chest CT scan looks for problems such as tumors, excess fluid around the lungs, and pulmonary embolism (a blood clot in the lungs). The scan also checks for other conditions, such as tuberculosis, emphysema, and pneumonia. Your doctor may recommend a chest CT scan if a standard chest x-ray does not help diagnose the problem. The chest CT scan can provide more detailed pictures of your lungs and other chest structures than a standard chest x-ray, find the exact location of a tumor or other problem, or show something that is not visible on a chest x-ray.

Contrast Dye

Your doctor may inject a substance called contrast dye into a vein in your arm for the test. You may feel some discomfort when the needle is inserted. As the dye is injected, you also may feel warm and have a metallic taste in your mouth. These feelings last only a few minutes. The contrast dye highlights areas inside your chest, which helps create clearer pictures. Your doctor may ask you to not eat or drink for a few hours before the test, especially if contrast dye is part of the test.

Some people are allergic to the contrast dye. If you have allergic symptoms, such as itching or hives, tell the technician or doctor right away. He or she can give you medicine to relieve the symptoms. The most common type of contrast dye used in CT scans contains iodine. Let your doctor know if you are allergic to iodine.

If you are breast feeding, ask your doctor how long you should wait after the test before you breast feed. The contrast dye can be passed to your baby through your breast milk. You may want to prepare for the test by pumping and saving milk for 24 to 48 hours in advance. You can bottle feed your baby in the hours after the CT scan.

What to Expect during a Chest CT Scan

A chest CT scan takes about 30 minutes, which includes preparation time. The actual scanning time is much shorter, only a few minutes or less. The CT scanner is a large, tunnel-like machine that has a hole in the middle. You will lie on a narrow table that moves through the hole. While you are inside the scanner, an x-ray tube moves around your body. You will hear soft buzzing, clicking, or whirring noises as the scanner takes pictures. The CT scan technician who controls the machine will be in the next room. He or she can see you through a glass window and talk to you through a speaker.

Moving your body can cause the pictures to blur. The technician will ask you to lie still and hold your breath for short periods. This will help make the pictures as clear as possible. The scan itself doesn't hurt, but you may feel anxious if you get nervous in tight or closed spaces. Your doctor may give you medicine to help you relax.

What to Expect after a Chest CT Scan

You usually can return to your normal routine right after a chest CT scan. If you got medicine to help you relax during the CT scan, your doctor will tell you when you can return to your normal routine. The medicine may make you sleepy, so you will need someone to drive you home.

If contrast dye was used during the test, you may have a bruise where the needle was inserted. Your doctor may give you special instructions, such as drinking plenty of liquids to flush out the contrast dye.

What Does a Chest CT Scan Show?

A chest CT scan provides detailed pictures of the size, shape, and position of your lungs and other structures in your chest. Doctors use this test to do the following:

- Follow up on abnormal results from standard chest x-rays.

- Find the cause of lung symptoms, such as shortness of breath or chest pain.

- Find out whether you have a lung problem, such as a tumor, excess fluid around the lungs, or a pulmonary embolism (a blood clot in the lungs). The test also is used to check for other conditions, such as tuberculosis, emphysema, and pneumonia.

What Are the Risks of a Chest CT Scan?

Radiation: Chest CT scans use radiation. The amount of radiation will vary based on the type of CT scan. On average, though, the amount of radiation will not exceed the amount you're naturally exposed to over three years. The radiation from the test is gone from the body within a few days. Children are more sensitive to radiation because they're smaller than adults and still growing. Exposure to radiation is associated with a risk of cancer. However, it's not known whether the amount of radiation from a chest CT scan increases your risk of cancer. You and your doctor will decide whether the benefits of the CT scan outweigh any possible risks. Your doctor also will try to avoid ordering repeated CT scans over a short period.

Allergic reaction: The contrast dye used in some chest CT scans can cause an allergic reaction, such as hives or trouble breathing. The risk of this happening is slight. If you have an allergic reaction, your doctor can give you medicine to relieve it. The most common contrast dye used in CT scans contains iodine. Tell your doctor if you are allergic to iodine.

Section 23.3

Coronary Calcium Scan

Excerpted from "Coronary Calcium Scan,"
National Heart, Lung, Blood Institute (NHLBI), November 2009.

A coronary calcium scan is a test that can help show whether you have coronary heart disease (CHD), also called coronary artery disease. CHD is the most common type of heart disease in both men and women. In CHD, a substance called plaque builds up inside your coronary arteries. These arteries supply your heart muscle with oxygen-rich blood. Plaque is made up of fat, cholesterol, calcium, and other substances found in the blood. Plaque narrows your coronary arteries and reduces blood flow to your heart muscle. It also makes it more likely that blood clots will form in your coronary arteries. Blood clots can partly or completely block blood flow to part of your heart muscle. This can cause chest pain or discomfort called angina or a heart attack. CHD also can lead to heart failure or arrhythmias. Heart failure is a condition in which your heart cannot pump enough blood to meet your body's needs. Arrhythmias are problems with the rate or rhythm of your heartbeat.

A coronary calcium scan looks for specks of calcium (called calcifications) in the walls of the coronary arteries. Calcifications are an early sign of CHD. The test can show whether you're at increased risk for a heart attack or other heart problems before other signs and symptoms occur. Two machines can show calcium in the coronary arteries—electron beam computed tomography (EBCT) and multi-detector computed tomography (MDCT). Both use an x-ray machine to make detailed pictures of your heart. Doctors study the pictures to see whether you're at risk for heart problems in the next 2–10 years.

What to Expect during a Coronary Calcium Scan

Coronary calcium scans are done in a hospital or outpatient office. The x-ray machine used is called a computed tomography (CT) scanner. The technician who runs the scanner will clean areas of your chest and apply sticky patches called electrodes. The patches are attached to an EKG (electrocardiogram) machine to record your heart's electrical activity during the scan. This makes it possible to take pictures of your heart when it's relaxed, between beats.

The CT scanner is a large machine that has a hollow, circular tube in the center. You will lie on your back on a sliding table. The table can move up and down, and it goes inside the tunnel-like machine. The table will slowly slide into the opening in the machine. Inside the scanner, an x-ray tube moves around your body to take pictures of your heart. The technician controls the CT scanner from the next room. He or she can see you through a glass window and talk to you through a speaker. You'll be asked to lie still and hold your breath for short periods while each picture is taken. You may be given medicine to slow down a fast heart rate. This helps the machine take better pictures of your heart. The medicine will be given by mouth or injected into a vein.

A coronary calcium scan takes about 10–15 minutes, although the actual scanning takes only a few seconds. During the test, the machine makes clicking and whirring sounds as it takes pictures. It causes no discomfort, but the exam room may be chilly to keep the machine working properly. If you become nervous in enclosed spaces, you may need to take medicine to stay calm. This is not a problem for most people, because the head will remain outside the opening in the machine. You will be able to return to your normal activities after the coronary calcium scan is done. Your doctor will discuss the results of the calcium scan with you.

What Does a Coronary Calcium Scan Show?

After a coronary calcium scan, you will get a calcium score called an Agatston score. The score is based on the amount of calcium found in your coronary (heart) arteries. You may get an Agatston score for each major artery and a total score.

The test is negative if no calcium deposits (calcifications) are found in your arteries. This means your chance of having a heart attack in the next 2–5 years is low.

The test is positive if calcifications are found in your arteries. Calcifications are a sign of atherosclerosis and coronary heart disease (CHD). (Atherosclerosis is a condition in which the arteries harden and narrow due to plaque buildup.) The higher your Agatston score is, the more severe the atherosclerosis. An Agatston score of 0 is normal. In general, the higher your score, the more likely you are to have CHD. If your score is high, your doctor may recommend more tests.

Section 23.4

Virtual Colonoscopy

Excerpted from "Virtual Colonoscopy," National Institute of Diabetes
and Digestive and Kidney Diseases (NIDDK), November 2008.

Virtual colonoscopy is a procedure used to look for signs of pre-
cancerous growths called polyps, cancer, and other diseases of the large
intestine. Images of the large intestine are taken using computerized
tomography (CT) or, less often, magnetic resonance imaging (MRI).
A computer puts the images together to create an animated, three-
dimensional view of the inside of the large intestine.

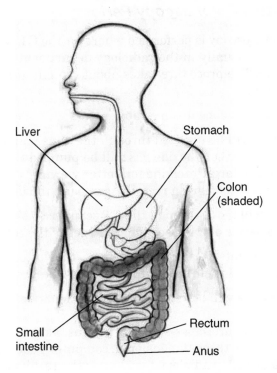

*Figure 23.1. The colon and rectum are the two main parts of the large
intestine.*

How to Prepare for Virtual Colonoscopy

The doctor will provide instructions about how to prepare for virtual colonoscopy. The process is called bowel prep. The bowel prep for virtual colonoscopy is almost identical to the bowel prep for conventional colonoscopy. Generally, all solids must be emptied from the gastrointestinal (GI) tract by following a clear liquid diet for 1–3 days before the procedure. Acceptable liquids include fat-free bouillon or broth, strained fruit juice, water, plain coffee, plain tea, sports drinks (such as Gatorade), and gelatin.

A laxative will be required the night before virtual colonoscopy. A laxative is medicine that loosens stool and increases bowel movements. Laxatives are usually swallowed in pill form or as a powder dissolved in water.

After the bowel prep, patients undergoing CT drink a liquid called contrast media that causes the large intestine to appear very bright during CT. Contrast media helps the doctor identify abnormal tissues.

How Is Virtual Colonoscopy Performed?

Virtual colonoscopy is performed wherever the CT scanner or MRI unit is located—usually in the radiology department of a hospital or medical center. The procedure takes about ten minutes and does not require sedation.

- Patients will lie face up on a table.

- A thin tube will be inserted through the anus and into the rectum. For CT, carbon dioxide gas will be pumped through the tube to expand the large intestine for better viewing. For MRI, contrast media will be given rectally to expand the large intestine.

- The table will move through the CT scanner or MRI unit to produce a series of cross-sectional images of the colon.

- At various points during the procedure, the doctor may ask patients to hold their breath to steady the images.

- The procedure will be repeated while patients lie face down.

After the procedure, cross-sectional images taken by CT or MRI are processed to create three-dimensional, computer-generated images of the large intestine. A radiologist evaluates the results to identify any abnormalities. If abnormalities are found, conventional colonoscopy may be performed the same day or at a later time.

How Is Virtual Colonoscopy Different from Conventional Colonoscopy?

The main difference between virtual and conventional colonoscopy is how the doctor sees inside the colon. Conventional colonoscopy uses a long, lighted, flexible tube called a colonoscope to view the inside of the colon, whereas virtual colonoscopy uses CT or MRI.

Virtual colonoscopy has several advantages over other procedures:

- Virtual colonoscopy does not require the insertion of a colonoscope into the entire length of the colon. Instead, a thin tube is inserted through the anus and into the rectum to expand the large intestine with air.

- No sedation is needed. A patient can return to usual activities or go home after the procedure without the aid of another person.

- Virtual colonoscopy provides clearer, more detailed images than a conventional x-ray using a barium enema—sometimes called a lower gastrointestinal (GI) series.

- Virtual colonoscopy takes less time than either conventional colonoscopy or a lower GI series.

- Virtual colonoscopy can see inside a colon that is narrowed due to inflammation or the presence of an abnormal growth.

Virtual colonoscopy has several disadvantages:

- As with conventional colonoscopy, virtual colonoscopy requires bowel prep and the insertion of a tube into the rectum for expanding the large intestine with gas or liquid.

- Virtual colonoscopy does not allow the doctor to remove tissue samples or polyps.

- Virtual colonoscopy does not detect pre-cancerous polyps smaller than ten millimeters.

- Medicare and many health insurance plans do not pay for virtual colonoscopy cancer screening.

- Virtual colonoscopy is a newer technology and is not as widely available as conventional colonoscopy.

Section 23.5

Full Body CT Scans: What You Need to Know

Excerpted from "Full Body CT Scans: What You Need to Know,"
U.S. Food and Drug Administration (FDA), April 6, 2010.

Using a technology that takes a look at people's insides and promises early warnings of cancer, cardiac disease, and other abnormalities, clinics and medical imaging facilities nationwide are touting a new service for health-conscious people—whole-body computed tomography (CT) screening. This typically involves scanning the body from the chin to below the hips with a form of x-ray imaging that produces cross-sectional images.

CT is recognized as an invaluable medical tool for the diagnosis of disease, trauma, or abnormality in patients with signs or symptoms of disease. It's also used for planning, guiding, and monitoring therapy. What's new is that CT is being marketed as a preventive or proactive health care measure to healthy individuals who have no symptoms of disease.

No Proven Benefits for Healthy People

Taking preventive action, finding unsuspected disease, uncovering problems while they are treatable, these all sound great, almost too good to be true. In fact, at this time the Food and Drug Administration (FDA) knows of no scientific evidence demonstrating that whole-body scanning of individuals without symptoms provides more benefit than harm to people being screened. The FDA is responsible for assuring the safety and effectiveness of such medical devices, and it prohibits manufacturers of CT systems to promote their use for whole-body screening of asymptomatic people. The FDA, however, does not regulate practitioners and they may choose to use a device for any use they deem appropriate.

Compared to most other diagnostic x-ray procedures, CT scans result in relatively high radiation exposure. The risks associated with such exposure are greatly outweighed by the benefits of diagnostic and therapeutic CT. However, for whole-body CT screening of asymptomatic people, the benefits are questionable:

- Can it effectively differentiate between healthy people and those who have a hidden disease?

- Do suspicious findings lead to additional invasive testing or treatments that produce additional risk with little benefit?

- Does a "normal" finding guarantee good health?

Many people do not realize that getting a whole body CT screening exam will not necessarily give them the peace of mind they are hoping for, or the information that would allow them to prevent a health problem. An abnormal finding, for example, may not be a serious one, and a normal finding may be inaccurate. CT scans, like other medical procedures, will miss some conditions, and "false" leads can prompt further, unnecessary testing.

Points to consider if you are thinking of having a whole-body screening:

- Whole-body CT screening has not been demonstrated to meet generally accepted criteria for an effective screening procedure.

- Medical professional societies have not endorsed whole-body CT scanning for individuals without symptoms.

- CT screening of high-risk individuals for specific diseases such as lung cancer or colon cancer is currently being studied.

- The radiation from a CT scan may be associated with a very small increase in the possibility of developing cancer later in a person's life.

FDA's recommendation: Before having a CT screening procedure, carefully investigate and consider the potential risks and benefits and discuss them with your physician.

Chapter 24

Magnetic Resonance Imaging (MRI)

Chapter Contents

Section 24.1

Introduction to MRI

Excerpted from "MRI (Magnetic Resonance Imaging),
U.S. Food and Drug Administration (FDA), March 2011.

Magnetic resonance imaging (MRI) is a medical imaging procedure that uses strong magnetic fields and radio waves to produce cross-sectional images of organs and internal structures in the body. Because the signal detected by an MRI machine varies depending on the water content and local magnetic properties of a particular area of the body, different tissues or substances can be distinguished from one another in the study image.

MRI can give different information about structures in the body than can be obtained using a standard x-ray, ultrasound, or computed tomography (CT) exam. For example, an MRI exam of a joint can provide detailed images of ligaments and cartilage, which are not visible using other study types. In some cases, a magnetically active material (called a contrast agent) is used to show internal structures or abnormalities more clearly.

In most MRI devices, an electric current is passed through coiled wires to create a temporary magnetic field around a patient's body. (In open-MRI devices, permanent magnets are used.) Radio waves are sent from and received by a transmitter/receiver in the machine, and these signals are used to produce digital images of the area of interest.

Using MRI scans, physicians can diagnose or monitor treatments for a variety of medical conditions, including the following:

- Abnormalities of the brain and spinal cord
- Tumors, cysts, and other abnormalities in various parts of the body
- Injuries or abnormalities of the joints
- Certain types of heart problems
- Diseases of the liver and other abdominal organs
- Causes of pelvic pain in women (for example: fibroids, endometriosis)

- Suspected uterine abnormalities in women undergoing evaluation for infertility

Risks/Benefits

MRI does not use ionizing radiation (high-energy radiation that can potentially cause damage to deoxyribonucleic acid [DNA], like the x-rays used in CT scans). There are no known harmful side-effects associated with temporary exposure to the strong magnetic field used by MRI scanners. However, there are important safety concerns to consider before performing or undergoing an MRI scan:

- The magnet may cause pacemakers, artificial limbs, and other implanted medical devices that contain metal to malfunction or heat up during the exam.

- Any loose metal object may cause damage or injury if it gets pulled toward the magnet.

- If a contrast agent is used, there is a slight risk of an allergic reaction. MRI contrast agents can cause problems in patients with significant kidney disease.

- Dyes from tattoos or tattooed eyeliner can cause skin or eye irritation.

- Medication patches can cause a skin burn.

- The wire leads used to monitor an electrocardiogram (ECG) trace or respiration during a scan must be placed carefully to avoid causing a skin burn.

- Prolonged exposure to radio waves during the scan could lead to slight warming of the body.

Section 24.2

MRI of the Brain

"Magnetic Resonance Imaging (MRI): Brain," January 2009, reprinted with permission from www.kidshealth.org. Copyright © 2009 The Nemours Foundation. This information was provided by KidsHealth, one of the largest resources online for medically reviewed health information written for parents, kids, and teens. For more articles like this one, visit www .KidsHealth.org, or www.TeensHealth.org.

What It Is

Magnetic resonance imaging (MRI) of the brain is a safe and painless test that uses a magnetic field and radio waves to produce detailed images of the brain and the brain stem. An MRI doesn't use radiation, which is one way it differs from a CAT scan (also called a CT scan or a computed axial tomography scan).

An MRI scanner consists of a large doughnut-shaped magnet that often has a tunnel in the center. Patients are placed on a table that slides into the tunnel. Some centers have open MRI machines that have larger openings and are helpful for patients with claustrophobia. MRI machines are located in hospitals and radiology centers.

During the exam, radio waves manipulate the magnetic position of the atoms of the body, which are picked up by a powerful antenna and sent to a computer. The computer performs millions of calculations, resulting in clear, cross-sectional black and white images of the body. These images can be converted into three-dimensional (3-D) pictures of the scanned area. This helps pinpoint problems in the brain and the brain stem when the scan focuses on those areas.

Why It's Done

MRI can detect a variety of conditions of the brain such as cysts, tumors, bleeding, swelling, developmental and structural abnormalities, infections, inflammatory conditions, or problems with the blood vessels. It can determine if a shunt is working and detect damage to the brain caused by an injury or a stroke.

MRI of the brain can be useful in evaluating problems such as persistent headaches, dizziness, weakness, and blurry vision or seizures, and it can help to detect certain chronic diseases of the nervous system, such as multiple sclerosis.

In some cases, MRI can provide clear images of parts of the brain that can't be seen as well with an x-ray, CAT scan, or ultrasound, making it particularly valuable for diagnosing problems with the pituitary gland and brain stem.

Preparation

In many cases, a brain MRI requires no special preparation. However, the technician will have your child remove any objects containing metal (such as eyeglasses and jewelry) because they can produce a bright or blank spot on the diagnostic film (but braces and dental fillings won't interfere with the scan). You'll also be asked questions to make sure your child doesn't have any internal metal clips from previous surgery or anything else that might cause a problem near a strong magnetic field. Electronic devices aren't permitted in the MRI room.

To obtain the highest quality MRI results, your child will need to stay still during the scan. For this reason, sedation may be required, especially for infants and young kids, who are likely to have difficulty staying still for the test. If sedation is needed, food and liquids will be stopped at a certain point before the MRI to allow your child's stomach to empty. It's important to notify the MRI technician of any illness, allergy, previous drug reactions, or pregnancy.

Sedation medications are usually given through an IV line (small tube in a vein) to help a child stay asleep during the entire test. Sedation is also helpful for kids who are claustrophobic. To relieve anxiety before and during the test, some patients take an oral sedative on the way to the hospital or radiology center.

You can stay in the MRI room with your child until the test begins, and in some centers you may be able to stay throughout the test. Otherwise, you'll join the technician in an outer room or be asked to stay in a waiting room. If you're nearby you'll be able to watch through a large window and talk to your child through an intercom during breaks between the scans. This can soothe your child if he or she is awake in the MRI machine.

Procedure

An MRI of the brain usually takes 30–45 minutes to perform. Your child will lie on the movable scanning table while the technologist places him or her into position. A special plastic device called a coil may be placed around your child's head. The table will slide into the tunnel and the technician will take images of the head. Each scan takes a few minutes.

To detect specific problems, your child may be given a contrast solution through an IV. The solution, which is painless as it goes into the vein, highlights certain areas of the brain, such as blood vessels, so doctors can see more detail in specific areas. The contrast solution used in MRI tests is safe and allergic reactions are very rare. The technician will ask if your child is allergic to any medications or food before the contrast solution is given.

As the exam proceeds, your child will hear repetitive sounds from the machine, which are normal. Your child may be given headphones to listen to music or earplugs to block the noise, and will have access to a call button in case he or she becomes uneasy during the test. If sedated, your child will be monitored at all times and will be hooked up to a machine that checks the heartbeat, breathing, and oxygen level.

Once the exam is over, the technician will help your child off the table; if sedation was used, your child may be moved to a recovery area.

What to Expect

An MRI exam is painless. Your child may have to lie still on the MRI table for 30–45 minutes during the procedure, but there are brief breaks between each scan. If your child feels cold lying on the MRI table, a blanket can be provided.

Unless sedation was used or you are told otherwise, your child can immediately return to normal routines and diet. Most sedation wears off within 1–2 hours, and any contrast material given should pass through the body in about 24 hours.

Getting the Results

The MRI images will be viewed by a radiologist who is specially trained in interpreting the scans. The radiologist will send a report to your doctor, who will discuss the results with you and explain what they mean. In most cases, results can't be given directly to the patient or family at the time of the test. If the MRI was done on an emergency basis, the results can be made available quickly.

Risks

MRIs are safe and relatively easy. No health risks are associated with the magnetic field or radio waves, since the low-energy radio waves use no radiation. The procedure can be repeated without side effects.

If your child requires sedation, there's a slight chance of slowed breathing due to the medications. If there are any problems with the sedation, the MRI staff will treat them right away. Allergic reactions to the contrast solution are rare, and the technician and other staff are prepared to handle such cases.

Helping Your Child

You can help your child prepare for an MRI by explaining the test in simple terms before the examination. Make sure to explain that pictures of the head will be taken and that the equipment will probably make knocking and buzzing noises.

It may also help to remind your child that you'll be nearby during the entire test.

If an injection of contrast fluid or sedation is required, you can tell your child that the initial sting of the needle will be brief and that the test itself is painless.

If your child will be awake for the test, be sure to explain the importance of lying still. Your doctor may suggest that you and your child take a tour of the MRI room before the test.

If You Have Questions

If you have questions about the MRI procedure, speak with your doctor. You can also talk to the MRI technician before the exam.

Section 24.3

Cardiac MRI

Excerpted from "Cardiac MRI," National Heart,
Lung, and Blood Institute (NHLBI), July 2009.

Cardiac magnetic resonance imaging (MRI) creates pictures of your heart as it is beating, producing both still and moving pictures of your heart and major blood vessels. Doctors use cardiac MRI to get pictures of the beating heart and to look at its structure and function. These pictures can help them decide how to treat people who have heart problems. Cardiac MRI is a common test. It is used to diagnose and evaluate a number of diseases and conditions.

What to Expect before Cardiac MRI

You will be asked to fill out a screening form before having cardiac MRI. The form may ask whether you have had previous surgeries, have any metal objects in your body, or have any medical devices (like a cardiac pacemaker) surgically implanted in your body.

MRI can seriously affect some types of implanted medical devices:

- Implanted cardiac pacemakers and defibrillators can malfunction.

- Cochlear (inner-ear) implants can be damaged. Cochlear implants are small electronic devices that help people who are deaf or who cannot hear well understand speech and the sounds around them.

- Brain aneurysm clips can move due to MRI's strong magnetic field. This can cause severe injury.

Your doctor will let you know if you should not have a cardiac MRI because of a medical device. If this happens, consider wearing a medical identification (ID) bracelet or necklace or carrying a medical alert card that states that you shouldn't have an MRI.

Tell your doctor if being in a fairly tight or confined space causes you anxiety or fear. This fear is called claustrophobia. If you have this condition, your doctor might give you medicine to help you relax. Your doctor may ask you to fast (not eat) for six hours before you take this medicine on the day of the test. Some of the newer cardiac MRI machines are open on all sides. Ask your doctor to help you find a facility that has an open MRI machine if you are fearful in tight or confined spaces.

What to Expect during Cardiac MRI

MRI machines usually are located at hospitals or special medical imaging facilities. A radiologist or other doctor who has special training in medical imaging oversees MRI testing. Cardiac MRI usually takes 45 to 90 minutes, depending on how many pictures are needed. The test may take less time with some newer MRI machines.

The MRI machine will be located in a specially constructed room. This will prevent radio waves from disrupting the machine. It also will prevent the MRI machine's strong magnetic fields from interfering with other equipment. Traditional MRI machines look like a long, narrow tunnel. Newer MRI machines, called short-bore systems, are shorter, wider, and do not completely surround you. Some of the newer machines are open on all sides. Your doctor will help decide which type of machine is best for you.

Cardiac MRI is painless and harmless. You will lie on your back on a sliding table that goes inside the tunnel-like machine. The technician will control the machine from the next room. He or she will be able to see you through a glass window and talk to you through a speaker. Tell the technician if you have a hearing problem. The MRI machine makes loud humming, tapping, and buzzing noises. Earplugs may help lessen the noises made by the MRI machine. Some facilities let you listen to music during the test.

You will need to remain very still during the test. Any movement may blur the pictures. If you're unable to lie still, you may be given medicine to help you relax. You may be asked to hold your breath for 10–15 seconds at a time while the technician takes pictures of your heart. Researchers are studying ways that will allow someone having a cardiac MRI to breathe freely during the exam, while achieving the same image quality.

A contrast agent, such as gadolinium, may be used to highlight your blood vessels or heart in the pictures. Contrast agent usually is injected into a vein in your arm with a needle. You may feel a cool sensation during the injection and discomfort where the needle was inserted. Gadolinium does not contain iodine, so it will not cause problems for people who are allergic to iodine. Your cardiac MRI may include a stress test to detect blockages in your coronary arteries. If so, you will get other medicines to increase the blood flow in your heart or to increase your heart rate.

What Does Cardiac MRI Show?

The doctor supervising your scan will provide your doctor with the results of your cardiac MRI. Your doctor will discuss the findings with you. Cardiac MRI can reveal various heart conditions and disorders, such as the following:

- Coronary heart disease
- Damage caused by a heart attack
- Heart failure
- Heart valve problems
- Congenital heart defects
- Pericarditis (a condition in which the membrane, or sac, around your heart is inflamed)
- Cardiac tumors

Cardiac MRI is a fast, accurate tool that can help diagnose a heart attack. The test does this by detecting areas of the heart that do not move normally, have poor blood supply, or are scarred. Cardiac MRI can show whether any of the coronary arteries are blocked, causing reduced blood flow to your heart muscle. Currently, coronary angiography is the most common procedure for looking at blockages in the coronary arteries. Coronary angiography is an invasive procedure that uses x-rays and iodine-based dyes. Researchers have found that cardiac MRI can replace coronary angiography in some cases, avoiding the need to use x-ray radiation and iodine-based dyes. This use of MRI is called MRI angiography.

What Are the Risks of Cardiac MRI?

Cardiac MRI produces no side effects from the magnetic fields and radio waves. This method of taking pictures of organs and tissues does not carry a risk of causing cancer or birth defects. Serious reactions to the contrast agent used for MRI are very rare. However, side effects are possible and include the following:

- Headache
- Nausea (feeling sick to your stomach)

- Dizziness

- Changes in taste

- Allergic reactions

Rarely, the contrast agent can be harmful in people who have severe kidney or liver disease. It may cause a disease called nephrogenic systemic fibrosis.

If your cardiac MRI includes a stress test, more medicines will be used during the test. These medicines may have other side effects that aren't expected during a regular MRI scan, such as arrhythmias (irregular heartbeats), chest pain, shortness of breath, and palpitations (feelings that your heart is skipping a beat, fluttering, or beating too hard or fast).

Section 24.4

Chest MRI

Excerpted from "Chest MRI," National Heart, Lung, and Blood Institute (NHLBI), March 2008.

Chest MRI (magnetic resonance imaging) is a safe, noninvasive test. This test creates detailed pictures of the structures in your chest, such as your chest wall, heart, and blood vessels. Chest MRI uses radio waves, magnets, and a computer to create these pictures.

What to Expect before Chest MRI

Your doctor or an MRI technician will ask you some questions before the test, such as these:

- Are you pregnant or do you think you could be? Generally, you should not have a chest MRI if you are pregnant, especially during the first trimester.

- Have you had any surgery? If so, what kind?

- Do you use transdermal patches (patches that stick to the skin) to take any of your medicines? Some medicine patches contain aluminum and other metals. These metals can cause skin burns during an MRI.

- Do you have any metal objects in your body, like metal screws or pins in a bone?

- Do you have any medical devices in your body, such as a pacemaker, an implantable cardioverter defibrillator, cochlear (inner-ear) implants, or brain aneurysm clips? The strong magnets in the MRI machine can damage these devices.

The MRI machine looks like a long, narrow tunnel. During the MRI, you lie on your back on a sliding table. The table passes through the scanner as it takes pictures of your chest. Newer machines are shorter and wider and do not completely surround you; others are open on all sides.

Tell your doctor if you are afraid of tight or closed spaces. He or she may give you medicine to help you relax, or find you a place that has an open MRI machine. If you receive medicine to relax you, your doctor may ask you to stop eating about six hours before you take it. This medicine may make you tired, so you will need someone to drive you home.

Contrast dye: Your doctor may inject a substance called contrast dye into a vein in your arm before the MRI. You may feel some discomfort where the needle is inserted. You also may have a cool feeling as the dye is injected. Contrast dye allows the MRI to take more detailed pictures of the structures in your chest. The dye used for chest MRIs does not contain iodine, so it will not create problems for people who are allergic to iodine. Rarely, people develop allergic symptoms from the dye, such as hives and itchy eyes. If this happens, your doctor can give you medicine to relieve your symptoms.

If you are breast feeding, ask your doctor how long you need to wait after the test before you breast feed. The contrast dye can be passed to your baby through your breast milk. You may want to prepare for the test by pumping and saving milk for 24 to 48 hours in advance. You can bottle feed your baby in the hours after the test.

What to Expect during Chest MRI

Chest MRI usually is done at a hospital or at a special medical imaging facility. A radiologist or other doctor with special training in this type of test oversees the testing. Chest MRI usually takes 45 to 90 minutes, depending on how many pictures are needed. The test may take less time with some newer MRI machines.

How the Test Is Done

Chest MRI is painless and has few risks. During the test, you lie on your back on a sliding table as it passes through the MRI machine. A technician will control the machine from the next room. He or she will be able to see you through a glass window and talk to you through a speaker. Tell the technician if you have a hearing problem.

You will hear loud humming, tapping, and buzzing noises from the MRI machine. You may be able to use earplugs or listen to music during the test. Moving your body can cause the pictures to blur. The technician will ask you to remain very still during the test. If you cannot lie still, you may be given medicine to help you relax. The technician also may ask you to hold your breath for 10–15 seconds at a time, while he or she takes pictures of the structures in your chest.

What Does Chest MRI Show?

The pictures from chest MRI may show a tumor, problems in the blood vessels (such as an aneurysm or blood clot), abnormal lymph nodes, or another chest condition (such as a pleural disorder).

What Are the Risks of Chest MRI?

The magnetic fields and radio waves used during chest MRI pose no risk. Serious reactions to the contrast dye used for some MRI tests are very rare. However, side effects are possible and include headache, nausea, dizziness, changes in taste, and allergic reactions. Rarely, contrast dye is harmful to people who have moderate to severe kidney disease.

Section 24.5

MRI of the Spine

What It Is

Magnetic resonance imaging (MRI) of the lumbar spine is a safe and painless test that uses a magnetic field and radio waves to produce detailed pictures of the lumbar spine (the bones, disks, and other structures in the lower back).

An MRI doesn't use radiation, which is one way it differs from a CAT scan (also called a CT scan or a computed axial tomography scan). An MRI scanner consists of a large doughnut-shaped magnet that often has a tunnel in the center. Patients are placed on a table that slides into the tunnel. Some centers have open MRI machines that have larger openings and are helpful for patients with claustrophobia. MRI machines are located in hospitals and radiology centers.

During the examination, radio waves manipulate the magnetic positions of the atoms of the body, which are picked up by a powerful antenna and sent to a computer. The computer performs millions of calculations used to create cross-sectional, black and white images of the body. These images can be reconstructed into three-dimensional (3-D) pictures of the scanned area. This helps to pinpoint problems in the lumbar spine when the scan focuses on that area.

Why It's Done

MRI can detect a variety of conditions of the lumbar spine, including problems with the bones (vertebrae), soft tissues (such as the spinal cord), nerves, and disks.

An MRI sometimes is performed to assess the anatomy of the lumbar spine, to help plan surgery on the spine, or to monitor changes in the spine after an operation. For example, it can find areas of the spine where the spinal canal (which contains the spinal cord) is abnormally narrowed and might require surgery. It can assess the disks to see whether they are bulging, ruptured, or pressing on the spinal cord or nerves.

MRI of the lumbar spine can be useful in evaluating symptoms such as lower back pain, leg pain, numbness, tingling or weakness, or problems with bladder and bowel control. It can also help to diagnose tumors, bleeding, swelling, developmental or structural abnormalities, and infections or inflammatory conditions in the vertebrae or surrounding tissues.

Preparation

A lumbar spine MRI usually doesn't require any special preparation. However, the technician will have your child remove any objects containing metal (such as eyeglasses and jewelry) because they can produce a bright or blank spot on the diagnostic film (but braces and dental fillings won't interfere with the scan). You'll also be asked questions to make sure your child doesn't have any internal metal clips from previous surgery or anything else that might cause a problem near a strong magnetic field. Electronic devices aren't permitted in the MRI room.

To obtain the highest quality MRI results, your child will need to stay still during the scan. For this reason, sedation may be required, especially for infants and young kids, who are likely to have difficulty staying still for the test. If sedation is needed, food and liquids will be stopped at a certain point before the MRI to allow your child's stomach to empty. It's important to notify the MRI technician of any illness, allergy, previous drug reactions, or pregnancy.

Sedation medications are usually given through an IV line (small tube in a vein) to help a child stay asleep during the entire test. Sedation is also helpful for kids who are claustrophobic. To relieve anxiety before and during the test, some patients take an oral sedative on the way to the hospital or radiology center.

You can stay in the MRI room with your child until the test begins, and in some centers you may be able to stay throughout the test. Otherwise, you'll join the technician in an outer room or be asked to stay in a waiting room.

If you're nearby, you'll be able to watch through a large window and talk to your child through an intercom during breaks between the scans. This can soothe your child if he or she is awake in the MRI machine.

Procedure

A lumbar spine MRI usually takes about 30–60 minutes to perform. Your child will lie on the movable scanning table while the technologist places him or her into position. A special plastic device called a coil may be placed around your child's head. The table will slide into the tunnel and the technician will take images of the lumbar spine. Each scan takes a few minutes.

As the exam proceeds, your child will hear repetitive sounds from the machine, which are normal. Your child may be given headphones to listen to music or earplugs to block the noise, and will have access to a call button in case he or she becomes uneasy during the test. If sedated, your child will be monitored at all times and will be hooked up to a machine that checks the heartbeat, breathing, and oxygen level.

Once the exam is over, the technician will help your child off the table; if sedation was used, your child may be moved to a recovery area.

What to Expect

MRIs are painless. Your child may have to lie still on the MRI table for 30–60 minutes during this procedure, but there are brief breaks between each scan. If your child feels cold lying on the MRI table, a blanket can be provided.

Unless sedation is used or you are told otherwise, your child can immediately return to normal routine and diet. Most sedation will wear off within 1–2 hours.

Getting the Results

The MRI images will be looked at by a radiologist who's specially trained in interpreting the scans. The radiologist will send a report to your doctor, who will discuss the results with you and explain what they mean. In most cases, results can't be given directly to the patient or family at the time of the test.

If the MRI was done on an emergency basis, the results can be made available quickly.

Risks

MRIs are safe and easy. No health risks have been associated with the magnetic field or low-energy radio waves that are used for the test. The procedure can be repeated without side effects.

If your child requires sedation, there's a slight chance of slowed breathing due to the medications. If there are any problems with the sedation, the MRI staff will treat them right away.

Helping Your Child

You can help your child prepare for an MRI by explaining the test in simple terms before the examination. Make sure you explain that the lower back will be examined and that the equipment will probably make knocking and buzzing noises.

It may also help to remind your child that you'll be nearby during the entire test.

If your child is going to be awake for the test, be sure to explain the importance of lying still. Your doctor may suggest that you and your child take a tour of the MRI room before the test.

If You Have Questions

If you have questions about the MRI procedure, speak with your doctor. You can also talk to the MRI technician before the exam.

Chapter 25

Nuclear Imaging

Chapter Contents

Section 25.1

Imaging Molecular Change

Reprinted by permission of the Society of Nuclear Medicine from: "What is Molecular Imaging," http://www.molecularimagingcenter.org/ docs/fact_sheets/What%20is%20Molecular%20Imaging.pdf

Molecular imaging is a type of medical imaging that provides detailed pictures of what is happening inside the body at the molecular and cellular level. Where other diagnostic imaging procedures—such as x-rays, computed tomography (CT), and ultrasound—predominantly offer anatomical pictures, molecular imaging allows physicians to see how the body is functioning and to measure its chemical and biological processes.

Molecular imaging offers unique insights into the human body that enable physicians to personalize patient care. In terms of diagnosis, molecular imaging is able to:

- provide information that is unattainable with other imaging technologies or that would require more invasive procedures such as biopsy or surgery; and

- identify disease in its earliest stages and determine the exact location of a tumor, often before symptoms occur or abnormalities can be detected with other diagnostic tests.

As a tool for evaluating and managing the care of patients, molecular imaging studies help physicians:

- determine the extent or severity of the disease, including whether it has spread elsewhere in the body;

- select the most effective therapy based on the unique biologic characteristics of the patient and the molecular properties of a tumor or other disease;

- determine a patient's response to specific drugs;

- accurately assess the effectiveness of a treatment regimen;

- adapt treatment plans quickly in response to changes in cellular activity;

- assess disease progression;

- identify recurrence of disease and help manage ongoing care.

Molecular imaging procedures, which are noninvasive, safe, and painless, are used to diagnose and manage the treatment of:

- cancer;

- heart disease;

- brain disorders, such as Alzheimer disease;

- gastrointestinal disorders;

- lung disorders;

- bone disorders; and

- kidney and thyroid disorders.

How does molecular imaging work?

When disease occurs, the biochemical activity of cells begins to change. For example, cancer cells multiply at a much faster rate and are more active than normal cells. Brain cells affected by dementia consume less energy than normal brain cells. Heart cells deprived of adequate blood flow begin to die.

As disease progresses, this abnormal cellular activity begins to affect body tissue and structures, causing anatomical changes that may be seen on CT or magnetic resonance imaging (MRI) scans. For example, cancer cells may form a mass or tumor. With the loss of brain cells, overall brain volume may decrease or affected parts of the brain may appear different in density than the normal areas. Similarly, the heart muscle cells that are affected stop contracting and the overall heart function deteriorates.

Molecular imaging excels at detecting the cellular changes that occur early in the course of disease, often well before structural changes can be seen on CT and MR images. Most molecular imaging procedures involve an imaging device and an imaging agent, or probe. A variety of imaging agents are used to visualize cellular activity, such as the chemical processes involved in metabolism, oxygen use or blood flow. In nuclear medicine, which is a branch of molecular imaging, the imaging agent is a radiotracer, a compound that includes a radioactive atom, or isotope. Other molecular imaging modalities, such as optical imaging and molecular ultrasound, use a variety of different agents. Magnetic resonance (MR) spectroscopy is able to measure chemical levels in the body, without the use of an imaging agent.

Once the imaging agent is introduced into the body, it accumulates in a target organ or attaches to specific cells. The imaging device detects the imaging agent and creates pictures that show how it is distributed in the body. This distribution pattern helps physicians discern how well organs and tissues are functioning.

How is molecular imaging performed?

Molecular imaging procedures are often performed on an outpatient basis. If an imaging agent is needed, it is injected, swallowed, or inhaled. Imaging is performed, depending on the procedure, immediately or hours or even days afterward, depending on the type of procedure. Images created by the device and a computer are reviewed and interpreted by a qualified imaging professional such as a nuclear medicine physician or radiologist who shares the results with the patient's physician.

What molecular imaging technologies are used today?

Gamma camera: A gamma camera is a specialized camera that is capable of detecting a radiotracer. The gamma camera creates two-dimensional pictures of the inside of the body from different angles.

Single-photon emission-computed tomography (SPECT): A SPECT scan uses a gamma camera that rotates around the patient to detect a radiotracer in the body. Working with a computer, SPECT creates three-dimensional images of the area being studied. SPECT may also be combined with CT for greater accuracy.

Positron emission tomography (PET): PET involves the use of an imaging device (PET scanner) and a radiotracer that is injected into the patient's bloodstream. A frequently used PET radiotracer is 18F-fluorodeoxyglucose (FDG), a compound derived from a simple sugar and a small amount of radioactive fluorine.

Once the FDG radiotracer accumulates in the body's tissues and organs, its natural decay includes emission of tiny particles called positrons that react with electrons in the body. This reaction, known as annihilation, produces energy in the form of a pair of photons. The PET scanner, which is able to detect these photons, creates three-dimensional images that show how the FDG is distributed in the area of the body being studied.

Areas where a large amount of FDG accumulates, called hot spots because they appear more intense than surrounding tissue, indicate that a high level of chemical activity or metabolism is occurring there. Areas of low metabolic activity appear less intense and are sometimes referred to as cold spots. Using these images and the information they provide, physicians are able to evaluate how well organs and tissues are working and to detect abnormalities.

PET-CT is a combination of PET and CT that produces highly detailed views of the body. The combination of two imaging techniques—called co-registration, fusion imaging or hybrid imaging—allows information from two different types of scans to be viewed in a single set of images. CT imaging uses advanced x-ray equipment and in some cases a contrast-enhancing material to produce three-dimensional images.

A combined PET-CT study is able to provide detail on both the anatomy and function of organs and tissues. This is accomplished by superimposing the precise location of abnormal metabolic activity (from PET) against the detailed anatomic image (from CT).

Magnetic resonance (MR) spectroscopy: Magnetic resonance (MR) imaging uses a magnetic field, radio waves, and a computer to create detailed images of the body. MR spectroscopy uses MR to measure metabolites, which are substances produced by chemical reactions in the brain and other areas of the body. MR spectroscopy provides information on the location of specific chemicals in the body and on biochemical activity within cells.

Optical imaging: In optical imaging, light-producing proteins are designed to attach to specific molecules—such as brain chemicals or molecules on the surface of cancer cells. Highly sensitive detectors are able to detect low levels of light emitted by these molecules from inside the body. The two major types of optical imaging are:

- bioluminescent imaging, which uses a natural light-emitting protein (luciferase, for example, the substance that produces the glow of fireflies) to trace the movement of certain cells or to identify the location of specific chemical reactions within the body; and

- fluorescence imaging, which uses proteins that produce light when activated by an external light source such as a laser.

Molecular ultrasound imaging: Traditional ultrasound imaging uses high-frequency sound waves to produce pictures of the inside of the body. As sound waves directed through the body bounce back when they encounter different tissues, echoes are measured with the help of a computer and are converted into real-time images of organs and tissues. Molecular ultrasound uses targeted micro-bubbles, extremely small, hollow structures that serve as a contrast agent during an ultrasound exam.

How safe is molecular imaging?

Molecular imaging procedures are noninvasive and very safe. When used, the amount of radioactivity used in nuclear medicine procedures is very small. The radiation risk is very low compared with the potential benefits. There are no known long-term side effects from nuclear medicine procedures, which have been performed for more than 50 years. Allergic reactions may occur but are extremely rare and usually mild. Imaging agents are approved by the U.S. Food and Drug Administration (FDA).

Is molecular imaging covered by insurance?

Medicare and private insurance companies cover the cost of many molecular imaging technologies. Check with your insurance company for specific information on your plan.

What is the future of molecular imaging?

In addition to increasing our understanding of the underlying causes of disease, molecular imaging is improving the way disease is detected and treated. Molecular imaging technologies are also playing an important role in the development of:

- screening tools, by providing a non-invasive and highly accurate way to assess at-risk populations;

- new and more effective drugs, by helping researchers quickly understand and assess new drug therapies; and

- personalized medicine, in which medical treatment is based on a patient's unique genetic profile.

In the future, molecular imaging will include an increased use of:

- fusion or hybrid imaging, in which two imaging technologies are combined to produce one image;

- optical imaging;

- new probes for imaging critical cancer processes; and

- reporter-probe pairs that will facilitate molecular-genetic imaging.

Section 25.2

Molecular Imaging and Alzheimer Disease

Reprinted by permission of the Society of Nuclear Medicine from: "Molecular Imaging and Alzheimer's Disease," http://www.molecularimaging center.org/docs/fact_sheets/Molecular%20Imaging%20and%20Alzheimers %20Disease.pdf

Alzheimer disease (AD) is an irreversible, progressive brain disease that slowly destroys memory and thinking skills and, eventually, the ability to carry out the simplest tasks of daily living. Although treatment can slow the progression of the disease and help manage its symptoms, there is no cure for AD. The Alzheimer's Association estimates that more five million people are currently living with the disorder.

AD begins deep in the brain where healthy neurons begin to work less efficiently and eventually die. This process gradually spreads to the brain's learning and memory center—the hippocampus—and other areas of the brain, which also begin to shrink. At the same time, beta-amyloid plaques and neurofibrillary tangles begin to spread throughout the brain. Scientists believe these brain changes begin 10–20 years before the signs or symptoms of the disease appear.

What is molecular imaging?

Molecular imaging is a type of medical imaging that provides detailed pictures of what is happening inside the body at the molecular and cellular level. Where other diagnostic imaging procedures—such as x-rays, computed tomography (CT), and ultrasound—predominantly offer anatomical pictures, molecular imaging allows physicians to see how the body is functioning and to measure its chemical and biological processes.

Molecular imaging offers unique insights into the human body that enable physicians to personalize patient care. In terms of diagnosis, molecular imaging is able to:

- provide information that is unattainable with other imaging technologies or that would require more invasive procedures such as biopsy or surgery; and

- identify disease in its earliest stages and determine the exact location of a tumor, often before symptoms occur or abnormalities can be detected with other diagnostic tests.

As a tool for evaluating and managing the care of patients, molecular imaging studies help physicians:

- determine the extent or severity of the disease, including whether it has spread elsewhere in the body;

- select the most effective therapy based on the unique biologic characteristics of the patient and the molecular properties of a tumor or other disease;

- determine a patient's response to specific drugs;

- accurately assess the effectiveness of a treatment regimen;

- adapt treatment plans quickly in response to changes in cellular activity;

- assess disease progression; and

- identify recurrence of disease and help manage ongoing care.

Molecular imaging procedures are noninvasive, safe, and painless.

How does molecular imaging work?

When disease occurs, the biochemical activity of cells begins to change. For example, cancer cells multiply at a much faster rate and are more active than normal cells. Brain cells affected by dementia consume less energy than normal brain cells. Heart cells deprived of adequate blood flow begin to die.

As disease progresses, this abnormal cellular activity begins to affect body tissue and structures, causing anatomical changes that may be seen on CT or magnetic resonance imaging (MRI) scans. For example, cancer cells may form a mass or tumor. With the loss of brain cells, overall brain volume may decrease or affected parts of the brain may appear different in density than the normal areas. Similarly, the heart muscle cells that are affected stop contracting and the overall heart function deteriorates.

Molecular imaging excels at detecting the cellular changes that occur early in the course of disease, often well before structural changes can be seen on CT and MR images. Most molecular imaging procedures involve an imaging device and an imaging agent, or probe. A variety of imaging agents are used to visualize cellular activity, such as the chemical processes involved in metabolism, oxygen use, or blood flow. In nuclear medicine, which is a branch of molecular imaging, the imaging agent is a radiotracer, a compound that includes a radioactive atom, or isotope. Other molecular imaging modalities, such as optical imaging and molecular ultrasound, use a variety of different agents. Magnetic resonance (MR) spectroscopy is able to measure chemical levels in the body, without the use of an imaging agent.

Once the imaging agent is introduced into the body, it accumulates in a target organ or attaches to specific cells. The imaging device detects the imaging agent and creates pictures that show how it is distributed in the body. This distribution pattern helps physicians discern how well organs and tissues are functioning.

What molecular imaging technologies are used for Alzheimer disease?

Diagnosis of AD is currently a long process that may include a detailed patient history, physical and neurological exams, laboratory tests, and a lengthy process of eliminating other possible causes of mental decline. Although experienced practitioners can diagnose the disease with up to 90% accuracy, a definitive diagnosis of AD is still only possible by autopsy following a patient's death.

Researchers are exploring how positron emission tomography (PET) can help physicians diagnose AD earlier and more accurately and effectively manage patients with the disease. Early diagnosis and treatment of AD can slow the progression of disease and help preserve individual functioning for months to years.

What is PET?

PET involves the use of an imaging device (PET scanner) and a radiotracer that is injected into the patient's bloodstream. A frequently used PET radiotracer is 18F-fluorodeoxyglucose (FDG), a compound derived from a simple sugar and a small amount of radioactive fluorine.

Once the FDG radiotracer accumulates in the body's tissues and organs, its natural decay includes emission of tiny particles called positrons that react with electrons in the body. This reaction, known as annihilation, produces energy in the form of a pair of photons. The PET scanner, which is able to detect these photons, creates three-dimensional images that show how the FDG is distributed in the area of the body being studied.

Areas where a large amount of FDG accumulates, called hot spots because they appear more intense than surrounding tissue, indicate that a high level of chemical activity or metabolism is occurring there. Areas of low metabolic activity appear less intense and are sometimes referred to as cold spots. Using these images and the information they provide, physicians are able to evaluate how well organs and tissues are working and to detect abnormalities.

Because brain cells affected by dementia are less active, they consume, or metabolize less glucose than normal cells and will appear less bright on PET scans. Researchers are exploring the use of additional neuroimaging probes, which bind to the abnormal plaques and tangles associated with Alzheimer disease and allow them to be visualized on a PET scan.

PET-CT is a combination of PET and computed tomography (CT) that produces highly detailed views of the body. The combination of two imaging techniques—called co-registration, fusion imaging or hybrid imaging—allows information from two different types of scans to be viewed in a single set of images. CT imaging uses advanced x-ray equipment and in some cases a contrast-enhancing material to produce three dimensional images.

A combined PET-CT study is able to provide detail on both the anatomy and function of organs and tissues. This is accomplished by superimposing the precise location of abnormal metabolic activity (from PET) against the detailed anatomic image (from CT).

How is PET performed?

The procedure begins with an intravenous (IV) injection of a radiotracer, such as FDG, which usually takes between 30 and 60 minutes to distribute throughout the body. The patient is then placed in the PET scanner where special detectors are used to create a three dimensional image of the FDG distribution. Scans are reviewed and interpreted by a qualified imaging professional such as a nuclear medicine physician or radiologist who shares the results with the patient's physician.

How is PET used for Alzheimer disease?

Researchers are exploring the use of PET to:

- help diagnose AD early in the disease process,

- differentiate AD from other types of dementia,

- monitor the progression of the disease,

- determine the effectiveness of new therapies, and

- gain a better understanding of AD, including its causes and progression.

What are the advantages of PET for the brain?

- PET allows metabolic activity to be directly visualized, not inferred.

- PET studies allow abnormal brain function to be detected before structural changes resulting from brain cell death can be seen on CT or MRI.

- PET is highly useful in detecting specific types of dementia, such as Alzheimer disease and Pick disease, a type of frontotemporal dementia. In these disorders, early brain damage is too spread out, or diffuse, and may not impact brain volume or structure that is identifiable on CT or MR.

Is PET covered by insurance?

Insurance companies will cover the cost of most PET scans, however, coverage for PET scans that measure brain amyloid plaques is not yet available. Check with your insurance company for specific information on your plan.

Dementia and Alzheimer Disease

Important research underway includes the National Institute on Aging Alzheimer Disease Neuroimaging Initiative (ADNI), which is following hundreds of cognitively healthy individuals and others with mild cognitive impairment (MCI) and early Alzheimer disease over at least five years. Participants will undergo annual MRI and PET scans so that researchers can assess changes in both the normal aging brain and in individuals with MCI and AD to better understand when and where in the brain degeneration occurs.

By correlating these images with other test results from the study's participants, such as cognitive function tests and fluid and urine samples, researchers hope to identify valuable biomarkers of the disease process. Researchers hope that this study and future initiatives using the ADNI database will create imaging and biomarker standards for measuring the success of potential treatments.

While molecular imaging technologies such as beta-amyloid imaging with PET are currently only used as research tools, they may soon help physicians to:

- routinely diagnose AD at its earliest stages, which is critical for providing the best possible care;
- identify individuals who are at high risk of developing Alzheimer disease;
- monitor the progress of the disease;
- assess patient response to drug treatment;
- contribute to the development of targeted drugs and therapies for dementia and Alzheimer disease.

Section 25.3

Nuclear Heart Scan

Excerpted from "Nuclear Heart Scan,"
National Heart, Lung, and Blood Institute (NHLBI), January 2010.

A nuclear heart scan is a test that allows your doctor to get important information about the health of your heart. During a nuclear heart scan, a safe, radioactive substance called a tracer is injected into your bloodstream through a vein. The tracer travels to your heart and releases energy. Special cameras outside of your body detect the energy and use it to create pictures of your heart. Nuclear heart scans are used for three main purposes:

- to check how blood is flowing to the heart muscle,
- to look for damaged heart muscle, and
- to see how well your heart pumps blood to your body.

Types of Nuclear Heart Scanning

The two main types of nuclear heart scanning are single photon emission computed tomography (SPECT) and cardiac positron emission tomography (PET). SPECT is the most well-established and widely used type, while PET is newer. There are specific reasons for using each.

Single photon emission computed tomography (SPECT): SPECT is the most common nuclear scanning test for diagnosing coronary heart disease (CHD). Combining SPECT with a stress test can show problems with blood flow to the heart that only can be detected when the heart is working hard and beating fast. SPECT also is used to look for areas of damaged or dead heart muscle tissue. These areas may be the result of a previous heart attack or other cause. SPECT also can show how well the heart's lower left chamber (left ventricle) pumps blood to the body. Weak pumping ability may be the result of a heart attack, heart failure, or other causes. The most commonly used tracers in SPECT are called thallium-201, technetium-99m sestamibi (Cardiolite®), and technetium-99m tetrofosmin (Myoview™).

Positron emission tomography: PET uses different tracers than SPECT. PET can provide more detailed pictures of the heart. However, PET is newer and has some technical limits that make it less available than SPECT. Research into advances in SPECT and PET is ongoing. Right now, there is no clear cut advantage of using one over the other in all situations. PET can be used for the same purposes as SPECT— to diagnose CHD, check for damaged or dead heart muscle tissue, and check the heart's pumping strength. PET takes a clearer picture through thick layers of tissue (such as abdominal or breast tissue). PET also is better than SPECT at showing whether CHD is affecting more than one of your heart's blood vessels. A PET scan also may be used if a SPECT scan does not produce good pictures.

What to Expect before a Nuclear Heart Scan

A nuclear heart scan can take a lot of time. Most scans take between 2–5 hours, especially if two sets of pictures are needed. Discuss with your doctor how a nuclear heart scan is done. Talk with him or her about your overall health, including health problems such as asthma, COPD (chronic obstructive pulmonary disease), diabetes, and kidney disease. If you have lung disease or diabetes, your doctor will give you special instructions before the nuclear heart scan. If you are having a stress test as part of your nuclear heart scan, wear comfortable walking shoes and loose-fitting clothes for the test. You may be asked to wear a hospital gown during the test.

Let your doctor know about any medicines you take, including prescription and over-the-counter medicines, vitamins, minerals, and other supplements. Some medicines and supplements can interfere with the medicines that may be used during the stress test to increase your heart rate.

What to Expect during a Nuclear Heart Scan

Many, but not all, nuclear medicine centers are located in hospitals. A doctor who has special training in nuclear heart scans—a cardiologist or radiologist—will oversee the test. Cardiologists are doctors who specialize in diagnosing and treating heart problems. Radiologists are doctors who specialize in diagnostic techniques, such as nuclear scans.

Before the test begins, the doctor or a technician will use a needle to insert an intravenous (IV) line into a vein in your arm. Through this IV line, he or she will put the radioactive tracer into your bloodstream at the right time. You also will have EKG (electrocardiogram) patches attached to your body to check your heart rate during the test.

During the Stress Test

If you are having an exercise stress test as part of your nuclear scan, you will walk on a treadmill or pedal a stationary bicycle. You will be attached to EKG and blood pressure monitors. You will be asked to exercise until you are too tired to continue, short of breath, or having chest or leg pain. You can expect that your heart will beat faster, you will breathe faster, your blood pressure will increase, and you will sweat. Tell the doctor if you have any chest, arm, or jaw pain or discomfort. Also report any dizziness, lightheadedness, or other unusual symptoms.

If you are unable to exercise, your doctor may give you medicine to make your heart beat faster. This is called a pharmacological stress test. The medicine used may make you feel anxious, sick, dizzy, or shaky for a short time. If the side effects are severe, your doctor may give you other medicine for relief. Before the exercise or pharmacological stress test stops, the tracer is injected through the IV line.

During the Nuclear Heart Scan

The nuclear heart scan will start shortly after the stress test. You will lie very still on a padded table. The nuclear heart scan camera, called a gamma camera, is enclosed in a metal housing. The part of the camera that detects the tracer's radioactivity can be put in several positions around your body as you lie on the padded table. For some nuclear heart scans, the metal housing is shaped like a doughnut and you lie on a table that goes slowly through the doughnut hole. The computer used to collect the pictures of your heart is nearby or in another room.

Usually, two sets of pictures are taken. One will be taken right after the stress test and the other will be taken after a period of rest. The pictures may be taken all in one day or over two days. It takes about 15 to 30 minutes to take each set of pictures.

Some people find it hard to stay in one position for some time. Others may feel anxious while lying in the doughnut-shaped scanner. The table may feel hard. Sometimes, the room feels chilly because of the air conditioning needed to maintain the machines. Let the doctor or technician know how you are feeling during the test so he or she can respond as needed.

What to Expect after a Nuclear Heart Scan

Your doctor may ask you to return to the nuclear medicine center on a second day for more pictures. Outpatients will be allowed to go home after the scan or leave the nuclear medicine center between the two scans. Most people can go back to their daily activities after a nuclear heart scan. The radioactivity will naturally leave your body in your urine or stool. It's helpful to drink plenty of fluids after the test.

The cardiologist or radiologist will read and interpret the results of the test within one to three days. Results will be reported to your doctor, who will contact you to discuss them. Or, the cardiologist or radiologist may discuss the results directly with you.

What Does a Nuclear Heart Scan Show?

The results from a nuclear heart scan can help doctors do the following:

- Diagnose heart conditions, such as coronary heart disease (CHD), and decide the best course of treatment.

- Manage certain heart diseases, such as CHD and heart failure, and predict short-term or long-term survival.

- Determine your risk for a heart attack.

- Decide whether other heart tests or procedures will help you. Examples of these tests and procedures include coronary angiography and cardiac catheterization.

- Decide whether procedures that can increase blood flow to the coronary arteries will help you. Examples of these procedures include angioplasty and coronary artery bypass grafting (CABG).

- Monitor procedures or surgeries that have been done, such as CABG or a heart transplant.

What Are the Risks of a Nuclear Heart Scan?

The radioactive tracer used during a nuclear heart scan exposes the body to a very small amount of radiation. No long-term effects have been reported from these doses. Radiation dose might be a concern for people who need multiple scans. However, advances in hardware and software may greatly reduce the radiation dose people receive. Some people are allergic to the radioactive tracer, but this is very rare.

If you have coronary heart disease, you may have chest pain during the stress test when you exercise or are given medicine to increase your heart rate. Medicine can relieve this symptom. If you are pregnant, tell your doctor or technician before the scan. It may be postponed until after the pregnancy.

Section 25.4

Nuclear Breast Imaging (Scintimammography)

Excerpted from "Nuclear Medicine Breast Imaging (Scintimammography), © 2008 Imaginis Corporation (www.imaginis.com). Reprinted with permission.

Nuclear medicine breast imaging (also called scintimammography) is a supplemental breast exam that may be used in some patients to investigate a breast abnormality. A nuclear medicine test is not a primary investigative tool for breast cancer but can be helpful in selected cases after diagnostic mammography has been performed. Nuclear medicine breast imaging involves injecting a radioactive tracer (dye) into the patient. Since the dye accumulates differently in cancerous and non-cancerous tissues, scintimammography can help physicians determine whether cancer is present.

Currently, only the Miraluma Tc-99m sestamibi compound, manufactured by DuPont Pharmaceuticals, is approved by the Food and Drug Administration (FDA) for breast imaging in the United States. Therefore, the nuclear medicine breast imaging test may be referred to as a "Miraluma." Nuclear medicine may be appropriate in patients who have dense breast tissue that makes their mammograms difficult to interpret or in patients with palpable abnormalities (those able to be physically felt) but whose mammograms do not reveal any abnormalities.

Who is a candidate for nuclear medicine breast imaging?

Nuclear medicine breast imaging is not a screening tool for breast cancer. However, after a physical breast exam, mammography, and ultrasound are performed, nuclear medicine breast imaging may be appropriate for certain patients. Supplemental breast imaging helps determine whether a patient has a suspicious breast abnormality that would require a biopsy to confirm the presence of breast cancer.

Nuclear medicine breast imaging may be appropriate for patients with the following:

- Dense breast tissue

- Large, palpable (able to be felt) abnormalities that cannot be imaged well with mammography or ultrasound

- Breast implants

- When multiple tumors are suspected

- A lump at the surgical site after mastectomy (breast removal) since scar tissue may be difficult to distinguish from other tumors with other breast imaging exams

- To check the axillary (underarm) lymph nodes to determine whether they contain cancer cells (sentinel lymph node biopsy)

Like magnetic resonance imaging (MRI) of the breast, nuclear medicine may also be helpful to determine if multiple breast tumors are present. For instance, a mammogram or ultrasound (sonogram) of the breast may reveal breast cancer in one area. However, a nuclear medicine breast imaging test may show that the cancer is in fact multi-focal; tumors are present in several areas of the breast. Determining the extent of breast cancer with nuclear medicine can help indicate treatment: breast conserving surgery (lumpectomy) or breast removal (mastectomy). Mastectomy is indicated if there are multiple tumors.

Studies show that nuclear medicine breast imaging is only 40% to 60% accurate in imaging small breast abnormalities but more than 90% accurate in detecting abnormalities over one centimeter. However, mammography and physical exams are often very useful for detecting large abnormalities. It is the small abnormalities that tend to need additional imaging. Therefore, in this respect, nuclear medicine breast imaging is often of limited value.

How is nuclear medicine breast imaging performed?

The nuclear medicine breast imaging test takes approximately 45 minutes to one hour to perform and costs approximately $200 to $600 per exam. Nuclear medicine involves the use of radiation, but the dose is very low and is not harmful to patients. Most of the drug leaves the body within a few hours of the test.

To perform the exam, a radioactive tracer (Tc-99m sestamibi) is injected in the patient's arm opposite of the breast being studied. Patients may experience a brief metallic taste after the tracer is injected. The radioactive tracer travels throughout the body, including to the breast that needs to be imaged. Normal tissue will only accumulate a small amount of the radioactive tracer (dye). However, cancer cells tend to take up more of the dye.

After the radioactive tracer has been injected, the patient is instructed to lie face down on a special table while the breast hangs down through a hole in the table. Approximately five minutes after the injection, a special gamma camera is used to capture images of the breast from several angles. This takes several minutes for each image that is taken. During this time, the patient should try to lie as still as possible. After all of the images are taken while the patient is lying face down on the table, she may be asked to sit up or raise her arms while additional images of her breast are taken. Unlike mammography, no breast compression is necessary during a nuclear medicine test (although mammography is performed prior to the recommendation of a nuclear medicine breast imaging test).

Section 25.5

Positron Emission Tomography (PET) Imaging

This section begins with an excerpt from "2008 Progress Report on Alzheimer's Disease: Neuroimaging," National Institute on Aging (NIA), December 2009. It continues with "PET Imaging Information," © 2011 Alzheimer Disease Cooperative Study (www.adcs.org). Reprinted with permission.

In a positron emission tomography (PET) scan, a small amount of a short-lived radioactive substance is attached to another molecule and injected into the body. The radioactive molecule travels through the blood and becomes concentrated in the organs and tissues where it is normally found. The PET machine measures the energy given off by the radioactive material and translates that information into pictures that can be viewed on a computer screen. PET scans frequently are used in brain research because they allow researchers to observe and measure activity in different parts of the brain by monitoring blood flow and the concentrations of the radioactive material in different areas of the brain.

Alzheimer Disease Cooperative Study: Pet Imaging Information

PET scanning can produce high quality pictures of different processes in your body. For this research study, PET was used to take pictures of how the brain uses glucose, or sugar. Glucose is the source of energy for the brain. Scientists have learned that there are abnormal patterns of glucose use in the brains of patients with Alzheimer disease, and in some older people.

How does PET work?

Scientists at your PET center make a special form of glucose that is labeled with radioactivity. This is called fluorodeoxyglucose, or FDG. The FDG is injected through a small needle into a vein in your arm, and the PET scanner will take pictures of the glucose use by your brain. The information in these scans will be analyzed to see how glucose use is different in people with memory problems, and to see how scans change over time. The entire PET scan will take about an hour.

Before the Scan

You should use the restroom before the scan begins. A small needle will be inserted in a vein in your arm. A blood sample will be taken to check your blood sugar level and make sure it is in range. The FDG also will be injected into this needle. After the FDG is injected, you will sit in a quiet room for 30 minutes. You will be placed in the scanner and pictures will be taken for the next 30 minutes. Some people will have a slightly different PET scan, called a quantitative PET scan. In this scan, you will be placed in the scanner before injection of the FDG and pictures will be taken for one hour. Five small blood samples will be taken from your arm during the scan.

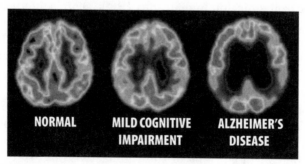

Figure 25.1. Brain Images Acquired with PET

During the Scan

The technologist will ask you to lie down on a cushioned table. This table will be moved into the scanner after you have been comfortably positioned for scanning. The technologist will leave the room but you will be in constant contact with him or her throughout the exam. The PET scan is quiet and does not make any noise. Most people do not find the scanner to be constricting or claustrophobic. It is very important to hold as still as possible during the scan and that you do not talk during the scan. When scanning is complete, the technologist will return to assist you off the table and ask you to go to the restroom.

Chapter 26

Digital Infrared Thermal Imaging

Chapter Contents

Section 26.1

Overview of Medical Digital Infrared Thermal Imaging

Editor's note: Thermography is being used in research settings for a number of purposes. Clinical use is more widespread among alternative medicine providers than mainstream physicians. Its overall role in medical diagnosis and treatment is still being defined.

Medical digital infrared thermal imaging (DITI) is a noninvasive diagnostic technique that allows the examiner to visualize and quantify changes in skin surface temperature. An infrared scanning device is used to convert infrared radiation emitted from the skin surface into electrical impulses that are visualized in color on a monitor. This visual image graphically maps the body temperature and is referred to as a thermogram. The spectrum of colors indicate an increase or decrease in the amount of infrared radiation being emitted from the body surface. Since there is a high degree of thermal symmetry in the normal body, subtle abnormal temperature asymmetries can be easily identified. Medical DITI's major clinical value is in its high sensitivity to pathology in the vascular, muscular, neural, and skeletal systems and as such can contribute to the pathogenesis and diagnosis made by the clinician.

Medical DITI has been used extensively in human medicine in the U.S.A., Europe, and Asia for the past 20 years. Until now, cumbersome equipment has hampered its diagnostic and economic viability. Current state of the art computer-based infrared technology designed specifically for clinical application has changed all this.

Clinical uses for DITI include:

1. To define the extent of a lesion of which a diagnosis has previously been made;

2. To localize an abnormal area not previously identified, so further diagnostic tests can be performed;

3. To detect early lesions before they are clinically evident;

4. To monitor the healing process before the patient is returned to work or training.

Skin blood flow is under the control of the sympathetic nervous system. In normal people there is a symmetrical dermal pattern which is consistent and reproducible for any individual. This is recorded in precise detail with a temperature sensitivity of 0.1° centigrade (C) by DITI.

The neuro-thermography application of DITI measures the somatic component of the sympathetic nervous system by assessing dermal blood flow. The sympathetic nervous system is stimulated at the same anatomical location as its sensory counterpart and produces a 'somato sympathetic response.' The somato sympathetic response appears on DITI as a localized area of altered temperature with specific features for each anatomical lesion.

The mean temperature differential in peripheral nerve injury is 1.5° C. In sympathetic dysfunctions (reflex sympathetic dystrophy [RSD], complex regional pain syndrome [CRPS]) temperature differentials ranging from 1°C to 10°C depending on severity are not uncommon.

Rheumatological processes generally appear as hot areas with increased temperature patterns. The pathology is generally an inflammatory process, for example, synovitis of joints and tendon sheaths, epicondylitis, capsular and muscle injuries, and so forth.

Both hot and cold responses may coexist if the pain associated with an inflammatory focus excites an increase in sympathetic activity. Also, vascular conditions are readily demonstrated by DITI including Raynaud disease, vasculitis, limb ischemia, and deep venous thrombosis.

Medical DITI Is Filling the Gap in Clinical Diagnosis

X-ray, computed tomography (CT), ultrasound, and magnetic resonance imaging are tests of anatomy. Electromyography is a test of motor physiology. DITI is unique in its capability to show physiological change and metabolic processes. It has also proven to be a very useful complementary procedure to other diagnostic modalities.

Unlike most diagnostic modalities DITI is non-invasive. It is a very sensitive and reliable means of graphically mapping and displaying skin surface temperature. With DITI you can diagnosis, evaluate, monitor, and document a large number of injuries and conditions, including soft tissue injuries and sensory/autonomic nerve fiber dysfunction.

Medical DITI can offer considerable financial savings by avoiding the need for more expensive investigation for many patients.

Medical DITI can graphically display the very subjective feeling of pain by objectively displaying the changes in skin surface temperature that accompany pain states.

Medical DITI can show a combined effect of the autonomic nervous system and the vascular system, down to capillary dysfunctions. The effects of these changes show as asymmetries in temperature distribution on the surface of the body.

Medical DITI is a monitor of thermal abnormalities present in a number of diseases and physical injuries. It is used as an aid for diagnosis and prognosis, as well as therapy follow up and rehabilitation monitoring, within clinical fields that include rheumatology, neurology, physiotherapy, sports medicine, oncology, pediatrics, orthopedics, and many others.

Results obtained with medical DITI systems are totally objective and show excellent correlation with other diagnostic tests.

Section 26.2

Breast Thermography

"What is breast thermography?" © 2002 American College of Clinical Thermology (www.thermologyonline.org). Reprinted with permission. Updated in April 2011 with an editorial note by David A. Cooke, MD, FACP.

Editor's note: Breast thermography for breast cancer screening and detection remains highly controversial. While some advocates view it as a very promising technology, others consider it unproven. The overall sensitivity (ability to detect) and specificity (ability to accurately distinguish cancer from non-cancerous conditions) of breast thermography remains unclear, and there has been conflicting data. For example, a 2010 study published in the *European Journal of Surgical Oncology* reported a breast thermography system to be up to 78% sensitive and 75% specific in detecting breast cancer in women under 50. However, a 2011 study published in *Clinical Radiology* found thermography to be only 25% sensitive and 85% specific when used for breast cancer screening. Studies of breast thermography to date have involved relatively small numbers of women, which may account for the widely differing conclusions.

Breast thermography is a 15-minute non-invasive test of physiology. It is a valuable procedure for alerting your doctor to changes that can indicate early stage breast disease. The benefit of breast thermography is that it offers the opportunity of earlier detection of breast disease than has been possible through breast self-examination, doctor examination, or mammography alone.

Thermography can detect the subtle physiologic changes that accompany breast pathology, whether it is cancer, fibrocystic disease, an infection, or a vascular disease. Your doctor can then plan accordingly and lay out a careful program to further diagnose and/or monitor you during and after any treatment.

Thermography is a painless, non-invasive, state of the art clinical test without any exposure to radiation and is used as part of an early detection program which gives women of all ages the opportunity to increase their chances of detecting breast disease at an early stage. It is particularly useful for women under 50 where mammography is less effective.

Thermography's role in breast cancer and other breast disorders is to help in early detection and monitoring of abnormal physiology and the establishment of risk factors for the development or existence of cancer. When used with other procedures, the best possible evaluation of breast health is made.

This test is designed to improve chances for detecting fast-growing, active tumors in the intervals between mammographic screenings or when mammography is not indicated by screening guidelines for women under 50 years of age. All patients' thermograms (breast images) are kept on record and form a baseline for all future routine evaluations. With the new ultra-sensitive, high resolution digital infrared cameras available today a technology that has been developing over the past 20 years is now becoming more accessible.

Thermography as a physiologic test, demonstrates heat patterns that are strongly indicative of breast abnormality, the test can detect subtle changes in breast temperature that indicate a variety of breast diseases and abnormalities and once abnormal heat patterns are detected in the breast, follow-up procedures including mammography are necessary to rule out or properly diagnose cancer and a host of other breast diseases such as fibrocystic syndrome and Paget disease.

Canadian researchers found that infrared imaging of breast cancers could detect minute temperature variations related to blood flow and demonstrate abnormal patterns associated with the progression of tumors. These images or thermograms of the breast were positive for 83% of breast cancers compared to 61% for clinical breast examination alone and 84% for mammography.

By performing thermography years before conventional mammography, a selected patient population at risk can be monitored more carefully, and then by accurately utilizing mammography or ultrasound as soon as is possible to detect the actual lesion—(once it has grown large enough and dense enough to be seen on mammographic film)—can increase the patients treatment options and ultimately improve the outcome.

It is in this role that thermography provides its most practical benefit to the general public and to the medical profession. It is certainly an adjunct to the appropriate usage of mammography and not a competitor. In fact, thermography has the ability to identify patients at the highest risk and actually increase the effective usage of mammographic imaging procedures.

Until such time as a cure has been found for this terrible disease, progress must be made in the fields of early detection and risk evaluation coupled with sound clinical decision making. Thermography, with its non-radiation, non-contact, and low-cost basis has been clearly demonstrated to be a valuable and safe early risk marker of breast pathology, and an excellent case management tool for the ongoing monitoring and treatment of breast disease when used under carefully controlled clinical protocols.

Chapter 27

Mammograms

A mammogram is a low-dose x-ray exam of the breasts to look for changes that are not normal. The results are recorded on x-ray film or directly into a computer for a doctor called a radiologist to examine.

A mammogram allows the doctor to have a closer look for changes in breast tissue that cannot be felt during a breast exam. It is used for women who have no breast complaints and for women who have breast symptoms, such as a change in the shape or size of a breast, a lump, nipple discharge, or pain. Breast changes occur in almost all women. In fact, most of these changes are not cancer and are called benign, but only a doctor can know for sure. Breast changes can also happen monthly, due to your menstrual period.

A high-quality mammogram plus a clinical breast exam, an exam done by your doctor, is the most effective way to detect breast cancer early. Finding breast cancer early greatly improves a woman's chances for successful treatment.

How is a mammogram done?

You stand in front of a special x-ray machine. The person who takes the x-rays, called a radiologic technician, places your breasts, one at a time, between an x-ray plate and a plastic plate. These plates are attached to the x-ray machine and compress the breasts to flatten them. This spreads the breast tissue out to obtain a clearer picture. You will feel pressure on

Excerpted from "Mammograms: Frequently Asked Questions," U.S. Department of Health and Human Services (HHS), November 17, 2010.

your breast for a few seconds. It may cause you some discomfort; you might feel squeezed or pinched. This feeling only lasts for a few seconds, and the flatter your breast, the better the picture. Most often, two pictures are taken of each breast—one from the side and one from above. A screening mammogram takes about 20 minutes from start to finish.

Screening mammograms are done for women who have no symptoms of breast cancer. It usually involves two x-rays of each breast. Screening mammograms can detect lumps or tumors that cannot be felt. They can also find microcalcifications or tiny deposits of calcium in the breast, which sometimes mean that breast cancer is present.

Diagnostic mammograms are used to check for breast cancer after a lump or other symptom or sign of breast cancer has been found. Signs of breast cancer may include pain, thickened skin on the breast, nipple discharge, or a change in breast size or shape. This type of mammogram also can be used to find out more about breast changes found on a screening mammogram, or to view breast tissue that is hard to see on a screening mammogram. A diagnostic mammogram takes longer than a screening mammogram because it involves more x-rays in order to obtain views of the breast from several angles. The technician can magnify a problem area to make a more detailed picture, which helps the doctor make a correct diagnosis.

A digital mammogram also uses x-rays to produce an image of the breast, but instead of storing the image directly on film, the image is stored directly on a computer. This allows the recorded image to be magnified for the doctor to take a closer look. Current research has not shown that digital images are better at showing cancer than x-ray film images in general. But, women with dense breasts who are pre- or perimenopausal, or who are younger than age 50, may benefit from having a digital rather than a film mammogram. Digital mammography may offer these benefits:

- Long-distance consultations with other doctors may be easier because the images can be shared by computer.

- Slight differences between normal and abnormal tissues may be more easily noted.

- The number of follow-up tests needed may be fewer.

- Fewer repeat images may be needed, reducing exposure to radiation.

How often should I get a mammogram?

The National Cancer Institute recommends that women 40 years and older should get a mammogram every one to two years. Women who have had breast cancer or other breast problems or who have a family history of breast cancer might need to start getting mammograms before age 40, or they might need to get them more often. Talk to your doctor about when to start and how often you should have a mammogram.

What if my screening mammogram shows a problem?

If you have a screening test result that suggests cancer, your doctor must find out whether it is due to cancer or to some other cause. Your doctor may ask about your personal and family medical history. You may have a physical exam. Your doctor also may order some of these tests:

- Diagnostic mammogram, to focus on a specific area of the breast.

- Ultrasound, an imaging test that uses sound waves to create a picture of your breast. The pictures may show whether a lump is solid or filled with fluid. A cyst is a fluid-filled sac. Cysts are not cancer. But a solid mass may be cancer. After the test, your doctor can store the pictures on video or print them out. This exam may be used along with a mammogram.

- Magnetic resonance imaging (MRI), which uses a powerful magnet linked to a computer. MRI makes detailed pictures of breast tissue. Your doctor can view these pictures on a monitor or print them on film. MRI may be used along with a mammogram.

- Biopsy, a test in which fluid or tissue is removed from your breast to help find out if there is cancer. Your doctor may refer you to a surgeon or to a doctor who is an expert in breast disease for a biopsy.

Where can I get a high-quality mammogram?

Women can get high-quality mammograms in breast clinics, hospital radiology departments, mobile vans, private radiology offices, and doctors' offices. The Food and Drug Administration (FDA) certifies mammography facilities that meet strict quality standards for their x-ray machines and staff and are inspected every year. You can ask your doctor or the staff at the mammography center about FDA certification before making your appointment. A list of FDA-certified facilities can be found in Chapter 68 of this book, or online at http://www.fda.gov/cdrh/mammography/certified.html.

Your doctor, local medical clinic, or local or state health department can tell you where to get no-cost or low-cost mammograms. You can also call the National Cancer Institute's Cancer Information Service toll-free at 800-422-6237, or search online at http://www.cancer.gov.

What if I have breast implants?

Women with breast implants should also have mammograms. A woman who had an implant after breast cancer surgery in which the entire breast was removed (mastectomy) should ask her doctor whether she needs a mammogram of the reconstructed breast.

If you have breast implants, be sure to tell your mammography facility that you have them when you make your appointment. The technician and radiologist must be experienced in x-raying patients with breast implants. Implants can hide some breast tissue, making it harder for the radiologist to see a problem when looking at your mammogram. To see as much breast tissue as possible, the x-ray technician will gently lift the breast tissue slightly away from the implant and take extra pictures of the breasts.

How do I get ready for my mammogram?

First, check with the place you are having the mammogram for any special instructions you may need to follow before you go. Here are some general guidelines to follow:

- If you are still having menstrual periods, try to avoid making your mammogram appointment during the week before your period. Your breasts will be less tender and swollen. The mammogram will hurt less and the picture will be better.

- If you have breast implants, be sure to tell your mammography facility that you have them when you make your appointment.

- Wear a shirt with shorts, pants, or a skirt. This way, you can undress from the waist up and leave your shorts, pants, or skirt on when you get your mammogram.

- Do not wear any deodorant, perfume, lotion, or powder under your arms or on your breasts on the day of your mammogram appointment. These things can make shadows show up on your mammogram.

- If you have had mammograms at another facility, have those x-ray films sent to the new facility so that they can be compared to the new films.

Are there any problems with mammograms?

Although they are not perfect, mammograms are the best method to find breast changes that cannot be felt. If your mammogram shows a breast change, sometimes other tests are needed to better understand it. Even if the doctor sees something on the mammogram, it does not mean it is cancer.

As with any medical test, mammograms have limits. These limits include:

- They are only part of a complete breast exam. Your doctor also should do a clinical breast exam. If your mammogram finds something abnormal, your doctor will order other tests.

- Finding cancer does not always mean saving lives. Even though mammography can detect tumors that cannot be felt, finding a small tumor does not always mean that a woman's life will be saved. Mammography may not help a woman with a fast growing cancer that has already spread to other parts of her body before being found.

- False negatives can happen. This means everything may look normal, but cancer is actually present. False negatives do not happen often. Younger women are more likely to have a false negative mammogram than are older women. The dense breasts of younger women make breast cancers harder to find in mammograms.

- False positives can happen. This is when the mammogram results look like cancer is present, even though it is not. False positives are more common in younger women, women who have had breast biopsies, women with a family history of breast cancer, and women who are taking estrogen, such as menopausal hormone therapy.

- Mammograms (as well as dental x-rays and other routine x-rays) use very small doses of radiation. The risk of any harm is very slight, but repeated x-rays could cause cancer. The benefits nearly always outweigh the risk. Talk to your doctor about the need for each x-ray. Ask about shielding to protect parts of the body that are not in the picture. You should always let your doctor and the technician know if there is any chance that you are pregnant.

Chapter 28

Neurological Imaging

Yesterday

Neurologists and neurosurgeons made clinical decisions based on first generation computed tomography (CT) scans. This was a quantum advance over the insensitive plain film x-ray techniques of previous generations. Early positron emission tomography (PET) and single photon emission computed tomography (SPECT) techniques utilized first generation radiographic tracers (or tags) to map brain function. Functional magnetic resonance imaging (fMRI) allowed researchers to measure blood oxygen level dependent (BOLD) changes in the brain of humans for the first time, and fMRI enabled the non-invasive study of everything from finger movements to thoughts and emotions.

Today

Advanced magnetic resonance imaging (MRI) is revolutionizing the care of patients with neurologic disorders, as well as research in understanding the brain. Magnetic resonance (MR) spectroscopy allows measurement of brain chemicals in living patients. PET imaging using compounds that bind to brain receptors now allows the study of molecular details not previously visualized.

The resolution of brain and spinal cord imaging has increased tremendously. For example, modern techniques allow the neuroimaging

---

Excerpted from "Neurological Imaging," National Institutes of Health (NIH), October 2010.

of subtle abnormalities of neurological development that give rise to seizures and enable many more persons to benefit from a surgical treatment of epilepsy. MRI can now identify spinal vascular malformations that are amenable to treatment. Many of these went undiagnosed 30 years ago.

Functional MRI BOLD imaging enables researchers not only to localize and measure important brain functions, but also to assess functional changes in the brain resulting from disease processes, injury, or response to treatment. fMRI is also being used to guide operative strategy in neurosurgery.

Diffusion tensor imaging, a technique that allows for the visualization and characterization of white matter tracts in the human brain, is allowing researchers to assess changes in the brain's maturation from childhood to adulthood, as well as to detect differences in white matter integrity between healthy and diseased populations.

Advanced diagnostics in many neurological diseases/disorders now are increasingly used as a means to monitor the progression of disease and response to treatment. For example, the development of Pittsburgh Compound B now permits the molecular imaging of the amyloid beta protein in patients with Alzheimer disease. In addition, MRI has become invaluable in the diagnosis of patients with multiple sclerosis and spinal cord disorders.

Advanced image processing allows clinicians and researchers to measure the subtle shrinkage of brain regions over time (from chronic disease progression) and use this information to test new therapies. Furthermore, neuroimaging has made it possible to detect, characterize, and monitor objective brain changes after insults such as traumatic brain injury.

Neuroimaging has played a crucial role in advancing understanding and treatment of stroke, and is now recommended by national guidelines for acute assessment and treatment decisions and for secondary prevention.

Tomorrow

Advanced neuroimaging techniques will allow researchers to understand all of the structural and functional pathways in the entire, living human brain. The National Institutes of Health (NIH) has launched the Human Connectome Project (http://www.humanconnectomeproject.org/), a $30 million multi-site project that aims to understand genetic and environmental influences on brain connectivity, as well as how dysfunction in connectivity can contribute to neurological and mental conditions.

Scientists will be able to use imaging to understand cognitive impairment in neurodegenerative diseases such as Alzheimer disease. The ongoing Alzheimer Disease Neuroimaging Initiative (ADNI) (http://www.adni-info.org/), a multi-site, longitudinal, prospective study of normal cognitive aging, mild cognitive impairment (MCI), and early Alzheimer disease (AD), will enable researchers to define rates of impairment, design improved methods for clinical trials, and develop more effective techniques to treat and prevent Alzheimer disease.

In the future, scientists will be able to use neuroimaging to determine consciousness states of individuals. A series of intriguing studies has improved the clinical assessment of states such as coma, vegetative state, minimally conscious state, and locked in syndrome, providing new information about evaluation of brain function, formation of diagnoses, and estimation of prognosis.

Chapter 29

Researching New Imaging Techniques

Chapter Contents

Section 29.1

Super-Cool Imaging Technique

Excerpted from "Super-Cool Imaging Technique Identifies
Aggressive Tumors," National Institute of Biomedical Imaging
and Bioengineering (NIBIB), December 28, 2009.

Each year nearly 200,000 men are diagnosed with prostate cancer. Although the prostate antigen specific (PSA) blood test has improved detection, it fails to indicate whether the cancer is aggressive or slow-growing. The current approach of active surveillance means that many patients spend years undergoing repeat blood tests and invasive biopsies to monitor the cancer's growth. Any changes in PSA results or biopsy samples may signal a need to alter treatment. "There are a lot of questions in prostate cancer like, 'Do you treat or not?'" says John Kurhanewicz, director of the Prostate Imaging Group and Biomedical Nuclear Magnetic Resonance (NMR) Lab, Department of Radiology and Biomedical Imaging, University of California, San Francisco (UCSF), who has tracked a cohort of men under active surveillance for the last decade. "Current [imaging] techniques fall short."

Unsatisfied with the lack of diagnostic precision in prostate cancer, Kurhanewicz and colleague Daniel Vigneron, associate director of the Surbeck Imaging Laboratory at UCSF, in collaboration with GE Healthcare, have applied a new method that can assess tumor aggressiveness rapidly and noninvasively. This technique, hyperpolarized carbon-13 magnetic resonance imaging, measures metabolic activity (the chemical reactions that sustain the tumor) within a tumor and homes in on specific chemical products produced by aggressive tumors.

Identifying Aggressive Prostate Tumors

Aggressive tumors are known to produce high levels of lactate. In a proof-of-concept study in mice with prostate tumors, the UCSF researchers tracked the tumor's uptake of hyperpolarized pyruvate (a compound known to convert to lactate) and the tumor's subsequent lactate production. Results showed that less aggressive tumors contained lower levels of lactate and more aggressive tumors had higher levels of lactate.

The researchers plan to begin a patient trial. The trial will examine dose safety of the imaging agent and how well carbon-13 magnetic resonance imaging (MRI) can characterize human prostate tumors. "This trial is critical because it takes metabolic probes that are inherently insensitive and makes them highly sensitive," explains Kurhanewicz. "It will give us a tool that gives a more direct assessment of disease in the clinic." Not only will diagnosis and treatment be more accurate, but the time it takes to perform a prostate staging exam is likely to decrease. Kurhanewicz suggests that the imaging technique could reduce the current one-hour prostate tumor staging exam to 30 minutes, lower the exam's cost, and be less stressful for the patient.

Moving Beyond Cancer

Although hyperpolarized compounds will play a key role in imaging metabolic activity associated with cancer, they will likely make diagnosis of other diseases more precise as well. These compounds are attractive because they do not alter cardiac function and the doses needed to image are similar to current MR contrast agents and less than computed tomography (CT) contrast doses. "If we can pave the way with one hyperpolarized agent in man, then more will follow," says Kurhanewicz.

In preclinical research, the hyperpolarized agents could increase understanding of how drugs interact with specific networks of molecules to alter cell function. "MRI alone is not good at targeting specific pathways," says Kurhanewicz. Because hyperpolarized agents greatly increase the sensitivity of MR spectroscopy, "they may allow us to track targeted agents to see if they are hitting the pathways they should."

Section 29.2

Blood Vessel Shape Reveals Disease

Excerpted from "Smooth or Wiggly Blood Vessel Shape
Reveals Disease," National Institute of Biomedical Imaging
and Bioengineering (NIBIB), August 31, 2009.

The human body contains a whopping 60,000 miles of blood vessels, and all of those tubes contain useful details about how well the body is functioning. For certain disease states, such as brain tumors, the size, shape, and number of vessels can reveal critical data on a tumor's progress or regression.

Describing the body's blood distribution system isn't easy. Angiography, the most common technique used to image vessels, only provides pictures (angiograms) of the vessels. However, by combining magnetic resonance angiography (MRA) with a set of powerful algorithms (mathematical equations), a research team led by Elizabeth Bullitt has hit on a method that defines blood vessels by describing their number and shape. The approach could lead to a noninvasive method of determining whether a tumor is malignant and of tracking how a tumor responds to treatment. It also may yield clues on how the brain ages.

"Blood vessels can provide an amazing amount of information," says Bullitt, the Van L. Weatherspoon Jr. Distinguished Professor of neurosurgery and head of the Computer-Assisted Surgery and Imaging Laboratory at the University of North Carolina (UNC), Chapel Hill. Bullitt has worked for over a decade to extract meaningful information from the often stunning images of blood vessels. She has been particularly interested in how cancer affects blood vessel networks because cancer can cause blood vessels to undergo tremendous changes. Although many groups have studied how to define vessels from three-dimensional images, Bullitt's approach gives flexibility when assessing the brain's blood vessel network. It can provide quantitative details for blood vessels over the entire brain, over a large or small region of interest, or over a connected set of vessels.

Bullitt analyzes ultrahigh-resolution three-dimensional images with specially designed software to make a computer model of the vessels that is so specific that she can count the number of vessels in a given location, map how vessels connect in their branching structures, and home in on each vessel's tortuosity—its wiggliness—a prominent characteristic in disease states.

Tracking Squiggly Vessels

In several different studies, Bullitt has assessed her computer-assisted MRA technique's ability to determine tumor malignancy and track a drug therapy's effect on tumor growth. "We've known for a long time that tumors have squiggly vessels," says Keith Smith, an associate professor of radiology at UNC Medical School and a Bullitt collaborator. The algorithm-enhanced MRA technique is "a way to put numbers on those squiggles."

In one study of 30 hard-to-diagnose cases, Bullitt's technique correctly identified whether a tumor was malignant in 29 of the cases. "These cases, which were all scheduled for gross tumor resection, were all scanned before surgery and included some really difficult cases where the presence of a malignancy could not be determined using conventional imaging," says Bullitt. Two of the tumors were just 0.3 cm^3, about the size of a coffee bean. Bullitt's technique also may give clinicians a more quantitative way of deciding whether a tumor is responding to treatment.

The Exercise Connection: Healthy Vessels, Healthy Brain

Preliminary research using computer-assisted magnetic resonance angiography (MRA) now suggests exercise may also keep your brain young. Bullitt's research may also give some insight into how the brain ages. The researchers discovered that, in older brains, smaller vessels tend to stop functioning over time. In addition, more pronounced wiggle patterns are often associated with conditions such as high blood pressure and diabetes.

Bullitt's technique offers radiologists another tool to assess healthy and diseased tissue. Whether an aging brain, a cancerous tumor, or a brain condition such as Alzheimer disease, the technique provides a noninvasive way to gather meaningful data on healthy and disease states. Because changes in blood vessel networks may directly affect or be caused by disease progression, accurately measuring those changes may make a difference in patient outcomes.

Section 29.3

Optical Coherence Tomography

Excerpted from "Optical Coherence Tomography Poised to Improve Diagnostics: October 23, 2008," National Institute of Biomedical Imaging and Bioengineering (NIBIB), July 14, 2009.

Just over 15 years ago, using technology that would revolutionize the telecommunications industry, researchers at the Massachusetts Institute of Technology (MIT) developed an elegant optical imaging technique—optical coherence tomography (OCT). The technique, analogous to ultrasound, uses near-infrared light rather than sound waves to create images. Light reflects off of tissue and is captured by a detector. Image analysis software combines the signals from the reflected light to form an image.

Initially, researchers used OCT to examine the fine structures of the eye's retina. Ophthalmologists embraced OCT because it gave them a noninvasive way to view the retina and at a relatively low cost compared with other techniques such as magnetic resonance imaging. Because every layer of the retina could be viewed by OCT, the technique could assist in tracking conditions such as glaucoma, macular holes (retinal tears), and nonvascular macular edema (swelling of the retina's center). The technique could also monitor how well retinal drug therapies were working. OCT is now considered the gold standard for retinal imaging.

Although OCT's image quality and image acquisition rates were adequate for ophthalmology studies, they were not good enough for use in other clinical fields. Since its introduction, researchers and engineers around the world have worked to improve OCT's image resolution and speed. The technique now can provide clear three-dimensional images taken in real time. With these advances, OCT is now poised to make a contribution in a number of fields including surgical oncology, cardiology, gastroenterology, and tissue engineering. OCT's ability to give immediate quantitative information may also make it an integral component of point-of-care diagnostics.

Better biopsies: Needle biopsies remove cells from a suspect area in the body, and those cells are then examined under a microscope to determine the extent of disease present. The procedure can have a high rate of nondiagnosis, which means captured tissue contains only normal cells even though another screening technique has shown an abnormal mass exists. In these cases, patients must undergo surgical biopsy. For breast cancer, roughly 10–15% of needle biopsies are nondiagnostic. For lung nodules, the nondiagnostic biopsy rate can be as high as 50% for nodules less than one centimeter. Often this nondiagnosis comes after hours of imaging to guide needle placement.

Image-guided needle biopsy and surgical tumor removal can benefit from imaging technologies capable of producing high-resolution images that show structural and, with the use of contrast agents or imaging dyes, molecular information about surrounding tissue. Boppart and his group have developed an OCT surgical system that allows surgeons to examine tumor beds, tissue margins, and lymph nodes during surgery and get a comprehensive picture of the patient's situation.

Improved stent placement: OCT offers cardiologists a nimble tool for examining the body's extensive network of blood vessels. In two areas, for instance, OCT comes out ahead of intravascular ultrasound (IVUS), a technology commonly used for imaging blood vessels. OCT can image the inner lining of a vessel well enough to pick up early stages of plaque development, and the OCT catheters are about five times smaller than the IVUS probes.

When it comes to placing stents (mesh tubes that expand to keep the vessel open), cardiologists would like to see what the stent looks like and how the stent has affected surrounding tissue. With OCT, clinicians can now see whether the stent is over-expanded and whether the blood vessel has been injured through placement.

Assessing the esophagus: Barrett's esophagus, a precancerous condition, arises when the cells lining the lower part of the esophagus become abnormal as a result of continued drenching by stomach acid. To monitor the condition, patients undergo regular biopsies. The standard of care for Barrett's is random quadrant biopsies, an approach that may miss areas that may be undergoing potentially harmful changes. In the future, OCT may offer these patients a less invasive way to monitor their condition. Clinicians would use OCT to survey the esophagus and detect suspicious lesions and then, based on those findings, biopsy dubious areas.

Visualizing tissue structure and function: Engineering tissue for the skin, eyes (in the form of corneas), and other organs is in its infancy. Often the tissue fails because it is a mechanical mismatch in the wound bed. By applying optical coherence techniques to microscopy, Boppart and his colleagues can noninvasively and nondestructively visualize in three dimensions the structural and functional properties of engineered tissue. This allows them to observe changes in the tissue over time and will help improve the design of engineered tissue.

Promise for point-of-care diagnostics: For outpatient procedures such as skin cancer removal and dental visits, OCT represents a quantum leap forward in point-of-care diagnostics. OCT's ability to pinpoint suspicious areas and give quantitative information about tissue could dramatically alter how and when clinicians decide on treatment. "OCT changes the process of diagnosis," says Boppart. "This will allow us to change the standard of care."

Section 29.4

Magnetic Resonance Elastography

Excerpted from "Picturing Liver Disease with Shear Waves,"
National Institute of Biomedical Imaging and Bioengineering
(NIBIB), August 28, 2008.

For the 170 million individuals worldwide who live with chronic hepatitis C, a major cause of liver disease, biopsies may be necessary to detect the development of fibrosis or scarring of liver tissue, which can impair liver function. Many other diseases also cause fibrosis of the liver, often without any symptoms. However, biopsies only provide information about one area of the liver. If fibrosis is not evenly distributed throughout the organ, the sample may under- or over-estimate the true extent of disease. Imaging is also used to diagnose diseases in the liver, but standard medical imaging technologies are not sensitive enough to diagnose fibrosis.

To overcome these limitations, Dr. Richard Ehman, professor of radiology at the Mayo Clinic in Rochester, Minnesota, and colleagues have developed a new imaging technique that gives precise data on the liver's stiffness or elasticity. Their noninvasive approach, called magnetic resonance elastography (MRE), uses a special magnetic resonance imaging (MRI) technique to capture snapshots of shear waves, a special type of sound wave, as they move through the tissue. The technology creates "elastograms" or images that show tissue stiffness. MRE allows sensitive measurement of changes in liver tissue stiffness that indicates the presence of early fibrosis, so the condition can be diagnosed reliably and treatment given before the disease progresses to irreversible cirrhosis."

The Mayo Clinic has been using MRE for patient care since early 2007, with over 600 patient examinations performed. In addition to monitoring fibrosis development, Ehman and his team have used MRE to characterize liver tumors, which typically are much stiffer than normal tissue. Their results showed that malignant tumors were stiffer than benign tumors and normal liver tissue.

New possibilities: Although Ehman and his team tested MRE on the liver initially, additional studies are underway in the brain, breast, kidney, and prostate. Ehman notes that measuring a tissue's mechanical properties such as stiffness can also help increase our understanding of what causes disease. "MRE opens a new window into our understanding of tumor biology," says Dr. Vivian Lee, professor of radiology, physiology, and neuroscience and senior vice president and chief scientific officer at New York University's Langone Medical Center. "We now have a tool to start to understand at a molecular level how and why fibrosis and increased stiffness develops as a property of tumors."

Part Four

Catheterization, Endoscopic, and Electrical Tests and Assessments

Chapter 30

Cardiac Catheterization

Cardiac catheterization is used to diagnose and/or treat many heart conditions. Doctors may recommend this procedure for various reasons. The most common reason is to evaluate chest pain. Chest pain may be a symptom of coronary heart disease (CHD). Cardiac catheterization can show whether plaque is narrowing or blocking your heart's arteries.

Doctors can treat CHD during cardiac catheterization with a procedure called angioplasty. During angioplasty, a tiny balloon is put through the catheter and into the blocked artery. When the balloon is inflated, it pushes the plaque against the artery wall. This creates a wider pathway for blood to flow to the heart. Sometimes a stent is placed in the artery during angioplasty. A stent is a small mesh tube that's used to treat narrowed or weakened arteries in the body.

Most people who have heart attacks have partly or completely blocked coronary arteries. Thus, cardiac catheterization may be done on an emergency basis while you are having a heart attack. When used with angioplasty, the procedure allows your doctor to open up blocked arteries and prevent more damage to your heart.

Cardiac catheterization also can help your doctor figure out the best treatment for your CHD if you:

- recently recovered from a heart attack, but are having chest pain;

- had a heart attack that caused major damage to your heart; or

Excerpted from "Cardiac Catheterization," National Heart, Lung, and Blood Institute (NHLBI), May 2009.

• had an EKG (electrocardiogram), stress test, or other test with results that suggested heart disease.

You also may need cardiac catheterization if your doctor suspects you have a heart defect or if you are about to have heart surgery. The procedure shows the overall shape of your heart and the four large spaces (heart chambers) inside it. This inside view of the heart will show certain heart defects and help your doctor plan your heart surgery.

Sometimes doctors do cardiac catheterization to see how well the valves at the openings and exits of the heart chambers are working. Valves control the flow of blood in the heart. To check your valves, your doctor will measure blood flow and oxygen levels in different parts of your heart. Cardiac catheterization also can check how well a man-made heart valve is working and how well your heart is pumping blood.

If your doctor thinks you have a heart infection or tumor, he or she may take samples of your heart muscle through the catheter. With the help of cardiac catheterization, doctors can even do minor heart surgery, such as repair certain heart defects.

What to Expect during Cardiac Catheterization

Cardiac catheterization is done in a hospital. During the procedure, you will be kept on your back and awake. This allows you to follow your doctor's instructions during the procedure. You will be given medicine to help you relax, which may make you sleepy.

Your doctor will numb the area on the arm, groin (upper thigh), or neck where the catheter will enter your blood vessel. A needle is used to make a small hole in the blood vessel. Through this hole your doctor will put a tapered tube called a sheath. Next, your doctor will put a thin, flexible wire through the sheath and into your blood vessel. This guide wire is then threaded through your blood vessel to your heart. The wire helps your doctor position the catheter correctly. Your doctor then puts a catheter through the sheath and slides it over the guide wire and into the coronary arteries.

Special x-ray movies are taken of the guide wire and the catheter as they are moved into the heart. The movies help your doctor see where to position the tip of the catheter. When the catheter reaches the right spot, your doctor will use it to do tests or treatments on your heart. For example, your doctor may do angioplasty and stenting.

During the procedure, your doctor may put a special dye in the catheter. This dye will flow through your bloodstream to your heart.

Once the dye reaches your heart, it will make the inside of your heart's arteries show up on an x-ray called an angiogram. This test is called coronary angiography. Coronary angiography can show how well blood is being pumped out of the heart's main pumping chambers, which are called ventricles. When the catheter is inside your heart, your doctor may use it to take blood samples from different parts of the heart or to do minor heart surgery.

To get a more detailed view of a blocked coronary artery, your doctor may do intracoronary ultrasound. For this test, your doctor will thread a tiny ultrasound device through the catheter and into the artery. This device gives off sound waves that bounce off the artery wall (and its blockage) to make an image of the inside of the artery. If the angiogram or intracoronary ultrasound shows blockages or other possible problems in the heart's arteries, your doctor may use angioplasty to open the blocked arteries.

After your doctor does all of the needed tests or treatments, he or she will pull back the catheter and take it out along with the sheath. The opening left in the blood vessel will then be closed up and bandaged. A small weight may be put on top of the bandage for a few hours to apply more pressure. This will help prevent major bleeding from the site.

What to Expect after Cardiac Catheterization

After cardiac catheterization, you will be moved to a special care area. You will rest there for several hours or overnight. During that time, your movement will be limited to avoid bleeding from the site where the catheter was inserted. While you recover in this area, nurses will check your heart rate and blood pressure regularly. They also will check for bleeding from the catheter insertion site.

A small bruise may develop on your arm, groin (upper thigh), or neck at the site where the catheter was inserted. That area may feel sore or tender for about a week. Let your doctor know if you develop problems such as:

- a constant or large amount of bleeding at the insertion site that cannot be stopped with a small bandage; or

- unusual pain, swelling, redness, or other signs of infection at or near the insertion site.

Talk to your doctor about whether you should avoid certain activities, such as heavy lifting, for a short time after the procedure.

What Are the Risks of Cardiac Catheterization?

Cardiac catheterization is a common medical procedure that rarely causes serious problems. However, complications can include:

- bleeding, infection, and pain where the catheter was inserted;

- damage to blood vessels (rarely, the catheter may scrape or poke a hole in a blood vessel as it's threaded to the heart);

- an allergic reaction to the dye used.

Other, less common complications of the procedure include:

- arrhythmias (irregular heartbeats) which often go away on their own, but may need treatment if they persist;

- damage to the kidneys caused by the dye used;

- blood clots that can trigger stroke, heart attack, or other serious problems;

- low blood pressure;

- a buildup of blood or fluid in the sac that surrounds the heart which can prevent the heart from beating properly.

As with any procedure involving the heart, complications can sometimes be fatal. However, this is rare with cardiac catheterization. The risk of complications with cardiac catheterization is higher if you have diabetes or kidney disease, or if you are aged 75 or older. The risk of complications also is greater in women and in people having cardiac catheterization on an emergency basis.

Chapter 31

Endoscopy

Chapter Contents

Section 31.1

Ten Questions to Ask Your Endoscopist

"Ten Questions to Ask Your GI Endoscopist," © 2011 American Society for Gastrointestinal Endoscopy. Reprinted with permission. All rights reserved. This material is regularly updated, check http://www.asge.org for the most recent information.

The answers to all of these should be "yes" and should reassure you that you are seeing a trained endoscopist who will safely and effectively perform your colonoscopy or other endoscopic procedure.

1. Are you a licensed medical doctor?

2. Have you had formal training in gastrointestinal (GI) endoscopy? (Not learned during a short 2–3 day course, or self-instruction without supervised experience)

3. Is your rate of cecal (total colon) intubation greater than 90%?

4. Do you perform more than 100 colonoscopies annually?

5. Do you have endoscopic privileges at a licensed health care facility or hospital?

6. Is polypectomy (polyp removal) routinely performed during elective colonoscopy?

7. Does your endoscopic facility have dedicated reprocessing (disinfection) personnel and equipment?

8. Do you offer intravenous sedation for colonoscopy?

9. Do you monitor blood pressure, pulse, and blood oxygen levels during sedation?

10. Do you employ a trained endoscopic assistant or nurse?

Section 31.2

Bronchoscopy

Excerpted from "Bronchoscopy," National Heart, Lung,
and Blood Institute (NHLBI), September 2009.

Bronchoscopy is a procedure used to look inside the lungs' airways, called the bronchi and bronchioles. The airways carry air from the trachea, or windpipe, to the lungs. The most common reason why your doctor may decide to do a bronchoscopy is if you have an abnormal chest x-ray or chest computed tomography (CT) scan. These tests may show a tumor, a pneumothorax (collapsed lung), or signs of an infection. Other reasons for bronchoscopy include if you are coughing up blood or if you have a cough that has lasted more than a few weeks. The procedure also can be done to remove something that is stuck in an airway (like a piece of food), to place medicine in a lung to treat a lung problem, or to insert a stent (small tube) in an airway to hold it open when a tumor or other condition causes a blockage.

What to Expect during Bronchoscopy

Your doctor will do the bronchoscopy in an exam room at a special clinic or in a hospital. The bronchoscopy itself usually lasts about 30 minutes. But the entire procedure, including preparation and recovery time, takes about four hours. Your doctor will give you medicine through an intravenous (IV) line in your bloodstream or by mouth to make you sleepy and relaxed. Your doctor also will squirt or spray a liquid medicine into your nose and throat to make them numb. This helps prevent coughing and gagging when the bronchoscope (long, thin tube) is inserted. Then, your doctor will insert the bronchoscope through your nose or mouth and into your airways. As the tube enters your mouth, you may gag a little. Once it enters your throat, that feeling will go away. Your doctor will look at your vocal cords and airways through the bronchoscope (which has a light and a small camera).

During the procedure, your doctor may take a sample of lung fluid or tissue for further testing. Samples can be taken using the following:

- **Bronchoalveolar lavage:** For this method, your doctor passes a small amount of salt water (a saline solution) through the bronchoscope and into part of your lung. He or she then suctions the salt water back out. The fluid picks up cells and bacteria from the airway, which your doctor can study.

- **Transbronchial lung biopsy:** For this method, your doctor inserts forceps into the bronchoscope and takes a small sample of tissue from inside the lung.

- **Transbronchial needle aspiration:** For this method, your doctor inserts a needle into the bronchoscope and removes cells from the lymph nodes in your lungs. These nodes are small, bean-shaped masses. They trap bacteria and cancer cells and help fight infection.

You may feel short of breath during bronchoscopy, but enough air is getting to your lungs. Your doctor will check your oxygen level. If the level drops, you will be given oxygen.

If you have a lot of bleeding in your lungs or a large object stuck in your throat, your doctor may use a bronchoscope with a rigid tube. The rigid tube, which is passed through the mouth, is wider. This allows your doctor to see inside it more easily, treat bleeding, and remove stuck objects. A rigid bronchoscopy usually is done in a hospital operating room using general anesthesia.

What to Expect after Bronchoscopy

After bronchoscopy, you will need to stay at the clinic or hospital for up to a few hours. If your doctor uses a bronchoscope with a rigid tube, the recovery time is longer. While you are at the clinic or hospital:

- You may have a chest x-ray if your doctor took a sample of lung tissue. This test will check for a pneumothorax and bleeding. A pneumothorax is a condition in which air or gas collects in the space around the lungs. This can cause one or both lungs to collapse. Usually, this condition is easily treated.

- A nurse will check your breathing and blood pressure.

- You cannot eat or drink until the numbness in your throat wears off. This takes 1–2 hours.

After recovery, you will need to have someone take you home. If samples of tissue or fluid were taken during the procedure, they will be tested in a lab. Talk to your doctor about when you'll get the lab results.

Recovery and Recuperation

Your doctor will let you know when you can return to your normal activities, such as driving, working, and physical activity. For the first few days, you may have a sore throat, cough, and hoarseness. Call your doctor right away if you:

* develop a fever,

* have chest pain,

* have trouble breathing,

* cough up more than a few tablespoons of blood.

Section 31.3

Capsule Endoscopy

"Capsule Endoscopy," © 2011 American Society for Gastrointestinal Endoscopy. Reprinted with permission. All rights reserved. This material is regularly updated, check http://www.asge.org for the most recent information.

What is capsule endoscopy?

Capsule endoscopy lets your doctor examine the lining of the middle part of your gastrointestinal tract, which includes the three portions of the small intestine (duodenum, jejunum, ileum). Your doctor will give you a pill-sized video camera for you to swallow. This camera has its own light source and takes pictures of your small intestine as it passes through. These pictures are sent to a small recording device you have to wear on your body. Your doctor will be able to view these pictures at a later time and might be able to provide you with useful information regarding your small intestine.

Why is capsule endoscopy done?

Capsule endoscopy helps your doctor evaluate the small intestine. This part of the bowel cannot be reached by traditional upper endoscopy or by colonoscopy. The most common reason for doing capsule endoscopy is to search for a cause of bleeding from the small intestine. It may also be useful for detecting polyps, inflammatory bowel disease (Crohn disease), ulcers, and tumors of the small intestine.

As is the case with most new diagnostic procedures, not all insurance companies are currently reimbursing for this procedure. You may need to check with your own insurance company to ensure that this is a covered benefit.

How should I prepare for the procedure?

An empty stomach allows for the best and safest examination, so you should have nothing to eat or drink, including water, for approximately twelve hours before the examination. Your doctor will tell you when to start fasting.

Tell your doctor in advance about any medications you take including iron, aspirin, bismuth subsalicylate products, and other over-the-counter medications. You might need to adjust your usual dose prior to the examination.

Discuss any allergies to medications as well as medical conditions, such as swallowing disorders and heart or lung disease.

Tell your doctor of the presence of a pacemaker or defibrillator, previous abdominal surgery, or previous history of bowel obstructions in the bowel, inflammatory bowel disease, or adhesions.

Your doctor may ask you to do a bowel prep/cleansing prior to the examination.

What can I expect during capsule endoscopy?

Your doctor will prepare you for the examination by applying a sensor device to your abdomen with adhesive sleeves (similar to tape). The pill-sized capsule endoscope is swallowed and passes naturally through your digestive tract while transmitting video images to a data recorder worn on your belt for approximately eight hours. At the end of the procedure you will return to the office and the data recorder is removed so that images of your small bowel can be put on a computer screen for physician review.

Most patients consider the test comfortable. The capsule endoscope is about the size of a large pill. After ingesting the capsule and until it is excreted you should not be near a magnetic resonance imaging (MRI) device or schedule an MRI examination.

What happens after capsule endoscopy?

You will be able to drink clear liquids after two hours and eat a light meal after four hours following the capsule ingestion, unless your doctor instructs you otherwise. You will have to avoid vigorous physical activity such as running or jumping during the study. Your doctor generally can tell you the test results within the week following the procedure; however, the results of some tests might take longer.

What are the possible complications of capsule endoscopy?

Although complications can occur, they are rare when doctors who are specially trained and experienced in this procedure perform the test. There is potential for the capsule to be stuck at a narrowed spot in the digestive tract resulting in bowel obstruction. This usually relates to a stricture (narrowing) of the digestive tract from inflammation, prior surgery, or tumor. It is important to recognize obstruction early. Signs of obstruction include unusual bloating, abdominal pain, nausea or vomiting. You should call your doctor immediately for any such concerns. Also, if you develop a fever after the test, have trouble swallowing or experience chest pain, tell your doctor immediately. Be careful not to prematurely disconnect the system as this may result in loss of pictures being sent to your recording device.

Capsule endoscopy may also be called capsule enteroscopy or wireless capsule endoscopy. Capsule endoscopy allows for examination of the small intestine, which cannot be easily reached by traditional methods of endoscopy.

Section 31.4

Colonoscopy

Excerpted from "Colonoscopy," National Institute of Diabetes and Digestive and Kidney Diseases (NIDDK), January 2010.

Colonoscopy is a procedure used to see inside the colon and rectum. Colonoscopy can detect inflamed tissue, ulcers, and abnormal growths. The procedure is used to look for early signs of colorectal cancer and can help doctors diagnose unexplained changes in bowel habits, abdominal pain, bleeding from the anus, and weight loss.

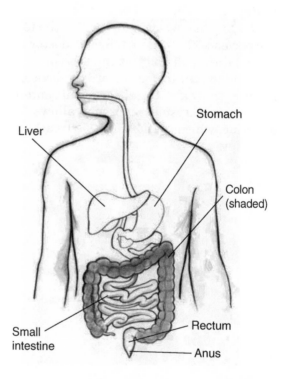

Figure 31.1. *The colon and rectum are the two main parts of the large intestine.*

How to Prepare for Colonoscopy

The doctor usually provides written instructions about how to prepare for colonoscopy. The process is called a bowel prep. Generally, all solids must be emptied from the gastrointestinal tract by following a clear liquid diet for 1–3 days before the procedure. Patients should not drink beverages containing red or purple dye. Acceptable liquids include fat-free bouillon or broth, strained fruit juice, water, plain coffee, plain tea, sports drinks such as Gatorade, and gelatin.

A laxative or an enema may be required the night before colonoscopy. A laxative is medicine that loosens stool and increases bowel movements. Laxatives are usually swallowed in pill form or as a powder dissolved in water. An enema is performed by flushing water, or sometimes a mild soap solution, into the anus using a special wash bottle.

Patients should inform the doctor of all medical conditions and any medications, vitamins, or supplements taken regularly, including aspirin, arthritis medications, blood thinners, diabetes medications, and vitamins that contain iron.

Driving is not permitted for 24 hours after colonoscopy to allow the sedative time to wear off. Before the appointment, patients should make plans for a ride home.

How Is Colonoscopy Performed?

During colonoscopy, patients lie on their left side on an examination table. In most cases, a light sedative, and possibly pain medication, helps keep patients relaxed. Deeper sedation may be required in some cases. The doctor and medical staff monitor vital signs and attempt to make patients as comfortable as possible.

The doctor inserts a long, flexible, lighted tube called a colonoscope, or scope, into the anus and slowly guides it through the rectum and into the colon. The scope inflates the large intestine with carbon dioxide gas to give the doctor a better view. A small camera mounted on the scope transmits a video image from inside the large intestine to a computer screen, allowing the doctor to carefully examine the intestinal lining. The doctor may ask the patient to move periodically so the scope can be adjusted for better viewing.

Once the scope has reached the opening to the small intestine, it is slowly withdrawn and the lining of the large intestine is carefully examined again. Bleeding and puncture of the large intestine are possible but uncommon complications of colonoscopy.

Removal of Polyps and Biopsy

A doctor can remove growths, called polyps, during colonoscopy and later test them in a laboratory for signs of cancer. Polyps are common in adults and are usually harmless. However, most colorectal cancer begins as a polyp, so removing polyps early is an effective way to prevent cancer. The doctor can also take samples from abnormal-looking tissues during colonoscopy. The procedure, called a biopsy, allows the doctor to later look at the tissue with a microscope for signs of disease.

The doctor removes polyps and takes biopsy tissue using tiny tools passed through the scope. If bleeding occurs, the doctor can usually stop it with an electrical probe or special medications passed through the scope. Tissue removal and the treatments to stop bleeding are usually painless.

Recovery

Colonoscopy usually takes 30 to 60 minutes. Cramping or bloating may occur during the first hour after the procedure. The sedative takes time to completely wear off. Patients may need to remain at the clinic for 1–2 hours after the procedure. Full recovery is expected by the next day. Discharge instructions should be carefully read and followed.

Patients who develop any of these rare side effects should contact their doctor immediately:

- Severe abdominal pain
- Fever
- Bloody bowel movements
- Dizziness
- Weakness

Section 31.5

Cystoscopy and Ureteroscopy

Excerpted from "Cystoscopy and Ureteroscopy," National Institute of
Diabetes and Digestive and Kidney Diseases (NIDDK), August 2009.

A cystoscopy is an examination of the inside of the bladder and
urethra, the tube that carries urine from the bladder to the outside of
the body. In men, the urethra is the tube that runs through the penis.
The doctor performing the examination uses a cystoscope—a long, thin
instrument with an eyepiece on the external end and a tiny lens and
a light on the end that is inserted into the bladder. The doctor inserts
the cystoscope into the patient's urethra, and the small lens magnifies the inner lining of the urethra and bladder, allowing the doctor to
see inside the hollow bladder. Many cystoscopes have extra channels
within the sheath to insert other small instruments that can be used
to treat or diagnose urinary problems.

A ureteroscopy is an examination or procedure using a ureteroscope.
A ureteroscope, like a cystoscope, is an instrument for examining the
inside of the urinary tract. A ureteroscope is longer and thinner than

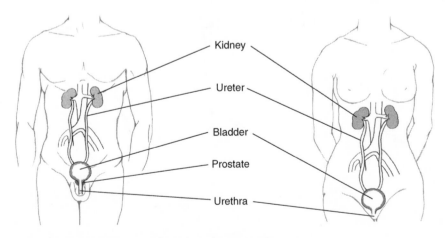

Figure 31.2. Male and female urinary tracts.

a cystoscope and is used to see beyond the bladder into the ureters, the tubes that carry urine from the kidneys to the bladder. Some uretero-scopes are flexible like a thin, long straw. Others are more rigid and firm. Through the ureteroscope, the doctor can see a stone in the ureter and then remove it with a small basket at the end of a wire inserted through an extra channel in the ureteroscope. Another way to treat a stone through a ureteroscope is to extend a flexible fiber through the scope up to the stone and then, with a laser beam shone through the fiber, break the stone into smaller pieces that can then pass out of the body in the urine. How and what the doctor will do is determined by the location, size, and composition of the stone.

How is a cystoscopy or ureteroscopy performed?

Usually, the patient lies on his or her back with knees raised and apart. A nurse or technician cleans the area around the urethral open-ing and applies a local anesthetic so the patient will not experience any discomfort during the test.

After anesthetic is used, the doctor gently inserts the tip of the cystoscope or ureteroscope into the urethra and slowly glides it up

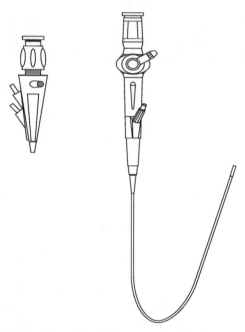

Figure 31.3. Rigid cystoscope (left) and semirigid ureteroscope (right).

into the bladder. A sterile liquid—water, or salt water called saline—flows through the scope to slowly fill the bladder and stretch it so the doctor has a better view of the bladder wall. As the bladder is filled with liquid, patients feel some discomfort and the urge to urinate. The doctor may then release some of the fluid, or the patient may empty the bladder as soon as the examination is over.

The time from insertion of the scope to removal may be only a few minutes, or it may be longer if the doctor finds a stone and decides to treat it. Taking a biopsy—a small tissue sample for examination with a microscope—will also make the procedure last longer. In most cases, the entire examination, including preparation, takes 15 to 30 minutes.

What happens after a cystoscopy or ureteroscopy?

Patients may have a mild burning feeling when they urinate, and they may see small amounts of blood in their urine. These problems should not last more than 24 hours. Patients should tell their doctor if bleeding or pain is severe or if problems last more than a day. To relieve discomfort, patients should drink two 8-ounce glasses of water each hour for two hours after the procedure. They may ask their doctor if they can take a warm bath to relieve the burning feeling. If not, they may be able to hold a warm, damp washcloth over the urethral opening. The doctor may prescribe an antibiotic to take to prevent an infection. Any signs of infection—including severe pain, chills, or fever—should be reported to a doctor.

Section 31.6

Endoscopic Ultrasound (EUS)

You've been referred to have an endoscopic ultrasonography, or EUS, which will help your doctor, evaluate or treat your condition.

What is EUS?

Endoscopic ultrasonography (EUS) allows your doctor to examine your esophageal and stomach linings as well as the walls of your upper and lower gastrointestinal tract. The upper tract consists of the esophagus, stomach, and duodenum; the lower tract includes your colon and rectum. EUS is also used to study other organs that are near the gastrointestinal tract, including the lungs, liver, gall bladder, and pancreas.

Endoscopists are highly trained specialists who welcome your questions regarding their credentials, training, and experience. Your endoscopist will use a thin, flexible tube called an endoscope that has a built-in miniature ultrasound probe. Your doctor will pass the endoscope through your mouth or anus to the area to be examined. Your doctor then will use the ultrasound to use sound waves to create visual images of the digestive tract.

Why is EUS done?

EUS provides your doctor with more information than other imaging tests by providing detailed images of your digestive tract. Your doctor can use EUS to diagnose certain conditions that may cause abdominal pain or abnormal weight loss.

EUS is also used to evaluate known abnormalities, including lumps or lesions, which were detected at a prior endoscopy or were seen on x-ray tests, such as a computed tomography (CT) scan. EUS provides a detailed image of the lump or lesion, which can help your doctor determine its origin and help treatment decisions. EUS can be used to diagnose diseases of the pancreas, bile duct, and gallbladder when other tests are inconclusive or conflicting.

Why is EUS used for patients with cancer?

EUS helps your doctor determine the extent of spread of certain cancers of the digestive and respiratory systems. EUS allows your doctor to accurately assess the cancer's depth and whether it has spread to adjacent lymph glands or nearby vital structures, such as major blood vessels. In some patients, EUS can be used to obtain a needle biopsy of a lump or lesion to help your doctor determine the proper treatment.

How should I prepare for EUS?

For EUS of the upper gastrointestinal tract, you should have nothing to eat or drink, usually for six hours before the examination. Your doctor will tell you when to start this fasting and whether it is advisable to take your regular prescription medications.

For EUS of the rectum or colon, your doctor will instruct you to either consume a colonic cleansing solution or to follow a clear liquid diet combined with laxatives or enemas prior to the examination. The procedure might have to be rescheduled if you don't follow your doctor's instructions carefully.

What about my current medications or allergies?

You can take most medications as usual until the day of the EUS examination. Tell your doctor about all medications that you're taking and about any allergies you have. Anticoagulant medications (blood thinners such as warfarin or heparin) and clopidogrel may need to be adjusted before the procedure. Insulin also needs to be adjusted on the day of EUS. In general, you can safely take aspirin and non-steroidal anti-inflammatory medications (ibuprofen, naproxen, and so forth.) before an EUS examination. Check with your doctor in advance regarding these recommendations.

Check with your doctor about which medications you should take the morning of the EUS examination, and take only essential medications with a small sip of water.

If you have an allergy to latex, you should inform your doctor prior to your test. Patients with latex allergies often require special equipment and may not be able to have a complete EUS examination.

Do I need to take antibiotics?

Antibiotics are not generally required before or after EUS examinations. However, your doctor might prescribe antibiotics if you are having specialized EUS procedures, such as to drain a fluid collection or a cyst using EUS guidance.

Should I arrange for help after the examination?

If you received sedatives, you will not be allowed to drive after the procedure, even if you do not feel tired. You should arrange a ride home in advance. You should also plan to have someone stay with you at home after the examination, because the sedatives could affect your judgment and reflexes for the rest of the day.

What can I expect during EUS?

Practices vary among doctors, but for an EUS examination of the upper gastrointestinal tract, some endoscopists spray your throat with a local anesthetic before the test begins. Most often you will receive sedatives intravenously to help you relax. You will most likely begin by lying on your left side. After you receive sedatives, your endoscopist will pass the ultrasound endoscope through your mouth, esophagus, and stomach into the duodenum. The instrument does not interfere with your ability to breathe. The actual examination generally takes less than 60 minutes. Many do not recall the procedure. Most patients consider it only slightly uncomfortable, and many fall asleep during it.

An EUS examination of the lower gastrointestinal tract can often be performed safely and comfortably without medications, but you'll receive a sedative if the examination will be prolonged or if the doctor will examine a significant distance into the colon. You will start by lying on your left side with your back toward the doctor. Most EUS examinations of the rectum generally take less than 45 minutes. You should know that if a needle biopsy of a lesion or drainage of a cyst is performed during the EUS, then the procedure will be longer and may take up to two hours.

What happens after EUS?

If you received sedatives, you will be monitored in the recovery area until most of the sedative medication's effects have worn off. If you had an upper EUS, your throat might be a little sore. You might feel bloated because of the air and water that were introduced during the examination. You'll be able to eat after you leave the procedure area, unless you're instructed otherwise. Your doctor generally can inform you of the preliminary results of the procedure that day, but the results of some tests, including biopsies, may take several days.

What are the possible complications of EUS?

Although complications can occur, they are rare when doctors with specialized training and experience perform the EUS examination. Bleeding might occur at a biopsy site, but it's usually minimal and rarely requires follow-up. You might have a slight sore throat for a day or so. Nonprescription anesthetic-type throat lozenges help soothe a sore throat.

Other potential but uncommon risks of EUS include a reaction to the sedatives used, aspiration of stomach contents into your lungs, infection, and complications from heart or lung diseases. One major but very uncommon complication of EUS is perforation. This is a tear through the lining of the intestine that might require surgery to repair.

The possibility of complications increases slightly if a needle biopsy is performed during the EUS examination, including an increased risk of pancreatitis or infection. These risks must be balanced against the potential benefits of the procedure and the risks of alternative approaches to the condition.

Additional Questions

If you have any questions about your need for EUS, alternative approaches to your problem, the cost of the procedure, methods of billing or insurance coverage, do not hesitate to speak to your doctor or doctor's office staff about it.

Section 31.7

Upper Endoscopy

Excerpted from "Upper GI Endoscopy," National Institute of Diabetes
and Digestive and Kidney Diseases (NIDDK), May 2009.

Upper gastrointestinal (GI) endoscopy is a procedure that uses a
lighted, flexible endoscope to see inside the upper GI tract. The upper
GI tract includes the esophagus, stomach, and duodenum—the first
part of the small intestine.

Upper GI endoscopy can be used to remove stuck objects, including
food, and to treat conditions such as bleeding ulcers. It can also be used
to biopsy tissue in the upper GI tract. During a biopsy, a small piece of
tissue is removed for later examination with a microscope.

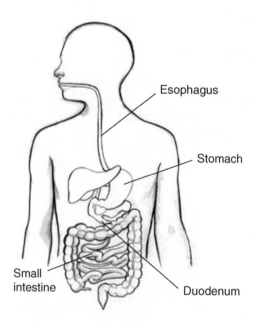

Figure 31.4. *Upper GI tract*

How to Prepare for Upper GI Endoscopy

The upper GI tract must be empty before upper GI endoscopy. Generally, no eating or drinking is allowed for 4–8 hours before the procedure. Smoking and chewing gum are also prohibited during this time.

Patients should tell their doctor about all health conditions they have—especially heart and lung problems, diabetes, and allergies—and all medications they are taking. Patients may be asked to temporarily stop taking medications that affect blood clotting or interact with sedatives, which are often given during upper GI endoscopy. Medications and vitamins may be restricted before and after upper GI endoscopy. Driving is not permitted for 12 to 24 hours after upper GI endoscopy to allow sedatives time to completely wear off. Before the appointment, patients should make plans for a ride home.

How Is Upper GI Endoscopy Performed?

Upper GI endoscopy is conducted at a hospital or outpatient center. Patients may receive a local, liquid anesthetic that is gargled or sprayed on the back of the throat. The anesthetic numbs the throat and calms the gag reflex. An intravenous (IV) needle is placed in a vein in the arm if a sedative will be given. Sedatives help patients stay relaxed and comfortable. While patients are sedated, the doctor and medical staff monitor vital signs.

During the procedure, patients lie on their back or side on an examination table. An endoscope is carefully fed down the esophagus and into the stomach and duodenum. A small camera mounted on the endoscope transmits a video image to a video monitor, allowing close examination of the intestinal lining. Air is pumped through the endoscope to inflate the stomach and duodenum, making them easier to see. Special tools that slide through the endoscope allow the doctor to perform biopsies, stop bleeding, and remove abnormal growths.

Recovery from Upper GI Endoscopy

After upper GI endoscopy, patients are moved to a recovery room where they wait about an hour for the sedative to wear off. During this time, patients may feel bloated or nauseated. They may also have a sore throat, which can stay for a day or two. Patients will likely feel tired and should plan to rest for the remainder of the day. Unless otherwise directed, patients may immediately resume their normal diet and medications.

Some results from upper GI endoscopy are available immediately after the procedure. The doctor will often share results with the patient after the sedative has worn off. Biopsy results are usually ready in a few days.

Patients who experience any of the following rare symptoms after upper GI endoscopy should contact their doctor immediately: swallowing difficulties; throat, chest, and abdominal pain that worsens; vomiting; bloody or very dark stool; or fever.

Section 31.8

Laryngoscopy

"Laryngoscopy," June 2009, reprinted with permission from www .kidshealth.org. Copyright © 2009 The Nemours Foundation. This information was provided by KidsHealth, one of the largest resources online for medically reviewed health information written for parents, kids, and teens. For more articles like this one, visit www .KidsHealth.org, or www.TeensHealth.org.

About Laryngoscopy

Laryngoscopy is a visual examination below the back of the throat, where the voice box (larynx) containing the vocal cords is located. The procedure is done by using mirrors and a light source at the back of the throat or by inserting a thin instrument (a laryngoscope) through the nose or mouth into the throat. This scope lights and magnifies images within the throat.

Laryngoscopy is an effective procedure for discovering the causes of voice and breathing problems, throat or ear pain, difficulty in swallowing, narrowing of the throat (strictures or stenosis), and airway blockages. It also can help diagnose problems in the vocal cords.

The procedure is relatively painless, but the idea of having a scope inserted into the throat can be a little scary for kids, so it helps to understand how a laryngoscopy is done.

The three kinds of laryngoscopy are:

- indirect laryngoscopy,

- fiber-optic (flexible) laryngoscopy, and
- direct laryngoscopy.

The indirect procedure can be performed in a doctor's office using a small hand mirror held at the back of the throat. The doctor will aim a light at the back of the throat, usually by wearing headgear that has a bright light attached, to examine the larynx, vocal cords, and hypopharynx. Indirect laryngoscopy is not typically used with kids because it tends to cause gagging.

Fiber-optic and direct laryngoscopy examinations, which see deeper into the throat via either a flexible or rigid telescope, usually are done by an ear, nose, and throat (ENT) specialist. Rigid telescopes are more often used as part of a surgical procedure in evaluating kids with stridor (a noisy, harsh breathing) and removing foreign objects in the throat and lower airway. They're also used in collecting tissue samples (biopsies), laser treatments, and in locating cancer of the larynx.

Why Is Laryngoscopy Performed?

Laryngoscopy is performed to:

- diagnose a persistent cough, throat pain, bleeding, hoarseness, or persistent bad breath;
- check for inflammation;
- discover a possible narrowing or blockage of the throat;
- visualize a mass or tumor in the throat or on the vocal cords;
- diagnose difficulty swallowing;
- diagnose suspected cancer;
- evaluate causes of persistent earache;
- diagnose voice problems, such as weak voice, hoarse voice, breathy voice, or no voice.

Laryngoscopy is also performed to remove foreign objects stuck in the throat or to biopsy a growth in the throat or on the vocal cords.

Preparation

Talk to your doctor about the kind of test being performed, how it will be done, the risks, and the results. Having your questions answered beforehand will help reduce your concerns and give you and your child a better understanding of how the procedure will go.

In many cases, the doctor will have the child undergo a physical exam, chest x-ray, or computed tomography (CT) scan (a type of x-ray that uses a computer to take pictures of the inside of the body). Your child also might be asked to swallow a liquid called barium while a series of x-rays of the larynx and esophagus are taken. Barium liquid is harmless and will pass through the body within a day or two. These measures will help your doctor further understand the physical symptoms your child is having.

For an office laryngoscopy in which local anesthesia is used, your child will not need to avoid eating or drinking beforehand.

If general anesthesia will be used, your doctor will give you instructions about your child not eating or drinking before the exam (this is to prevent vomiting). A direct laryngoscopy might be done if, for instance, your child gags easily or the airway below the vocal folds needs to be examined. This is done using general anesthesia, so it is important for your child to avoid eating or drinking within eight hours before the procedure.

During Laryngoscopy

Indirect laryngoscopy and fiber-optic laryngoscopies often are performed in the doctor's office, sometimes using local anesthetic. They usually take only five to ten minutes.

Indirect laryngoscopy will require your child to sit up straight in a high-backed chair with a headrest and open his or her mouth wide. The doctor will spray the throat with an anesthetic or numbing medication (which your child will gargle and spit out), then cover the tongue with gauze and hold it down.

The doctor will hold up a warm mirror to the back of the throat and, with a light attached to his or her headgear, will tilt the mirror to view various areas of the throat. Your child may be asked to make high-pitched or low-pitched sounds so that the doctor can view the larynx and see the vocal cords move.

Fiber-optic laryngoscopy uses a fiber-optic laryngoscope (a thin, flexible instrument that lights and magnifies images) for a better view of the larynx and vocal cords.

This might be done in an operating room under general anesthesia or in the doctor's office, and usually doesn't require a hospital stay. The flexible scope is inserted through a nostril or the mouth, then the doctor examines the throat area through the scope's eyepiece. Sometimes the images are displayed on a monitor so that family members can see what the doctor is seeing.

Direct laryngoscopy is done in an operating room and your child will be put under general anesthesia and not feel the scope in the throat. If needed, the doctor will remove foreign objects from the throat, collect tissue samples, perform laser treatment, or remove growths from the vocal cords. This can take as little as 15 to 30 minutes, but might take much longer if specific treatments are required.

After the Procedure

If a local anesthetic or topical numbing spray was used, it will wear off in about 30 minutes. Your child should not eat or drink anything until the spray has worn off and the throat is no longer numb.

After a direct laryngoscopy, your child will be watched by a nurse until fully awake and able to swallow. This usually takes about two hours. In some cases, an overnight hospital stay may be required. Your child may have some nausea, general muscle aches, and feel tired for a day or two.

Gargling and sucking on throat lozenges will help with the soreness, and pain medication will be given, if needed. Your child may sound hoarse or have noisy breathing for a few days after the procedure. This is normal. If the hoarseness persists or your child has difficulty breathing, contact your doctor.

Results

The doctor will explain the findings after the procedure. If a biopsy was taken, a laboratory will examine the tissue and report the results to your doctor, who will discuss the results and treatment options with you. Usually, biopsy results take about three to five days. Depending on the outcome of the exam, your doctor might schedule an office visit or a follow-up procedure for four to six weeks after the initial laryngoscopy.

When your child is having any kind of procedure, it's understandable to be a little uneasy. But it helps to know that a laryngoscopy is considered an extremely effective and routine medical exam and complications are rare. However, as with most procedures, there are some risks, which your doctor will review with you. If you have any questions about laryngoscopy, speak with your doctor.

Section 31.9

Flexible Sigmoidoscopy

Excerpted from "Flexible Sigmoidoscopy," National Institute of Diabetes and Digestive and Kidney Diseases (NIDDK), November 2008.

Flexible sigmoidoscopy is a procedure used to see inside the sigmoid colon and rectum. Flexible sigmoidoscopy can detect inflamed tissue, abnormal growths, and ulcers. The procedure is used to look for early signs of cancer and can help doctors diagnose unexplained changes in bowel habits, abdominal pain, bleeding from the anus, and weight loss.

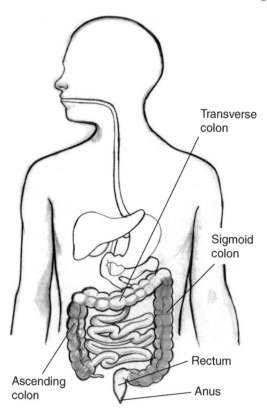

Transverse colon

Sigmoid colon

Rectum

Ascending colon

Anus

Figure 31.5. *The sigmoid colon is the last one-third of the colon.*

How Is Flexible Sigmoidoscopy Different from Colonoscopy?

Flexible sigmoidoscopy enables the doctor to see only the sigmoid colon, whereas colonoscopy allows the doctor to see the entire colon. Colonoscopy is the preferred screening method for cancers of the colon and rectum; however, to prepare for and perform a flexible sigmoidoscopy usually requires less time.

To prepare for a flexible sigmoidoscopy, one or more enemas are performed about two hours before the procedure to remove all solids from the sigmoid colon. In some cases, the entire gastrointestinal tract must be emptied by following a clear liquid diet for 1–3 days before the procedure—similar to the preparation for colonoscopy. A laxative or an enema may also be required the night before a flexible sigmoidoscopy.

Examination of the Sigmoid Colon

During a flexible sigmoidoscopy, patients lie on their left side on an examination table. The doctor inserts a long, flexible, lighted tube called a sigmoidoscope, or scope, into the anus and slowly guides it through the rectum and into the sigmoid colon. The scope inflates the colon with air to give the doctor a better view. A small camera mounted on the scope transmits a video image from inside the colon to a computer screen, allowing the doctor to carefully examine the tissues lining the sigmoid colon and rectum. The doctor may ask the patient to move periodically so the scope can be adjusted for better viewing. When the scope reaches the transverse colon, the scope is slowly withdrawn while the lining of the colon is carefully examined again.

Biopsy and Removal of Colon Polyps

The doctor can remove growths, called polyps, during flexible sigmoidoscopy using special tools passed through the scope. Polyps are common in adults and are usually harmless. However, most colon cancer begins as a polyp, so removing polyps early is an effective way to prevent cancer. If bleeding occurs, the doctor can usually stop it with an electrical probe or special medications passed through the scope.

During a flexible sigmoidoscopy, the doctor can also take samples from abnormal-looking tissues. Called a biopsy, this procedure allows the doctor to later look at the tissue with a microscope for signs of disease. Tissue removal and the treatments to stop bleeding are usually painless. If polyps or other abnormal tissues are found, the doctor may suggest examining the rest of the colon with a colonoscopy.

Recovery

A flexible sigmoidoscopy takes about 20 minutes. Cramping or bloating may occur during the first hour after the procedure. Bleeding and puncture of the large intestine are possible but uncommon complications. Discharge instructions should be carefully read and followed.

Patients who develop any of these rare side effects should contact their doctor immediately: severe abdominal pain, fever, bloody bowel movements, dizziness, or weakness.

Section 31.10

Endoscopic Retrograde Cholangiopancreatography (ERCP)

Excerpted from "ERCP (Endoscopic Retrograde Cholangiopancreatography)," National Institute of Diabetes and Digestive and Kidney Diseases (NIDDK), November 2004. Reviewed in April 2011 by David A. Cooke, MD, FACP.

Endoscopic retrograde cholangiopancreatography (ERCP) enables the physician to diagnose problems in the liver, gallbladder, bile ducts, and pancreas. ERCP is used primarily to diagnose and treat conditions of the bile ducts, including gallstones, inflammatory strictures (scars), leaks (from trauma and surgery), and cancer. ERCP combines the use of x-rays and an endoscope, which is a long, flexible, lighted tube. Through the endoscope, the physician can see the inside of the stomach and duodenum, and inject dyes into the ducts in the biliary tree and pancreas so they can be seen on x-rays.

For the procedure, you will lie on your left side on an examining table in an x-ray room. You will be given medication to help numb the back of your throat and a sedative to help you relax during the exam. You will swallow the endoscope, and the physician will then guide the scope through your esophagus, stomach, and duodenum until it reaches the spot where the ducts of the biliary tree and pancreas open into the duodenum. At this time, you will be turned to lie flat on your stomach, and the physician will pass a small plastic tube through the scope. Through the tube, the physician will inject a dye into the ducts to make them show up clearly on x-rays. X-rays are taken as soon as the dye is injected.

If the exam shows a gallstone or narrowing of the ducts, the physician can insert instruments into the scope to remove or relieve the obstruction. Also, tissue samples (biopsy) can be taken for further testing.

Possible complications of ERCP include pancreatitis (inflammation of the pancreas), infection, bleeding, and perforation of the duodenum. Except for pancreatitis, such problems are uncommon. You may have tenderness or a lump where the sedative was injected, but that should go away in a few days.

ERCP takes 30 minutes to two hours. You may have some discomfort when the physician blows air into the duodenum and injects the dye into the ducts. However, the pain medicine and sedative should keep you from feeling too much discomfort. After the procedure, you will need to stay at the hospital for 1–2 hours until the sedative wears off. The physician will make sure you do not have signs of complications before you leave. If any kind of treatment is done during ERCP, such as removing a gallstone, you may need to stay in the hospital overnight.

Preparation: Your stomach and duodenum must be empty for the procedure to be accurate and safe. You will not be able to eat or drink anything after midnight the night before the procedure, or for 6–8 hours beforehand, depending on the time of your procedure. Also, the physician will need to know whether you have any allergies, especially to iodine, which is in the dye. You must also arrange for someone to take you home—you will not be allowed to drive because of the sedatives. The physician may give you other special instructions.

Chapter 32

Electrocardiogram (EKG)

An electrocardiogram, also called an EKG or ECG, is a simple, painless test that records the heart's electrical activity. Your doctor may recommend an electrocardiogram (EKG) if you have signs or symptoms that suggest a heart problem.

You may need to have more than one EKG so your doctor can diagnose certain heart conditions. An EKG also may be done as part of a routine health exam. The test can screen for early heart disease that has no symptoms. You may have an EKG so your doctor can check how well heart medicine or a medical device, such as a pacemaker, is working. The test also may be used for routine screening before major surgery. Your doctor also may use EKG results to help plan your treatment for a heart condition.

What to Expect with an Electrocardiogram

You do not need to take any special steps before having an electrocardiogram (EKG). However, tell your doctor or his or her staff about the medicines you're taking. Some medicines can affect EKG results.

An electrocardiogram (EKG) is painless and harmless. A nurse or technician will attach soft, sticky patches called electrodes to the skin of your chest, arms, and legs. The patches are about the size of a quarter. Often, 12 patches are attached to your body. This helps detect your heart's electrical activity from many areas at the same time. The nurse may have to shave areas of your skin to help the patches stick. After the patches are

Excerpted from "Electrocardiogram," National Heart, Lung, and Blood Institute (NHLBI), November 2008.

placed on your skin, you will lie still on a table while the patches detect your heart's electrical signals. A machine will record these signals on graph paper or display them on a screen. The entire test will take about ten minutes.

Special Types of Electrocardiogram

The standard EKG described, called a resting 12-lead EKG, only records seconds of heart activity at a time. It will show a heart problem only if the problem occurs during the test. Many heart problems are present all the time, and a resting 12-lead EKG will detect them. But some heart problems, like those related to an irregular heartbeat, can come and go. They may occur only for a few minutes a day or only while you exercise. Doctors use special EKGs, such as stress tests and Holter and event monitors, to help diagnose these kinds of problems.

After an electrocardiogram: You may develop a rash or redness where the EKG patches were attached. This mild rash often goes away without treatment. You usually can go back to your normal daily routine after an EKG.

What Does an Electrocardiogram Show?

Many heart problems change the heart's electrical activity in distinct ways. An electrocardiogram (EKG) can help detect these heart problems. EKG recordings can help doctors diagnose heart attacks that are in progress or have happened in the past. This is especially true if doctors can compare a current EKG recording to an older one.

An EKG also can show the following:

- Lack of blood flow to the heart muscle (coronary heart disease)
- A heartbeat that is too fast, too slow, or irregular (arrhythmia)
- A heart that does not pump forcefully enough (heart failure)
- Heart muscle that is too thick or parts of the heart that are too big (cardiomyopathy)
- Birth defects in the heart (congenital heart defects)
- Problems with the heart valves (heart valve disease)
- Inflammation of the sac that surrounds the heart (pericarditis)

An EKG can reveal whether the heartbeat starts in the correct place in the heart. The test also shows how long it takes for electrical signals to travel through the heart. Delays in signal travel time may suggest heart block or long QT syndrome (LQTS).

Chapter 33

Electroencephalogram (EEG)

What It Is

An electroencephalogram (EEG) is a test used to detect abnormalities related to electrical activity of the brain. This procedure tracks and records brain wave patterns. Small metal discs with thin wires (electrodes) are placed on the scalp, and then send signals to a computer to record the results. Normal electrical activity in the brain makes a recognizable pattern. Through an EEG, doctors can look for abnormal patterns that indicate seizures and other problems.

Why It's Done

The most common reason an EEG is performed is to diagnose and monitor seizure disorders. EEGs can also help to identify causes of other problems such as sleep disorders and changes in behavior. EEGs are sometimes used to evaluate brain activity after a severe head injury or before heart or liver transplantation.

Preparation

If your child is having an EEG, preparation is minimal. Your child's hair should be clean and free of oils, sprays, and conditioner to help the electrodes stick to the scalp. Your doctor may recommend that your child stop taking certain medications before the test that can alter results. It's often recommended that kids avoid caffeine up to eight hours before the test. If it's necessary for your child to sleep during the EEG, the doctor will suggest ways to help make this easier.

The Procedure

An EEG can either be performed in an area near the doctor's office or at a hospital. Your child will be asked to lie on a bed or sit in a chair. The EEG technician will attach electrodes to different locations on the scalp using adhesive paste. Each electrode is connected to an amplifier and EEG recording machine. The electrical signals from the brain are converted into wavy lines on a computer screen. Your child will be asked to lie still because movement can alter the results.

If the goal of the EEG is to mimic or produce the problem your child is experiencing, he or she may be asked to look at a bright flickering light or breathe a certain way. The health care provider performing the EEG will know your child's medical history and will be prepared for any issues that may arise during the test.

Most EEGs take about an hour to perform. If your child is required to sleep during it, the test will take longer. You might be able to stay in the room with your child, or you can step outside to a waiting area.

What to Expect

An EEG isn't uncomfortable and patients do not feel any shocks on the scalp or elsewhere; however, having electrodes pasted to the scalp can be a little stressful for kids, as can lying still during the test.

Getting the Results

A neurologist (a doctor trained in nervous system disorders) will read and interpret the results. Though EEGs vary in complexity and duration, results are typically available in several days.

Risks

EEGs are very safe. If your child has a seizure disorder, your doctor might want to stimulate and record a seizure during the EEG. A seizure can be triggered by flashing lights or a change in breathing pattern.

Helping Your Child

You can help prepare your child for an EEG by explaining that the test won't be uncomfortable. You can describe the room and the equipment that will be used, and reassure your child that you'll be right there for support. For older kids, be sure to explain the importance of keeping still while the EEG is done so it won't have to be repeated.

If You Have Questions

If you have questions about the EEG procedure, speak with your doctor. You can also talk to the EEG technician before the exam.

Chapter 34

Electromyography and Nerve Conduction Velocities

Diagnosis of neuromuscular disease hinges on a doctor's ability to identify a specific defect of neuromuscular function. Sometimes, a doctor can infer this functional defect—and the disease associated with it—by giving a physical exam, doing a blood test, or looking at the anatomy of nerves and muscles. But other times, the doctor may have to directly evaluate the functions of nerves and muscles and the connections between them by using two complementary techniques—nerve conduction velocity testing (NCVs) and electromyography (EMGs).

Action Potentials

Both NCV and EMG rely on the fact that the activity of nerves and muscles produces electrical signals called action potentials. A nerve is actually a bundle of axons, cables that conduct action potentials from one end of a nerve cell (or neuron) to the other. In motor neurons (neurons that connect to muscle), these action potentials travel toward the muscle where they cause the release of a chemical called acetylcholine. Acetylcholine opens tiny pores in the muscle, and the flow of sodium and potassium ions through these pores creates action potentials in the muscle, leading to contraction. In NCV and EMG, these tiny electrical events are amplified electronically, then visualized on a TV-like monitor called an oscilloscope and can even be heard using audio equipment.

"Simply Stated...Electromyography and Nerve Conduction Velocities," reprinted by permission of the Muscular Dystrophy Association of the United States (www.mda.org), © 2000. Reviewed in April 2011 by David A. Cooke, MD, FACP.

NCV and Axons

NCV measures action potentials conducted by axons, so doctors use it for diagnosing diseases that primarily affect nerve function, such as different forms of Charcot-Marie-Tooth disease (CMT). It's done by placing surface electrodes (similar to those used for electrocardiograms) on the skin at various points over a nerve. One electrode delivers a mild electrical shock to the nerve, stimulating it to generate an action potential. The other electrodes record the action potential as it's conducted through the nerve.

Doctors often use NCV to determine the speed of nerve conduction (hence, its name). Conduction speed is influenced by a coating around axons, called myelin. Myelin insulates each axon and normally forces action potentials to "jump" quickly from one end of the axon to the other. If the myelin breaks down (as in CMT1), the action potential travels more slowly. NCV also can measure the strength of the action potential in the nerve, which is proportional to the number of axons that contribute to it. If axons degenerate (as in amyotrophic lateral sclerosis) or become clogged with debris (as in CMT2), the action potential becomes smaller.

EMG and Muscle

An electromyogram measures the action potentials produced by muscles, and is therefore useful for diagnosing diseases that primarily affect muscle function, including the muscular dystrophies. Also, some EMG data can reveal defects in nerve function. In EMG, the doctor inserts a needlelike electrode into a muscle. The electrode records action potentials that occur when the muscle is at rest and during voluntary contractions directed by the doctor.

While a healthy muscle appears quiet at rest, spontaneous action potentials are seen in damaged muscles or muscles that have lost input from nerve cells (as in amyotrophic lateral sclerosis [ALS] or myasthenia gravis). During voluntary contraction, dystrophic (wasted) muscles show very small action potentials, and myotonic (stiff) muscles show prolonged trains of action potentials. Altered patterns of muscle action potentials can indicate defects in nerve function.

A Little Discomfort

Though NCVs and EMGs are valuable tools for doctors, they can be distressing for patients. Some people find the electric shocks of the NCV or the needle penetration of the EMG uncomfortable or even painful. Young children might struggle during the tests, making it difficult for doctors to carefully monitor nerve and muscle activity. To ease discomfort, topical anesthetic can be applied to the skin—but it won't prevent muscle pain during the EMG. Sometimes sedating medications are needed to keep a child calm.

Partly because of these factors, NCVs and EMGs are generally used when it's not possible to gather the right information from other diagnostic tests. Muscle biopsy (excising and examining muscle tissue) can reveal hallmark anatomical features of some neuromuscular diseases, making EMG and NCV unnecessary. Genetic tests are now available for diagnosing some diseases, and in those cases, EMG and NCV usually can be bypassed.

Nonetheless, NCV and EMG remain the gold standards for evaluating the function of nerve and muscle. So, when a doctor suspects that a patient has a neuromuscular disease that isn't clearly associated with anatomical or genetic defects (like some types of CMT, or myasthenia gravis), NCV and EMG are among the most valuable diagnostic tools.

Chapter 35

Electronystagmography: Looking at Eye Movements

Electronystagmography is a test to look at voluntary and involuntary eye movements. It evaluates the acoustic nerve which runs from the brain to the ears (and control hearing and balance), and the occulomotor nerve which runs from the brain to the eyes.

How the Test Is Performed

Patches called electrodes (similar to those used with electrocardiogram [ECG], but smaller) are placed above, below, and to the side of each eye. They may be attached by adhesive or by a band around the head. Another electrode is attached to the forehead.

The electrodes record eye movements that occur when the inner ear and nearby nerves are stimulated by delivering cold and warm water to the ear canal at different times. Sometimes, the test is done using air instead of water. Each ear is tested separately.

When cold water enters the ear, it should cause rapid, side-to-side eye movements called nystagmus. The eyes should move rapidly away from the cold water and slowly back. Next, warm water is placed into the ear. The eyes should now move rapidly toward the warm water then slowly away.

Patients may also be asked to use their eyes to track objects, such as flashing lights. The electrodes detect the length and speed of eye movements, and a computer records the results. The test takes about 90 minutes.

"Electronystagmography," © 2011 A.D.A.M., Inc. Reprinted with permission.

Electronystagmography provides exact measurements of eye movements detected by the electrical changes the movements produce. It is more objective than simply watching the eyes after flushing warm or cold water into the ears. It can record behind closed eyelids or with the head in a variety of positions.

How to Prepare for the Test

No preparation is necessary. Check with your health care provider if you are taking any medications.

How the Test Will Feel

There is minimal discomfort. You may find cold water in the ear uncomfortable. Brief dizziness (vertigo) may occur during the test.

Why the Test Is Performed

The test is used to determine whether a balance or nerve disorder is the cause of dizziness or vertigo. Your doctor may order this test if you have dizziness or vertigo, impaired hearing, or suspected damage to the inner ear from certain medications.

Normal Results

Distinct involuntary eye movements should occur after instillation of warm or cold water into the ear canal. Normal value ranges may vary slightly among different laboratories. Talk to your doctor about the meaning of your specific test results.

What Abnormal Results Mean

Abnormal results may be a sign of damage to the nerve of the inner ear or other parts of the brain that control eye movements. Any disease or injury that damages the acoustic nerve can cause vertigo. This may include the following:

- Blood vessel disorders with bleeding (hemorrhage), clots, or atherosclerosis of the blood supply of the ear
- Cholesteatoma and other ear tumors
- Congenital disorders
- Injury

- Medications that are toxic to the ear nerves, including aminoglycoside antibiotics, some antimalarial drugs, loop diuretics, and salicylates

- Multiple sclerosis

- Movement disorders such as progressive supranuclear palsy

- Rubella

- Some poisons

Additional conditions under which the test may be performed:

- Acoustic neuroma

- Benign positional vertigo

- Labyrinthitis

- Ménière disease

Risks

There is a small risk associated with the caloric stimulation part of the test. Excessive water pressure can injure a previously damaged eardrum, but this rarely occurs. Caloric stimulation should not be performed if your eardrum has been perforated recently because of the risk of causing ear infection.

Chapter 36

Holter and Event Monitors

Holter and event monitors are medical devices that record the heart's electrical activity. Doctors most often use these monitors to diagnose arrhythmias. Holter and event monitors are similar to an EKG (electrocardiogram). An EKG is a simple test that detects and records the heart's electrical activity. It is the most common test for diagnosing a heart rhythm problem. However, a standard EKG only records the heartbeat for a few seconds. It will not detect heart rhythm problems that do not occur during the test. Although similar, Holter and event monitors are not the same. A Holter monitor records your heart's electrical activity the entire time you are wearing it. An event monitor only records your heart's electrical activity at certain times while you're wearing it.

Types of Holter and Event Monitors

Holter monitors are sometimes called continuous EKGs (electrocardiograms). This is because Holter monitors record your heart rhythm continuously for 24 to 48 hours. A Holter monitor is about the size of a large deck of cards. You can clip it to a belt or carry it in a pocket. Wires connect the device to sensors (called electrodes) that are stuck to your chest using sticky patches. These sensors detect your heart's electrical signals, and the monitor records your heart's rhythm.

Excerpted from "Holter and Event Monitors," National Heart, Lung, and Blood Institute (NHLBI), February 2010.

Wireless Holter monitors have a longer recording time than standard Holter monitors. Wireless monitors record your heart's electrical activity for a preset amount of time. These monitors use wireless cellular technology to send the recorded data to your doctor's office or a company that checks the data. This happens automatically at certain times. Wireless monitors still have wires that connect the device to the sensors stuck to your chest.

You can use a wireless Holter monitor for days or even weeks until signs or symptoms of a heart rhythm problem occur. These monitors usually are used to detect heart rhythm problems that do not occur often. Although wireless Holter monitors work for longer periods, they have a down side. You must remember to write down the time of symptoms so your doctor can match it to the heart rhythm recording. Also, the batteries in the wireless monitor must be changed every one to two days.

Event monitors are similar to Holter monitors. You wear one while you do your normal daily activities. Most event monitors have wires that connect the device to sensors. The sensors are stuck to your chest using sticky patches. Unlike Holter monitors, event monitors do not continuously record your heart's electrical activity. They only record when symptoms occur. For many event monitors, you need to start the monitor when you feel symptoms. Some event monitors start automatically if they detect abnormal heart rhythms. Event monitors tend to be smaller than Holter monitors because they don't need to store as much data.

Post-event recorders are among the smallest event monitors. You can wear a post-event recorder like a wristwatch or carry it in your pocket. The pocket version is about the size of a thick credit card. These monitors do not have wires that connect the device to chest sensors. When you feel a symptom, you start the recorder. A post-event recorder only records what happens after you start it. It may miss a heart rhythm problem that occurs before and during the onset of symptoms. Also, it may be hard to start the monitor when a symptom is in progress.

Presymptom memory loop recorders are the size of a small cell phone. They are also called continuous loop event recorders. You can clip this event monitor to your belt or carry it in your pocket. Wires connect the device to sensors on your chest. These recorders are always recording and erasing data. When you feel a symptom, you push a button on the device. The normal erase process stops. The recording will show a few minutes of the data from before, during, and after the symptom. This may make it possible for your doctor to see very brief changes in your heart rhythm.

Autodetect recorders are about the size of the palm of your hand. Wires connect the device to sensors on your chest. You do not need to start an autodetect recorder during symptoms. These recorders detect abnormal heart rhythms and automatically record and send the data to your doctor's office.

Implantable loop recorders: You may need an implantable loop recorder if other event monitors cannot provide enough data. Implantable loop recorders are about the size of a pack of gum. This type of event monitor is inserted under the skin on your chest. No wires or chest sensors are used. Your doctor can program the device to record when you start it during symptoms or automatically if it detects an abnormal heart rhythm. Devices may differ, so your doctor will tell you how to use your recorder. In some cases, a special card is held close to the recorder to start it.

What to Expect before Using a Holter or Event Monitor

Your doctor will do a physical exam before giving you a Holter or event monitor. You may have an EKG (electrocardiogram) test before your doctor sends you home with a Holter or event monitor.

A standard EKG will not detect heart rhythm problems that do not happen during the test. For this reason, your doctor may give you a Holter or event monitor. These monitors are portable. You can wear one while doing your normal daily activities. This increases the chance of recording symptoms that only occur once in a while. Your doctor will explain how to wear and use the Holter or event monitor. Usually, you will leave the office wearing it.

Each type of monitor is slightly different, but most have sensors (called electrodes) that are attached to the skin on your chest with sticky patches. It's important that the sensors have good contact with your skin. Poor contact can result in poor results. Oil, too much sweat, and hair can keep the patches from sticking to your skin. You may need to shave the area on your chest where your doctor will attach the patches. If you have to replace the patches, you will need to clean the area with a special prep pad that the doctor will provide. You may need to use a small amount of special paste or gel to help the patches stick to your skin. Some patches come with paste or gel on them.

What to Expect While Using a Holter or Event Monitor

Your experience while using a Holter or event monitor depends on the type of monitor you have. However, most monitors have some factors in common.

Recording the Heart's Electrical Activity

All monitors record the heart's electrical activity. So it is important to maintain a clear signal between the sensors (electrodes) and the recording device. In most cases, the sensors are attached to your chest with sticky patches. Wires connect the sensors to the monitor. You usually can clip the monitor to your belt or carry it in your pocket. (Postevent and implantable loop recorders do not have chest sensors.) A good stick between the patches and your skin helps provide a clear signal. Poor contact leads to a poor recording that is hard for your doctor to read.

When you have a symptom, stop what you are doing. This will ensure that the recording shows your heart's activity rather than your movement. Your doctor will tell you whether you need to adjust your activity level during the testing period.

Other everyday items also can disrupt the signal between the sensors and the monitor. These items include magnets, metal detectors, microwave ovens, and electric blankets, toothbrushes, and razors. Avoid using these items. Also avoid areas with high voltage. Cell phones and MP3 players (such as iPods) may interfere with the signal if they are too close to the monitor. When using any electronic device, try to keep it at least six inches away from the monitor.

Keeping a Diary

When using a Holter or event monitor, you need to keep a diary of your symptoms and activities. Write down when symptoms occur, what they are, and what you were doing at the time.

The most common symptoms of heart rhythm problems include:

• fainting or feeling dizzy; and

• palpitations (feelings that your heart is skipping a beat, fluttering, or beating too hard or fast which are felt in your chest, throat, or neck).

It is important to note the time that symptoms occur, because your doctor matches the data with the information in your diary. This allows your doctor to see whether certain activities trigger changes in your heart rate and rhythm. You also should include details in your diary about when you take any medicine or if you feel stress at certain times during the testing period.

What Does a Holter or Event Monitor Show?

A Holter or event monitor may show what is causing symptoms of an arrhythmia. An arrhythmia is a problem with the rate or rhythm of the heartbeat. A Holter or event monitor also can show whether a heart rhythm problem is harmless or requires treatment. The monitor may alert your doctor to medical conditions that can result in heart failure, stroke, or sudden cardiac arrest.

If the symptoms of a heart rhythm problem occur often, a Holter or event monitor has a good chance of capturing them. You may not have symptoms while using a monitor. Even so, your doctor may learn more about your heart rhythm from the test results.

Sometimes, Holter and event monitors cannot help doctors diagnose heart rhythm problems. If this happens, talk with your doctor about other steps you can take. One option may be to try a different type of monitor. Wireless Holter monitors and implantable loop recorders have longer recording periods. This may allow the monitor to get the data that your doctor needs to make a diagnosis.

Chapter 37

Diagnostic Laparoscopy

Diagnostic laparoscopy is a procedure that allows a health care provider to look directly at the contents of a patient's abdomen or pelvis, including the fallopian tubes, ovaries, uterus, small bowel, large bowel, appendix, liver, and gallbladder.

How the Test Is Performed

The procedure is usually done in the hospital or outpatient surgical center under general anesthesia (while the patient is unconscious and pain-free). However, very rarely, this procedure may also be done using local anesthesia, which numbs only the area affected by the surgery and allows you to stay awake.

A surgeon makes a small cut below the belly button (navel) and inserts a needle into the area. Carbon dioxide gas is passed into the area to help move the abdominal wall and any organs out of the way, creating a larger space to work in. This helps the surgeon see the area better.

A tube is placed through the cut in your abdominal area. A tiny video camera (laparoscope) goes through this tube and is used to see the inside of your pelvis and abdomen. Additional small cuts may be made if other instruments are needed to get a better view of certain organs. In the case of gynecologic laparoscopy, dye may be injected into your cervix area so the surgeon can better see your fallopian tubes.

After the exam, the laparoscope and instruments are removed, and the cuts are closed. You will have bandages over those areas.

To Prepare for the Test

Do not eat or drink anything for eight hours before the test. You must sign a consent form.

How the Test Will Feel

If you are given general anesthesia, you will feel no pain during the procedure, although the surgical cuts may throb and be slightly painful afterward. Your doctor may prescribe medicine to relieve pain.

With local anesthesia, you may feel a prick and a burning sensation when the local anesthetic is given. The laparoscope may cause pressure, but there should be no pain during the procedure. Afterward, you may also feel soreness at the site of the surgical cut. A pain reliever may be prescribed by your doctor.

You may also have shoulder pain for a few days, because the gas used during the procedure can irritate the diaphragm, which shares some of the same nerves as the shoulder. You may also have an increased urge to urinate, since the gas can put pressure on the bladder.

Why the Test Is Performed

The examination helps identify the cause of pain in the abdomen and pelvic area. It is done after other, noninvasive tests. Laparoscopy may detect or diagnose appendicitis, cancer (such as ovarian cancer), ectopic pregnancy, endometriosis, inflammation of the gallbladder (cholecystitis), and pelvic inflammatory disease. The procedure may also be done instead of open surgery after an accident to see if there is any injury to the abdomen.

Major procedures to treat cancer, such as surgery to remove an organ, may begin with laparoscopy to rule out the presence of cancer spread (metastatic disease), which would change the course of treatment.

Normal Results

There is no blood in the abdomen, no hernias, no intestinal obstruction, and no cancer in any visible organs. The uterus, fallopian tubes, and ovaries are of normal size, shape, and color. The liver is normal.

Abnormal Results Mean

Abnormal results may be due to a number of different conditions, including the following:

- Adhesions
- Appendicitis
- Cholecystitis
- Endometriosis
- Ovarian cysts
- Pelvic inflammatory disease
- Signs of injury
- Spread of cancer
- Tumors
- Uterine fibroids

Risks

There is some risk of infection. Antibiotics may be given to prevent this complication. There is a risk of puncturing an organ, which could cause leakage of intestinal contents, or bleeding into the abdominal cavity. Such a complication could lead to immediate open surgery (laparotomy).

Chapter 38

Stress Testing

Stress testing gives your doctor information about how your heart works during physical stress. Some heart problems are easier to diagnose when your heart is working hard and beating fast. During a stress test, you exercise (walk or run on a treadmill or pedal a bicycle) to make your heart work hard and beat fast. Tests are done on your heart while you exercise. Doctors usually use stress testing to help diagnose coronary heart disease (CHD), also called coronary artery disease. They also use stress testing to see how severe CHD is in people who have it.

You may not have any signs or symptoms of CHD when your heart is at rest. But when your heart has to work harder during exercise, it needs more blood and oxygen. Narrowed arteries cannot supply enough blood for your heart to work well. As a result, signs and symptoms of CHD may only occur during exercise. A stress test can detect the following problems, which may suggest that your heart is not getting enough blood during exercise:

- Abnormal changes in your heart rate or blood pressure

- Symptoms such as shortness of breath or chest pain, which are particularly important if they occur at low levels of exercise

- Abnormal changes in your heart's rhythm or electrical activity

Excerpted from "Stress Testing," National Heart, Lung, and Blood Institute (NHLBI), June 2009.

During a stress test, if you cannot exercise for as long as what is considered normal for someone your age, it may be a sign that not enough blood is flowing to your heart. However, other factors besides CHD can prevent you from exercising long enough (for example, lung disease, anemia, or poor general fitness). A stress test also may be used to assess other problems, such as heart valve disease or heart failure.

Types of Stress Testing

Standard Exercise Stress Test

A standard exercise stress test uses an EKG (electrocardiogram) to detect and record the heart's electrical activity. An EKG shows how fast your heart is beating and the heart's rhythm (steady or irregular). It also records the strength and timing of electrical signals as they pass through each part of your heart.

During a standard stress test, your blood pressure will be checked. You also may be asked to breathe into a special tube during the test. This allows your doctor to see how well you're breathing and measure the gases that you breathe out. A standard stress test shows changes in your heart's electrical activity. It also may show signs that your heart is not getting enough blood during exercise.

Imaging Stress Test

Some stress tests take pictures of the heart when you exercise and when you are at rest. These imaging stress tests can show how well blood is flowing in various parts of your heart and/or how well your heart squeezes out blood when it beats. One type of imaging stress test involves echocardiography (echo). This test uses sound waves to create a moving picture of your heart. An exercise stress echo can show how well your heart's chambers and valves are working when your heart is under stress. The test can identify areas of poor blood flow to your heart, dead heart muscle tissue, and areas of the heart muscle wall that are not contracting normally. These areas may have been damaged during a heart attack, or they may not be getting enough blood.

Other imaging stress tests use radioactive dye to create pictures of the blood flow to your heart. The dye is injected into your bloodstream before the pictures of your heart are taken. The pictures show how much of the dye has reached various parts of your heart during exercise and while you are at rest. Tests that use radioactive dye include a thallium or sestamibi stress test and a positron emission tomography (PET) stress test. The amount of radiation in the dye is thought to be safe and not a danger to you or those around you. However, if you're pregnant, you should not have this test because of risks it might pose to your unborn child.

Imaging stress tests tend to be more accurate at detecting CHD than standard (nonimaging) stress tests. Imaging stress tests also can predict the risk of a future heart attack or premature death. An imaging stress test may be done first (as opposed to a standard exercise stress test) if any of the following apply to you:

- Cannot exercise for enough time to get your heart working at its hardest. (Medical problems, such as arthritis or leg arteries clogged by plaque, may prevent you from exercising enough.)

- Have abnormal heartbeats or other problems that will cause a standard exercise stress test to be inaccurate.

- Had a heart procedure in the past, such as coronary artery by-pass grafting or placement of a stent in a coronary artery.

Who Needs Stress Testing?

You may need stress testing if you have had chest pains, shortness of breath, or other symptoms of limited blood flow to your heart. Imaging stress tests, particularly, can show whether you have coronary heart disease (CHD) or a heart valve problem. (Heart valves are like doors that let blood flow between the heart's chambers and into the heart's arteries. So, like CHD, faulty heart valves can limit the amount of blood reaching your heart.) If you have been diagnosed with CHD or recently had a heart attack, a stress test can show whether you can tolerate an exercise program. If you have had angioplasty with or without stents or coronary artery bypass grafting, a stress test can show how well the treatment relieves your CHD symptoms.

You also may need a stress test if, during exercise, you feel faint, get a rapid heartbeat or a fluttering feeling in your chest, or have other symptoms of an arrhythmia (an abnormal heartbeat). If you do not have chest pain when you exercise, but still get short of breath, you may need a stress test. The test can help show whether a heart problem, rather than a lung problem or being out of shape, is causing your breathing problems.

Stress testing is not used as a routine screening test for CHD. Usually, you have to have symptoms of CHD before a doctor will recommend stress testing. However, your doctor may want to use a stress test to screen for CHD if you have diabetes. This disease increases your risk for CHD.

What to Expect before Stress Testing

Standard stress testing often is done in a doctor's office. Imaging stress testing usually is done at a hospital. Be sure to wear athletic or other shoes in which you can exercise comfortably. You may be asked to wear comfortable clothes, or you may be given a gown to wear during the test. Your doctor may ask you not to eat or drink anything but water for a short time before the test. If you are diabetic, ask your doctor whether you need to adjust your medicines on the day of your test.

For some stress tests, you cannot drink coffee or other caffeinated drinks for a day before the test. Certain over-the-counter or prescription medicines also may interfere with some stress tests. Discuss with your doctor whether you need to avoid certain drinks or food or change how you take your medicine before the test. If you use an inhaler for asthma or other breathing problems, bring it to the test. Make sure you let the doctor know that you use it.

What to Expect during Stress Testing

During all types of stress testing, a technician or nurse will always be with you to closely check your health status. Before you start the stress part of a stress test, the technician or nurse will put sticky patches called electrodes on the skin of your chest, arms, and legs. To help an electrode stick to the skin, the technician or nurse may have to shave a patch of hair where the electrode will be attached. The electrodes are connected to an EKG (electrocardiogram) machine. This machine records your heart's electrical activity and shows how fast your heart is beating and the heart's rhythm (steady or irregular). An EKG also records the strength and timing of electrical signals as they pass through each part of your heart. The technician or nurse will put a blood pressure cuff on your arm to check your blood pressure during the stress test. (The cuff will feel tight on your arm when it expands every few minutes.) Also, you may be asked to breathe into a special tube so the gases you breathe out can be measured.

After these preparations, you will exercise on a treadmill or stationary bicycle. If such exercise poses a problem for you, you may instead turn a crank with your arms. During the test, the exercise level will get harder. You can stop whenever you feel the exercise is too much for you.

If you cannot exercise, medicine may be injected into a vein in your arm or hand. This medicine will increase blood flow through your coronary arteries and/or make your heart beat fast, as would exercise.

366

The stress test can then be done. The medicine may make you flushed and anxious, but the effects go away as soon as the test is over. The medicine also may give you a headache. While you are exercising or getting medicine to make your heart work harder, the technician will frequently ask you how you are feeling. You should tell him or her if you feel chest pain, short of breath, or dizzy.

The exercise or medicine infusion will continue until you reach a target heart rate, or until you:

- feel moderate to severe chest pain,

- get too out of breath to continue,

- develop abnormally high or low blood pressure or an arrhythmia (an abnormal heartbeat), or

- become dizzy.

The technician will continue to check your heart functions and blood pressure after the test until they return to your normal levels.

The stress part of a stress test (when you're exercising or given medicine that makes your heart work hard) usually lasts about 15 minutes or less. However, there is prep time before the test and monitoring time afterward. Both extend the total test time to about an hour for a standard stress test, and up to three hours or more for some imaging stress tests.

Exercise Stress Echocardiogram Test

For an exercise stress echocardiogram (echo) test, the technician will take pictures of your heart using echocardiography before you exercise and as soon as you finish. A sonographer (a person who specializes in using ultrasound techniques) will apply gel to your chest. Then, he or she will briefly put a transducer (a wand-like device) against your chest and move it around. The transducer sends and receives high-pitched sounds that you usually cannot hear. The echoes from the sound waves are converted into moving pictures of your heart on a screen.

You may be asked to lie on your side on an exam table for this test. Some stress echo tests also use a dye to improve imaging. This dye is injected into your bloodstream while the test occurs.

Sestamibi or Other Imaging Stress Tests Involving Radioactive Dye

For a sestamibi stress test, or other imaging stress tests that use radioactive dye, the technician will inject a small amount of dye (such as sestamibi) into your bloodstream. This is done through a needle placed in a vein in your arm or hand.

You are usually given the dye about a half-hour before you start exercising or take medicine to make your heart work hard. The amount of radiation in the dye is thought to be safe and not a danger to you or those around you. However, if you are pregnant, you should not have this test because of risks it might pose to your unborn child.

Pictures will be taken of your heart at least two times: when it is at rest and when it is working its hardest. You'll lie down on a table, and a special camera or scanner that can see the dye in your bloodstream will take pictures of your heart. Some pictures may not be taken until you lie quietly for a few hours after the stress test. Some patients may even be asked to return in a day or so for more pictures.

What Does Stress Testing Show?

Stress testing gives your doctor information about how your heart works during physical stress (exercise) and how healthy your heart is. A standard exercise stress test uses an EKG (electrocardiogram) to monitor changes in your heart's electrical activity. Imaging stress tests take pictures of blood flow in various parts of your heart. They also show your heart valves and the movement of your heart muscle. Both types of stress tests are used to look for signs that your heart is not getting enough blood flow during exercise. Abnormal test results may be due to coronary heart disease (CHD) or other factors, such as a lack of physical fitness.

If you have a standard exercise stress test and the results are normal, no further testing or treatment may be needed. But if your test results are abnormal, or if you are physically unable to exercise, your doctor may want you to have an imaging stress test or other tests.

Even if your standard exercise stress test results are normal, your doctor may want you to have an imaging stress test if you continue having symptoms (such as shortness of breath or chest pain). Imaging stress tests are more accurate than standard exercise stress tests, but they're much more expensive. Imaging stress tests show how well blood is flowing in the heart muscle and reveal parts of the heart that aren't contracting strongly. They also can show the parts of the heart that are not getting enough blood, as well as dead tissue in the heart, where no blood flows. (A heart attack can cause some tissue in the heart to die.) If your imaging stress test suggests significant CHD, your doctor may want you to have more testing and/or treatment.

What Are the Risks of Stress Testing?

There is little risk of serious harm from any type of stress testing. The chance of these tests causing a heart attack or death is about one in 5,000. More common, but less serious side effects linked to stress testing include these:

- Arrhythmia (an abnormal heartbeat). Often, an arrhythmia will go away quickly once you're at rest. But if it persists, you may need monitoring or treatment in a hospital.

- Low blood pressure, which can cause you to feel dizzy or faint. This problem may go away once your heart stops working hard; it usually does not require treatment.

- Jitteriness or discomfort while getting medicine to make your heart work harder (you may be given medicine if you cannot exercise). These side effects usually go away shortly after you stop getting the medicine. In some cases, the symptoms may last a few hours.

Also, some of the medicines used for pharmacological stress tests can cause wheezing, shortness of breath, and other asthma-like symptoms. In some cases, these symptoms may be severe and require treatment.

Part Five

Screening and Assessments for Specific Conditions and Diseases

Chapter 39

Allergy Testing

Allergy tests are any of several tests used to determine the substances to which a person is allergic.

How the Test Is Performed

There are many methods of allergy testing. Among the more common are skin tests, elimination-type tests, and blood tests (including the radioallergosorbent, or RAST, test).

Skin Tests

Skin tests are the most common. Specific methods vary. One of the most common methods is the prick test. This test involves placing a small amount of suspected allergy-causing substances on the skin, usually the forearm, upper arm, or the back. Then, the skin is pricked so the allergen goes under the skin's surface. The health care provider closely watches the skin for signs of a reaction, usually swelling and redness of the site. Results are usually seen within 15–20 minutes. Several allergens can be tested at the same time.

A similar method involves injecting a small amount of allergen into the skin and watching for a reaction at the site. This is called an intradermal skin test. It is more likely to be used when testing is

This chapter begins with "Allergy Testing," © 2011 A.D.A.M., Inc. Reprinted with permission; and concludes with an excerpt from "Food Allergy," National Institute of Allergy and Infectious Diseases (NIAID), December 2, 2010.

being done to find out if you are allergy to something specific, such as bee venom or penicillin.

Patch testing is a method to diagnose allergic reactions on the skin. Possible allergens are taped to the skin for 48 hours. The health care provider will look at the area in 24 hours, and then again 48 hours later.

Skin tests are most useful for diagnosing:

- food allergy;
- mold, pollen, animal, and other allergies that cause allergic rhinitis and asthma;
- penicillin allergy;*
- venom allergy;
- allergic contact dermatitis.

Elimination Tests

An elimination diet can be used to check for food allergies. An elimination diet is one in which foods that may be causing symptoms are removed from the diet for several weeks and then slowly re-introduced one at a time while the person is watched for signs of an allergic reaction.

Blood Tests

Blood tests can be done to measure the amount of immunoglobulin (Ig) E antibodies to a specific allergen in the blood. This test may be used when skin testing is not helpful or cannot be done. Other blood tests include the absolute eosinophil count and total IgE level.

Provocation Testing

Provocation (challenge) testing involves exposing a person to a suspected allergen under controlled circumstances. This may be done in the diet or by breathing in the suspected allergen. This type of test may provoke severe allergic reactions. Challenge testing should only be done by a doctor.

Another method is the double-blind test. This method involves giving foods and harmless substances in a disguised form. The person being tested and the provider are both unaware of whether the substance tested in that session is the harmless substance or the suspected food. A third party knows the identity of the substances and identifies them with some sort of code. This test requires several sessions if more than one substance is under investigation.

While the double-blind strategy is useful and practical for mild allergic reactions, it must be done carefully in individuals with suspected severe reactions to foods. Blood tests may be a safer first approach.

How to Prepare for the Test

Before any allergy testing, the health care provider will ask for a very detailed medical history. This may include questions about such things as illnesses, emotional and social conditions, work, entertainment, lifestyle, foods, and eating habits.

If skin testing will be performed, you should not take antihistamines before the test. This may lead to a false-negative result, falsely reassuring you that a substance is unlikely to cause a severe allergic reaction. Your doctor will tell you which medicines to avoid and when to stop taking them before the test.

How the Test Will Feel

Skin tests may cause very mild discomfort when the skin is pricked. Itching may occur if you have a positive reaction to the allergen.

Why the Test Is Performed

Allergy tests are done to determine the specific substances that cause an allergic reaction in a person. Your doctor may order allergy tests if you have:

- allergic rhinitis and asthma symptoms that are not easily controlled with medications,

- angioedema and hives,

- food allergies,

- contact dermatitis,

- penicillin allergy.*

***Note:** Allergies to penicillin and closely related medications are the only drug allergies that can be tested using skin tests. Skin tests for allergies to other drugs can be dangerous.

The prick skin test may also be used to diagnose food allergies. Intradermal tests are not used to test for food allergies because of high false positive results and the danger of causing a severe allergic reaction.

Normal Results

In a non-allergic person, allergy tests should be negative (no response to the allergen).

What Abnormal Results Mean

A positive result means you reacted to a specific substance. Often, but not always, a positive result means the symptoms that you are having are due to exposure to the substance in question. In general, a stronger response means you are more sensitive to the substance. People can have a positive response with allergy skin testing, but not have any problems with the specific substance in everyday life. The skin tests are generally reliable. However, if the dose of allergen is excessive, a positive reaction will occur even in persons who are not allergic.

Risks

Risks related to skin and food allergy tests may include allergic reaction or life-threatening anaphylactic reaction.

Considerations

The accuracy of allergy testing varies quite a bit. Even the same test performed at different times on a person may give different results. A person may react to a substance during testing, but never react during normal exposure. Rarely, a person may also have a negative allergy test and still be allergic to the substance.

Food Allergy

After ruling out food intolerances and other health problems, your health care provider will use several steps to find out if you have an allergy to specific foods.

Detailed History

Your health care professional will begin by taking a detailed medical history to find out if your symptoms are caused by an allergy to specific foods, food intolerance, or other health problems. A detailed history is the most valuable tool used for diagnosing food allergy. Your healthcare professional will ask you several questions, including the following:

- Did your reaction come on quickly, usually within several minutes after eating the food?

- Is your reaction always associated with a certain food?

- How much of this potentially allergenic food did you eat before you had a reaction?

- Have you eaten this food before and had a reaction?

- Did anyone else who ate the same food get sick?

- Did you take allergy medicines, and if so, did they help? (Antihistamines should relieve hives, for example.)

Diet Diary

Sometimes your health care professional cannot make a diagnosis based only on your history. You may be asked to keep a diet diary containing details about the foods you eat and whether you have a reaction. Based on the diary record, you and your health care professional may be able to identify a consistent pattern in your reactions.

Elimination Diet

The next step some health care professionals use is a limited elimination diet, in which the food that is suspected of causing an allergic reaction is removed from your diet to see whether that stops your allergic reactions. For example, if you suspect you are allergic to egg, your health care professional will instruct you to eliminate egg from your diet. The limited elimination diet is done under the direction of your health care professional.

Skin Prick Test

If your history, diet diary, or elimination diet suggests a specific food allergy is likely, then your healthcare professional will use the skin prick test to confirm the diagnosis. With a skin prick test, your health care professional uses a needle to place a tiny amount of food extract just below the surface of the skin on your lower arm or back. If you are allergic, there will be swelling or redness at the test site. This is a positive result. It means that there are immunoglobulin E (IgE) molecules on the skin's mast cells that are specific to the food being tested.

The skin prick test is simple and relatively safe, and results are ready in minutes. You can have a positive skin test to a food, however, without having an allergic reaction to that food. A health care professional often makes a diagnosis of food allergy when someone has both a positive skin test to a specific food and a history of reactions that suggests an allergy to the same food.

Blood Test

Instead of the skin prick test, your health care professional can take a blood sample to measure the levels of food-specific IgE antibodies. As with skin testing, positive blood tests do not necessarily mean that you have a food allergy. Your health care professionals must combine these test results with information about your history of reactions to food to make an accurate diagnosis of food allergy.

Oral Food Challenge

Caution: Because oral food challenges can cause a severe allergic reaction, they should always be conducted by a health care professional who has experience performing them. An oral food challenge is the final method health care professionals use to diagnose food allergy. This method includes the following steps:

- Your health care professional gives you individual doses of various foods (masked so that you do not know what food is present), some of which are suspected of starting an allergic reaction. Initially, the dose of food is very small, but the amount is gradually increased during the challenge.

- You swallow the individual dose.

- Your health care professional watches you to see if a reaction occurs.

To prevent bias, oral food challenges are often double blinded. In a true double-blind challenge, neither you nor your health care professional knows whether the substance you eat contains the likely allergen. Another medical professional has made up the individual doses. In a single-blind challenge, your health care professional knows what you are eating but you do not. A reaction only to suspected foods and not to the other foods tested confirms the diagnosis of a food allergy.

Chapter 40

Bladder and Kidney Function Tests

Section 40.1

Urodynamics

This section includes excerpts from "Urodynamic Testing," National Institute of Diabetes and Digestive and Kidney Diseases (NIDDK), November 2006. Reviewed in April 2011 by David A. Cooke, MD, FACP. The section concludes with text from "National Guideline Clearinghouse–SOGC Committee Opinion on Urodynamics Testing," Agency for Healthcare Research and Quality (AHRQ), March 25, 2009.

If you have a problem with urine leakage or blocked urine flow, your doctor or nurse may be able to help. One of the tools they may use to evaluate the cause of your symptoms is urodynamic testing.

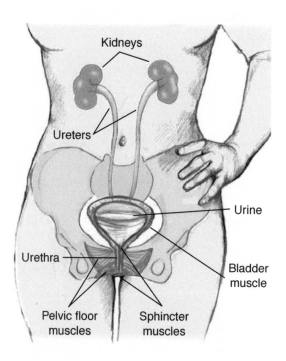

Figure 40.1. Urinary Tract

Several muscles, organs, and nerves are involved in collecting, storing, and releasing urine. The kidneys form urine by filtering wastes and extra water from the bloodstream. The ureters are tubes that carry urine from the kidneys to the bladder. Normally urine flows in one direction. If urine backs up toward the kidneys, infections and kidney damage can occur.

The bladder, a hollow muscular organ shaped like a balloon, sits in the pelvis and is held in place by ligaments attached to other organs and to the pelvic bones. The bladder stores urine until you are ready to empty it. It swells into a round shape when it is full and gets smaller as it empties. A healthy bladder can hold up to 16 ounces (two cups) of urine comfortably. How frequently it fills depends on how much excess water your body is trying to get rid of.

The bladder opens into the urethra, the tube that allows urine to pass outside the body. Circular muscles called sphincters close tightly to keep urine from leaking. The involuntary leakage of urine is called incontinence. Nerves in the bladder tell you when it is time to empty your bladder. When the bladder begins to fill with urine, you may notice a feeling that you need to urinate. The sensation becomes stronger as the bladder continues to fill and reaches its limit. At that point, nerves in the bladder send a message to the brain, and your urge to urinate intensifies. When you are ready to urinate, the brain signals the sphincter muscles to relax. At the same time, the brain signals the bladder muscles to squeeze, thus allowing urine to flow through the urethra. When these signals occur in the correct order, normal urination occurs.

Problems in the urinary system can be caused by aging, illness, or injury. The muscles in and around your bladder and urethra tend to become weaker with age. Weak bladder muscles may result in your not being able to empty your bladder completely, leaving you at a higher risk for urinary tract infections. Weak muscles of the sphincters and pelvis can lead to urinary incontinence because the sphincter muscles cannot remain tight enough to hold urine in the bladder, or the bladder does not have enough support from the pelvic muscles to stay in its proper position.

Urodynamics is a study that assesses how the bladder and urethra are performing their job of storing and releasing urine. Urodynamic tests help your doctor or nurse see how well your bladder and sphincter muscles work and can help explain symptoms such as:

- incontinence,

- frequent urination,

- sudden, strong urges to urinate,
- problems starting a urine stream,
- painful urination,
- problems emptying your bladder completely,
- recurrent urinary tract infections.

These tests may be as simple as urinating behind a curtain while a doctor or nurse listens or more complicated, involving imaging equipment that films urination and pressure monitors that record the pressures of the bladder and urethra.

Seeing Your Doctor or Nurse

The first step in solving a urinary problem is to talk with your doctor or nurse. He or she should ask you about your general medical history, including any major illnesses or surgeries. You should talk about the medicines you take, both prescription and nonprescription, because they might be part of the problem. You should talk about how much fluid you drink a day and whether you use alcohol or caffeine. Give as many details as you can about the problem and when it started. The doctor or nurse may ask you to keep a voiding diary, which is a record of fluid intake and trips to the bathroom, plus any episodes of leakage.

If leakage is the problem, the doctor or nurse may ask you to do a pad test. This test is a simple way to measure how much urine leaks out. You will be given a number of absorbent pads and plastic bags of a standard weight. You will be told to wear the pad for one or two hours while in the clinic or to wear a series of pads at home during a specific period of time. The pads are collected and sealed in a plastic bag. Your health care team will then weigh the bags to see how much urine has been caught in the pad. A simpler but less precise method is to change pads as often as you need to and keep track of how many pads you use in a day.

A physical exam will also be performed to rule out other causes of urinary problems. This exam usually includes an assessment of the nerves in the lower part of your body. It will also include a pelvic exam in women to assess the pelvic muscles and the other pelvic organs. In men, a rectal exam is given to assess the prostate. Your doctor will also want to check your urine for evidence of infection or blood.

Preparing for the Test

If the doctor or nurse recommends bladder testing, usually no special preparations are needed, but make sure you understand any instructions you do receive. Depending on the test, you may be asked to come with a full bladder or an empty one. Also, ask whether you should change your diet or skip your regular medicines and for how long.

Taking the Test

Any procedure designed to provide information about a bladder problem can be called a urodynamic test. The type of test you take depends on your problem. Most urodynamic testing focuses on the bladder's ability to empty steadily and completely. It can also show whether the bladder is having abnormal contractions that cause leakage. Your doctor will want to know whether you have difficulty starting a urine stream, how hard you have to strain to maintain it, whether the stream is interrupted, and whether any urine is left in your bladder when you are done. The remaining urine is called the postvoid residual. Urodynamic tests can range from simple observation to precise measurement using sophisticated instruments.

Uroflowmetry (measurement of urine speed and volume): A uroflowmeter automatically measures the amount of urine and the flow rate—that is, how fast the urine comes out. You may be asked to urinate privately into a toilet that contains a collection device and scale. This equipment creates a graph that shows changes in flow rate from second to second so the doctor or nurse can see the peak flow rate and how many seconds it took to get there. Results of this test will be abnormal if the bladder muscle is weak or urine flow is obstructed.

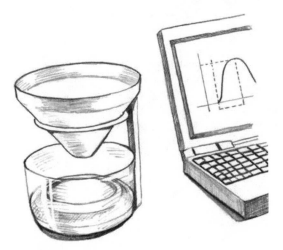

Figure 40.2. Uroflowmeter Equipment

Your doctor or nurse can also get some idea of your bladder function by using a stopwatch to time you as you urinate into a graduated container. The volume of urine is divided by the time to see what your average flow rate is. For example, 330 milliliters (mL) of urine in 30 seconds means that your average flow rate is 11mL per second.

Measurement of postvoid residual: After you have finished, you may still have some urine, usually only an ounce or two, remaining in your bladder. To measure this postvoid residual, the doctor or nurse may use a catheter, a thin tube that can be gently glided into the urethra. He or she can also measure the postvoid residual with ultrasound equipment that uses harmless sound waves to create a picture of the bladder. A postvoid residual of more than 200mL, about half a pint, is a clear sign of a problem. Even 100mL, about half a cup, requires further evaluation. However, the amount of postvoid residual can be different each time you urinate.

Cystometry (measurement of bladder pressure): A cystometrogram (CMG) measures how much your bladder can hold, how much pressure builds up inside your bladder as it stores urine, and how full it is when you feel the urge to urinate. The doctor or nurse will use a catheter to empty your bladder completely. Then a special, smaller catheter will be placed in the bladder. This catheter has a pressure-measuring device called a manometer. Another catheter may be placed in the rectum to record pressure there as well. Your bladder will be filled slowly with warm water. During this time you will be asked how your bladder feels and when you feel the need to urinate. The volume of water and the bladder

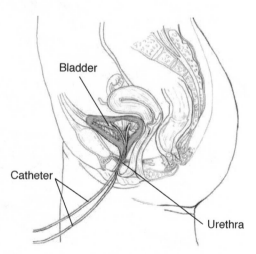

Figure 40.3. *Cystometry in a Female Patient*

pressure will be recorded. You may be asked to cough or strain during this procedure. Involuntary bladder contractions can be identified.

Measurement of leak point pressure: While your bladder is being filled for the CMG, it may suddenly contract and squeeze some water out without warning. The manometer will record the pressure at the point when the leakage occurred. This reading may provide information about the kind of bladder problem you have. You may also be asked to apply abdominal pressure to the bladder by coughing, shifting position, or trying to exhale while holding your nose and mouth. These actions help the doctor or nurse evaluate your sphincter muscles.

Pressure flow study: After the CMG, you will be asked to empty your bladder. The catheter can measure the bladder pressures required to urinate and the flow rate a given pressure generates. This pressure flow study helps to identify bladder outlet obstruction that men may experience with prostate enlargement. Bladder outlet obstruction is less common in women but can occur with a fallen bladder or rarely after a surgical procedure for urinary incontinence. Most catheters can be used for both CMG and pressure flow studies.

Electromyography (measurement of nerve impulses): If your doctor or nurse thinks that your urinary problem is related to nerve or muscle damage, you may be given an electromyography. This test measures the muscle activity in and around the urethral sphincter by using special sensors. The sensors are placed on the skin near the urethra and rectum or they are located on the urethral or rectal catheter. Muscle activity is recorded on a machine. The patterns of the impulses will show whether the messages sent to the bladder and urethra are coordinated correctly.

Video urodynamics: Urodynamic tests may be performed with or without equipment to take pictures of the bladder during filling and emptying. The imaging equipment may use x-rays or sound waves. If x-ray equipment is used, the bladder will be filled with a contrast medium that will show up on the x-ray instead of the warm water. The pictures and videos show the size and shape of the urinary tract and help your doctor or nurse understand your problem.

After the Test

You may have mild discomfort for a few hours after these tests when you urinate. Drinking an 8-ounce glass of water each half-hour for two hours should help. Ask your doctor whether you can take a warm bath. If not, you may be able to hold a warm, damp washcloth over the urethral opening to relieve the discomfort. Your doctor may give you an antibiotic to take for one or two days to prevent an infection. If you have signs of infection—including pain, chills, or fever—call your doctor at once.

Getting the Results

Results for simple tests can be discussed with your doctor or nurse immediately after the test. Results of other tests may take a few days. You will have the chance to ask questions about the results and possible treatments for your problem.

Recommendations of the Society of Obstetricians and Gynecologists of Canada (SOGC) Committee on Urodynamics Testing

Controversies remain with respect to the indications for urodynamic testing. Urodynamics is an objective tool that is invaluable, when used by experts trained in its interpretation, in clarifying confusing or complex urinary tract symptoms. It is also invasive and can be embarrassing for patients. It is not cost-effective to apply a universal policy of urodynamic testing. Experts agree that it is not necessary to perform urodynamic testing on patients prior to instituting conservative management but that it is necessary to perform these tests on any patient undergoing repeat incontinence surgery. To date, no published studies have demonstrated that the performance of urodynamic testing improves clinical outcomes; however, it is undoubtedly true that urodynamic testing is an indispensable tool in the evaluation of urinary tract complaints. Further research is needed to better elucidate the most appropriate patient criteria for urodynamic testing.

Potential benefits: Appropriate urodynamic testing for the evaluation of abnormal bladder function.

Potential harms: Urodynamic testing has a number of pitfalls: (1) lack of standardization of values and parameters being evaluated; (2) the artificial testing settings may not represent what happens to the patient during normal daily activities; (3) inconsistent reproducibility within the same patient; (4) the wide range of physiologic values in normal asymptomatic patients; (5) false negatives, the absence of a specific abnormality during urodynamic testing, does not necessarily exclude its existence; and (6) not all abnormalities found during urodynamic testing are clinically significant.

Section 40.2

Screening for Kidney Disease

Excerpted from "About Kidney Disease," National Kidney
Disease Education Program (NKDEP), June 30, 2010.

Chronic kidney disease—called kidney disease here for short—is a
condition in which the small blood vessels in the kidneys are damaged,
making the kidneys unable to do their job. Waste then builds up in the
blood, harming the body.

Testing for Kidney Disease

Early kidney disease does not have symptoms, so testing is the only
way to know how your kidneys are working. It's important for you to
get tested for kidney disease if you have the key risk factors—diabetes,
high blood pressure, cardiovascular (heart) disease, or a family history
of kidney failure.

A blood test and a urine test are used to check for kidney disease:

- The blood test helps to measure your glomerular filtration rate
  (GFR). GFR measures how much blood your kidneys filter each
  minute. You cannot raise your GFR, but you can try to keep it
  from going lower. GFR is reported as a number.

  - A GFR of 60 or higher is in the normal range.

  - A GFR below 60 may mean you have kidney disease.

  - A GFR of 15 or lower may mean kidney failure.

- The urine test looks for high amounts of protein or albumin,
  a specific type of protein. Albumin is too big to pass through a
  healthy kidney. If your kidneys are damaged, albumin can pass
  into the urine. You cannot see or feel albumin in your urine. So,
  a urine albumin test is important. In general, the less albumin
  in your urine, the better. Your provider may give you medicines
  to lower the amount of albumin in your urine and to keep your
  kidneys healthy.

When to Get Tested

The earlier kidney disease is found, the earlier it can be treated.

Keep Your Kidneys Healthy

If you are at risk for kidney disease, the most important steps you can take to keep your kidneys healthy are these:

- Get your blood and urine checked for kidney disease.

- Manage your diabetes, high blood pressure, and heart disease.

What Should I Tell My Family about Kidney Disease?

- Diabetes and high blood pressure are the leading causes of kidney failure.

- Managing your blood sugar and blood pressure may help the kidneys stay healthy.

- Get tested for kidney disease because it runs in families.

- Blood and urine tests are the only way to find out if you have kidney disease because there are no early warning signs.

- Finding kidney disease early and treating it can slow kidney damage and may prevent kidney failure.

Table 40.1. When to Test for Kidney Disease

If you have...	Get your kidneys checked...
Type 1 Diabetes	Every year, starting five years after diabetes diagnosis
Type 2 Diabetes	Every year
Other risk factors (cardiovascular disease, family history)	Regularly–talk to your provider about how often

Section 40.3

Tracking Chronic Kidney Disease

Excerpted from "Chronic Kidney Disease," National Kidney
Disease Education Program (NKDEP), April 2010.

You've been told that you have chronic kidney disease (CKD). What
does that mean? And what does it mean for your health and your life?
CKD means that your kidneys are damaged and cannot filter blood like
they should. This damage can cause wastes to build up in your body.
It can also cause other problems that can harm your health. CKD is
often a progressive disease, which means it can get worse over time.
CKD may lead to kidney failure. The only treatment options for kidney
failure are dialysis or a kidney transplant.

What tests will help track my CKD?

Track your blood pressure. In most cases, you should keep it below
130/80. If you have diabetes, monitor your blood glucose and keep it in
your target range. Like high blood pressure, high blood glucose can be
harmful to your kidneys. Know your test results and track them over
time to see how your kidneys are doing.

Blood pressure: The most important thing you can do to slow
down CKD is keep your blood pressure below 130/80. This can delay
or prevent kidney failure.

Glomerular filtration rate (GFR): The GFR tells you how well
your kidneys are filtering blood. You cannot raise your GFR. The goal is
to keep your GFR from going down to prevent or delay kidney failure.
See the Figure 40.4.

Urine albumin: Albumin is a protein in your blood that can pass into
the urine when kidneys are damaged. You cannot undo kidney damage,
but you may be able to lower the amount of albumin in your urine with
treatment. Lowering your urine albumin is good for your kidneys.

A1C: A1C test is a lab test that shows your average blood glucose
level over the last three months. The goal is less than seven for most

people with diabetes. Lowering your A1C can help you to stay healthy. (For people with diabetes only.)

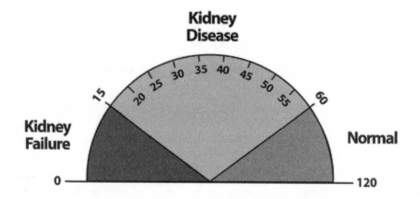

Figure 40.4. *Glomerular Filtration Rate (GFR)*

Chapter 41

Cancer Screening Tests

Section 41.1

Cancer Screening Overview

Excerpted from PDQ® Cancer Information Summary. National Cancer Institute: Bethesda, MD. "Cancer Screening Overview (PDQ®)–Patient Version." Updated September 2010. Available at http://cancer.gov. Accessed April 2, 2011.

Cancer screening is looking for cancer before a person has any symptoms. Screening tests can help find cancer at an early stage, before symptoms appear. When abnormal tissue or cancer is found early, it may be easier to treat or cure. By the time symptoms appear, the cancer may have grown and spread. This can make the cancer harder to treat or cure.

It is important to remember that when your doctor suggests a screening test, it does not always mean he or she thinks you have cancer. Screening tests are done when you have no cancer symptoms.

Screening tests include the following:

- **Physical exam and history:** An exam of the body to check general signs of health, including checking for signs of disease, such as lumps or anything else that seems unusual. A history of the patient's health habits and past illnesses and treatments will also be taken.

- **Laboratory tests:** Medical procedures that test samples of tissue, blood, urine, or other substances in the body.

- **Imaging procedures:** Procedures that make pictures of areas inside the body.

- **Genetic tests:** Tests that look for certain gene mutations (changes) that are linked to some types of cancer.

Screening tests have risks: Not all screening tests are helpful and most have risks. It is important to know the risks of the test and whether it has been proven to decrease the chance of dying from cancer.

- Some screening tests cause serious problems.

- Some screening procedures can cause bleeding or other problems. For example, colon cancer screening with sigmoidoscopy or colonoscopy can cause tears in the lining of the colon.

False-positive test results are possible: Screening test results may appear to be abnormal even though there is no cancer. A false-positive test result (one that shows there is cancer when there really isn't) can cause anxiety and is usually followed by more tests and procedures, which also have risks.

False-negative test results are possible: Screening test results may appear to be normal even though there is cancer. A person who receives a false-negative test result (one that shows there is no cancer when there really is) may delay seeking medical care even if there are symptoms.

Finding the cancer may not improve the person's health or help the person live longer: Some cancers never cause symptoms or become life-threatening, but if found by a screening test, the cancer may be treated. There is no way to know if treating the cancer would help the person live longer than if no treatment were given. Also, treatments for cancer have side effects. For some cancers, finding and treating the cancer early does not improve the chance of a cure or help the person live longer. It can be hard to make decisions about screening tests. Before having any screening test, you may want to discuss the test with your doctor.

What are the goals of screening tests?

A screening test that works the way it should and is helpful does the following:

- Finds cancer before symptoms appear.
- Screens for a cancer that is easier to treat and cure when found early.
- Has few false-negative test results and false-positive test results.
- Decreases the chance of dying from cancer.

Screening tests are not meant to diagnose cancer: Screening tests usually do not diagnose cancer. If a screening test result is abnormal, more tests may be done to check for cancer. For example, a screening mammogram may find a lump in the breast. A lump may be cancer or something else. More tests need to be done to find out if the lump is cancer. These are called diagnostic tests. Diagnostic tests may include a biopsy, in which cells or tissues are removed so a pathologist can check them under a microscope for signs of cancer.

Does screening help people live longer?

- Finding some cancers at an early stage (before symptoms appear) may help decrease the chance of dying from those cancers.

- Screening studies are done to see whether deaths from cancer decrease when people are screened.

- Certain factors may cause survival times to look like they are getting better when they are not.

Section 41.2

Bladder and Other Urothelial Cancers Screening

Excerpted from PDQ® Cancer Information Summary. National Cancer Institute: Bethesda, MD. "Bladder and Other Urothelial Cancers Screening (PDQ®)–Patient Version." Updated July 2010. Available at: http://cancer .gov. Accessed April 1, 2011.

Bladder and other urothelial cancers are diseases in which malignant (cancer) cells form in the urothelium. The bladder holds urine until it is passed out of the body. Urine is the liquid waste that is made by the kidneys as they clean the blood. The urine passes from the two kidneys into the bladder through two tubes called ureters. When the bladder is emptied during urination, the urine goes from the bladder to the outside of the body through another tube called the urethra.

The urothelium is a layer of tissue that lines the urethra, bladder, ureters, prostate, and renal pelvis. Cancer that begins in the urothelium of the bladder is much more common than cancer that begins in the urothelium of the urethra, ureters, prostate, or renal pelvis. Because it is the most common form of urothelial cancer, bladder cancer is the focus of this summary.

There are three types of cancer that begin in the urothelial cells of the bladder. These cancers are named for the type of cells that become malignant (cancerous):

- **Transitional cell carcinoma:** Cancer that begins in cells in the innermost layer of the bladder urothelium. These cells are able to stretch when the bladder is full and shrink when it is emptied. Most bladder cancers begin in the transitional cells.

- **Squamous cell carcinoma:** Cancer that forms in squamous cells, which are thin, flat cells that may form in the bladder urothelium after long-term infection or irritation.

- **Adenocarcinoma:** Cancer that begins in glandular (secretory) cells. Glandular cells in the bladder urothelium make substances such as mucus.

Most newly diagnosed bladder cancers occur in people 60 years and older. In the United States (U.S.), bladder cancer occurs more often in men than in women, and more often in whites than in blacks. As the U.S. population has gotten older, the number of people diagnosed with bladder cancer has increased, but the number of deaths from bladder cancer has decreased. This is true for men and women of all races over the last 30 years. However, blacks and women with bladder cancer are more likely to die from the disease than white men with bladder cancer are. Smoking, gender, and diet can affect the risk of developing bladder cancer.

Screening for Bladder and Other Urothelial Cancers

There is no standard or routine screening test for bladder cancer. Two tests may be used to screen for bladder cancer in patients who have had bladder cancer in the past:

Cystoscopy is a procedure to look inside the bladder and urethra to check for abnormal areas. A cystoscope (a thin, lighted tube) is inserted through the urethra into the bladder. Tissue samples may be taken for biopsy.

Urine cytology is the examination of urine under a microscope to check for abnormal cells. Hematuria tests may also be used to screen for bladder cancer. Hematuria (red blood cells in the urine) may be caused by cancer or by other conditions. A hematuria test is used to check for blood in a sample of urine by viewing it under a microscope or using a special test strip. The test may be repeated over time.

Risks of Screening for Bladder and Other Urothelial Cancers

Decisions about screening tests can be difficult. Not all screening tests are helpful and most have risks. Before having any screening test, you may want to discuss the test with your doctor. It is important to know the risks of the test and whether it has been proven to reduce the risk of dying from cancer.

False-positive test results can occur: Screening test results may appear to be abnormal even though no cancer is present. A false-positive test result (one that shows there is cancer when there really isn't) can cause anxiety and is usually followed by more tests (such as cystoscopy or other invasive procedures), which also have risks. False-positive results often occur with hematuria testing; blood in the urine is usually caused by conditions other than cancer.

False-negative test results can occur: Screening test results may appear to be normal even though bladder cancer is present. A person who receives a false-negative test result (one that shows there is no cancer when there really is) may delay seeking medical care even if there are symptoms. Your doctor can advise you about your risk for bladder cancer and your need for screening tests.

Section 41.3

Breast Cancer Screening

Excerpted from PDQ® Cancer Information Summary. National Cancer Institute: Bethesda, MD. "Breast Cancer Screening (PDQ®)–Patient Version." Updated March 2010. Available at http://cancer.gov. Accessed April 1, 2011.

Breast cancer is the second leading cause of death from cancer in American women. Women in the United States get breast cancer more than any other type of cancer except for skin cancer. Breast cancer is second only to lung cancer as a cause of cancer death in women. Breast cancer occurs in men also, but the number of cases is small.

Age and health history can affect the risk of developing breast cancer. Anything that increases your chance of getting a disease is called a risk factor. Having a risk factor does not mean that you will get cancer; not having risk factors doesn't mean that you will not get cancer. People who think they may be at risk should discuss this with their doctor.

Breast Cancer Screening

Two tests are commonly used by health care providers to screen for breast cancer:

- **Mammogram:** An x-ray of the breast. This test may find tumors that are too small to feel. A mammogram may also find ductal carcinoma in situ, abnormal cells in the lining of a breast duct, which may become invasive cancer in some women. The ability of a mammogram to find breast cancer may depend on the size of the tumor, the density of the breast tissue, and the skill of the radiologist. Mammograms are less likely to find breast tumors in women younger than 50 years than in older women. This may be because younger women have denser breast tissue that appears white on a mammogram. A tumor also appears white on a mammogram, which makes it hard to find.

- **Clinical breast exam (CBE):** An exam of the breast by a doctor or other health professional. The doctor will carefully feel the breasts and under the arms for lumps or anything else that seems unusual. It is important to know how your breasts usually look and feel.

If you feel any lumps or notice any other changes, talk to your doctor. If a lump or other change is found by mammogram or clinical breast exam, follow-up tests may be needed. If a lump or anything else that seems abnormal is found using one of these two tests, ultrasound may be used to learn more. Ultrasound is not used by itself as a screening test for breast cancer. This is a procedure in which high-energy sound waves (ultrasound) are bounced off internal tissues or organs and make echoes. The echoes form a picture of body tissues called a sonogram.

Other Screening Tests Being Studied in Clinical Trials

MRI (Magnetic Resonance Imaging)

MRI is a procedure that uses a magnet, radio waves, and a computer to make a series of detailed pictures of areas inside the body. This procedure is also called nuclear magnetic resonance imaging (NMRI). MRI does not use any x-rays.

In women with a high inherited risk of breast cancer, screening trials of MRI breast scans have shown that MRI is more sensitive than mammography for finding breast tumors. It is common for MRI breast scan results to appear abnormal even though no cancer is present. Screening studies of breast MRI in women at high inherited risk are ongoing.

In women at average risk for breast cancer, MRI scans may be done to help with diagnosis. MRI may be used to:

- Study lumps in the breast that remain after surgery or radiation therapy.

- Study breast lumps or enlarged lymph nodes found during a clinical breast exam or a breast self-exam that were not seen on mammography or ultrasound.

- Plan surgery for patients with known breast cancer.

Tissue Sampling

Breast tissue sampling is taking cells from breast tissue to examine under a microscope. Abnormal cells in breast fluid have been linked to an increased risk of breast cancer in some studies. Scientists are studying whether breast tissue sampling can be used to find breast cancer at an early stage or predict the risk of developing breast cancer. Three methods of tissue sampling are under study:

- **Fine-needle aspiration:** A thin needle is inserted into the breast tissue around the areola (darkened area around the nipple) to withdraw cells and fluid.

- **Nipple aspiration:** The use of gentle suction to collect fluid through the nipple. This is done with a device similar to the breast pumps used by nursing women.

- **Ductal lavage:** A hair-size catheter (tube) is inserted into the nipple and a small amount of salt water is released into the duct. The water picks up breast cells and is removed.

Risks of Breast Cancer Screening

The risks of breast cancer screening tests include the following:

Finding breast cancer may not improve health or help a woman live longer: Screening may not help you if you have fast-growing breast cancer or if it has already spread to other places in your body. Also, some breast cancers found on a screening mammogram may never cause symptoms or become life-threatening. When such cancers are found, treatment would not help you live longer and may instead cause serious treatment-related side effects. At this time, it is not possible to be sure which breast cancers found by screening will cause symptoms and which breast cancers will not.

False-negative test results can occur: Screening test results may appear to be normal even though breast cancer is present. A woman who receives a false-negative test result (one that shows there is no cancer when there really is) may delay seeking medical care even if she has symptoms.

One in five cancers may be missed by mammography. False-negatives occur more often in younger women than in older women because the breast tissue of younger women is more dense. The size of the tumor, the rate of tumor growth, the level of hormones, such as estrogen and progesterone, in the woman's body, and the skill of the radiologist can also affect the chance of a false-negative result.

False-positive test results can occur: Screening test results may appear to be abnormal even though no cancer is present. A false-positive test result (one that shows there is cancer when there really isn't) can cause anxiety and is usually followed by more tests (such as biopsy), which also have risks.

Most abnormal test results turn out not to be cancer. False-positives are more common in younger women, women who have had previous breast biopsies, women with a family history of breast cancer, and women who take hormones such as estrogen and progesterone. The skill of the doctor also can affect the chance of a false-positive result.

Mammograms expose the breast to radiation: Being exposed to radiation is a risk factor for breast cancer. The risk of developing breast cancer from radiation exposure, such as screening mammograms or x-rays, is greater with higher doses of radiation and in younger women. For women older than 40 years, the benefits of an annual screening mammogram may be greater than the risks from radiation exposure.

The benefits of breast cancer screening may vary among age groups:

- In women who have a life expectancy of five years or less, finding and treating early stage breast cancer may reduce their quality of life without helping them live longer.

- In women older than 65 years, the results of a screening test may lead to more diagnostic tests and anxiety while waiting for the test results. Also, the breast cancers found are usually not life-threatening.

- It has not been shown that women benefit from starting mammography at younger than 40 years.

Routine breast cancer screening is advised for women who have had radiation treatment to the chest, especially at a young age. The benefits and risks of mammograms and MRIs for these women are not known. There is no information on the benefits or risks of breast cancer screening in men.

No matter how old you are, if you have risk factors for breast cancer you should ask for medical advice about when to begin having mammograms and how often to be screened.

Section 41.4

Cervical Cancer Screening

Excerpted from PDQ® Cancer Information Summary. National Cancer Institute: Bethesda, MD. "Cervical Cancer Screening (PDQ®)–Patient Version." Updated May 2010. Available at http://cancer.gov. Accessed April 1, 2011.

Cervical cancer is a disease in which malignant (cancer) cells form in the cervix. The cervix is the lower, narrow end of the uterus (the hollow, pear-shaped organ where a fetus grows). The cervix leads from the uterus to the vagina (birth canal). Cervical cancer usually develops slowly over time. Before cancer appears in the cervix, the cells of the cervix go through changes known as dysplasia, in which cells that are not normal begin to appear in the cervical tissue. Later, cancer cells start to grow and spread more deeply into the cervix and to surrounding areas.

Screening for cervical cancer using the Pap test has decreased the number of new cases of cervical cancer and the number of deaths due to cervical cancer since 1950. Cervical dysplasia occurs more often in women who are in their 20s and 30s. Death from cervical cancer is rare in women younger than 30 years and in women of any age who have regular screenings with the Pap test. The Pap test is used to detect cancer and changes that may lead to cancer. The chance of death from cervical cancer increases with age. It is highest for white women between the ages of 45 and 70 years and for black women in their 70s. Deaths from cervical cancer occur more often in black women than in white women.

Human papillomavirus (HPV) infection is the major risk factor for development of cervical cancer. Although most women with cervical cancer have the human papillomavirus (HPV) infection, not all women with an HPV infection will develop cervical cancer. Many different types of HPV can affect the cervix and only some of them cause abnormal cells that may become cancer. Some HPV infections go away without treatment. HPV infections are spread mainly through sexual contact. Women who become sexually active at a young age and have many sexual partners are at increased risk for HPV infections.

Cervical Cancer Screening

Studies show that screening for cervical cancer helps decrease the number of deaths from the disease. Regular screening of women between the ages of 25 and 60 years with the Pap test decreases their chance of dying from cervical cancer. In women younger than 25 years, screening with the Pap test may show changes in the cells of the cervix that are not cancer but lead to further testing and possibly treatment. Screening with the Pap test is not helpful in women older than 60 years who have had recent negative Pap tests.

Pap Test

A Pap test is commonly used to screen for cervical cancer. A Pap test is a procedure to collect cells from the surface of the cervix and vagina. A piece of cotton, a brush, or a small wooden stick is used to gently scrape cells from the cervix and vagina. The cells are viewed under a microscope to find out if they are abnormal. This procedure is also called a Pap smear. A new method of collecting and viewing cells has been developed, in which the cells are placed into a liquid before being placed on a slide. It is not known if the new method will work better than the standard method to reduce the number of deaths from cervical cancer.

HPV Deoxyribonucleic Acid (DNA) Test

After certain positive Pap test results, an HPV DNA test may be done to find out if the HPV infection that is causing the abnormal cells is one that is linked to cervical cancer. In women aged 30 or older, the HPV DNA test and the Pap test are used to screen for HPV infection. In women younger than 30 years, HPV infections are common but usually do not last long or cause problems.

Risks of Cervical Cancer Screening

Screening tests have risks. The risks of cervical cancer screening include the following:

False-negative test results can occur: Screening test results may appear to be normal even though cervical cancer is present. A woman who receives a false-negative test result (one that shows there is no cancer when there really is) may delay seeking medical care even if she has symptoms.

False-positive test results can occur: Screening test results may appear to be abnormal even though no cancer is present. Also, some abnormal cells in the cervix never become cancer. A false-positive test result (one that shows there is cancer when there really isn't) can cause anxiety and is usually followed by more tests and procedures (such as colposcopy, cryotherapy, or loop electrosurgical excision procedure [LEEP]), which also have risks. The long-term effects of these procedures on fertility and pregnancy are not known.

Women aged 20 to 24 are most likely to have abnormal Pap test results that lead to further testing and treatment. Your doctor can advise you about your risk for cervical cancer and your need for screening tests.

Studies show that the number of cases of cervical cancer and deaths from cervical cancer are greatly reduced by screening with Pap tests. Many doctors recommend a Pap test be done every year. New studies have shown that after a woman has a Pap test and the results show no sign of abnormal cells, the Pap test can be repeated every two to three years.

The Pap test is not a helpful screening test for cervical cancer in the following groups of women:

- Women who are younger than 25 years.

- Women who have had a total hysterectomy (surgery to remove the uterus and cervix) for a condition that is not cancer.

- Women who are aged 60 years or older and have a Pap test result that shows no abnormal cells. These women are very unlikely to have abnormal Pap test results in the future.

The decision about how often to have a Pap test is best made by you and your doctor.

Section 41.5

Colorectal Cancer Screening

Excerpted from PDQ® Cancer Information Summary. National Cancer Institute: Bethesda, MD. "Colorectal Cancer Screening (PDQ®)–Patient Version." Updated April 2010. Available at http://cancer.gov. Accessed April 1, 2011.

Colorectal cancer is a disease in which malignant (cancer) cells form in the tissues of the colon or the rectum. The colon and rectum are parts of the body's digestive system. Colorectal cancer is the second leading cause of death from cancer in the United States. The number of new colorectal cancer cases and the number of deaths from colorectal cancer are decreasing a little bit each year. Colorectal cancer is found more often in men than in women. Age and health history can affect the risk of developing colon cancer.

Colorectal Cancer Screening

Five tests are commonly used to screen for colorectal cancer:

Fecal occult blood test: A fecal occult blood test is a test to check stool (solid waste) for blood that can only be seen with a microscope. Small samples of stool are placed on special cards and returned to the doctor or laboratory for testing. Blood in the stool may be a sign of polyps or cancer.

Sigmoidoscopy: A procedure to look inside the rectum and sigmoid (lower) colon for polyps, abnormal areas, or cancer. A sigmoidoscope is inserted through the rectum into the sigmoid colon. A sigmoidoscope is a thin, tube-like instrument with a light and a lens for viewing. It may also have a tool to remove polyps or tissue samples, which are checked under a microscope for signs of cancer. A sigmoidoscopy and a digital rectal exam (DRE) may be used together to screen for colorectal cancer.

Barium enema: A series of x-rays of the lower gastrointestinal tract. A liquid that contains barium (a silver-white metallic compound) is put into the rectum. The barium coats the lower gastrointestinal tract and x-rays are taken. This procedure is also called a lower gastrointestinal (GI) series.

Colonoscopy: A procedure to look inside the rectum and colon for polyps, abnormal areas, or cancer. A colonoscope is inserted through the rectum into the colon. A colonoscope is a thin, tube-like instrument with a light and a lens for viewing. It may also have a tool to remove polyps or tissue samples, which are checked under a microscope for signs of cancer.

Digital rectal exam (DRE): An exam of the rectum. The doctor or nurse inserts a lubricated, gloved finger into the lower part of the rectum to feel for lumps or anything else that seems unusual.

Screening Tests Being Studied in Clinical Trials

Virtual colonoscopy: A procedure that uses a series of x-rays called computed tomography to make a series of pictures of the colon. A computer puts the pictures together to create detailed images that may show polyps and anything else that seems unusual on the inside surface of the colon. This test is also called colonography or CT colonography. Clinical trials are comparing virtual colonoscopy with commonly used colorectal cancer screening tests. Other clinical trials are testing whether drinking a contrast material that coats the stool, instead of using laxatives to clear the colon, shows polyps clearly.

Deoxyribonucleic acid (DNA) stool test: This test checks DNA in stool cells for genetic changes that may be a sign of colorectal cancer.

Risks of Colorectal Cancer Screening

The following colorectal cancer screening tests have risks:

Fecal occult blood testing: The results of fecal occult blood testing may appear to be abnormal even though no cancer is present. A false-positive test result can cause anxiety and lead to more testing, including colonoscopy or barium enema with sigmoidoscopy.

Sigmoidoscopy: There can be discomfort or pain during sigmoidoscopy. Women may have more pain during the procedure, which may lead them to avoid future screening. Tears in the lining of the colon and bleeding also may occur.

Colonoscopy: Serious complications from colonoscopy are rare, but can include tears in the lining of the colon, bleeding, and problems with the heart or blood vessels. These complications may occur more often in older patients.

Virtual colonoscopy: This procedure often finds problems with organs other than the colon, including the kidneys, chest, liver, ovaries, spleen, and pancreas. Some of these findings lead to more testing. The risks and benefits of this follow-up testing are being studied.

Your doctor can advise you about your risk for colorectal cancer and your need for screening tests.

Section 41.6

Esophageal Cancer Screening

Excerpted from PDQ® Cancer Information Summary. National Cancer Institute: Bethesda, MD. "Esophageal Cancer Screening (PDQ®)– Patient Version." Updated May 2010. Available at: http://cancer.gov. Accessed April 1, 2011.

Esophageal cancer is a disease in which malignant (cancer) cells form in the tissues of the esophagus. The esophagus is the hollow, muscular tube that moves food and liquid from the throat to the stomach. The stomach and esophagus are part of the upper digestive system. The two most common types of esophageal cancer are named for the type of cells that become malignant (cancerous):

- **Squamous cell carcinoma:** Cancer that begins in squamous cells, the thin, flat cells lining the esophagus. This cancer is most often found in the upper and middle part of the esophagus but can occur anywhere along the esophagus. This is also called epidermoid carcinoma.

- **Adenocarcinoma:** Cancer that begins in glandular (secretory) cells. Glandular cells in the lining of the esophagus produce and release fluids such as mucus. Adenocarcinomas usually form in the lower part of the esophagus, near the stomach.

Esophageal cancer is found more often in men. Men are about three times more likely than women to have esophageal cancer. There are more new cases of esophageal adenocarcinoma each year and fewer new cases of squamous cell carcinoma. Squamous cell carcinoma of the esophagus is found more often in blacks than in whites. The chance of developing esophageal cancer increases with age. Smoking, heavy alcohol use, and Barrett esophagus can affect the risk of developing esophageal cancer.

Esophageal Cancer Screening

There is no standard or routine screening test for esophageal cancer. The following tests that may detect (find) esophageal cancer are being studied:

Esophagoscopy: A procedure to look inside the esophagus to check for abnormal areas. An esophagoscope is inserted through the mouth or nose and down the throat into the esophagus. An esophagoscope is a thin, tube-like instrument with a light and a lens for viewing. It may also have a tool to remove tissue samples, which are checked under a microscope for signs of cancer.

Biopsy: The removal of cells or tissues so they can be viewed under a microscope by a pathologist to check for signs of cancer. Taking biopsy samples from several different areas in the lining of the lower part of the esophagus may detect early Barrett esophagus. This procedure may be used for patients who have risk factors for Barrett esophagus.

Brush cytology: A procedure in which cells are brushed from the lining of the esophagus and viewed under a microscope to see if they are abnormal. This may be done during an esophagoscopy.

Balloon cytology: A procedure in which cells are collected from the lining of the esophagus using a deflated balloon that is swallowed by the patient. The balloon is then inflated and pulled out of the esophagus. Esophageal cells on the balloon are viewed under a microscope to see if they are abnormal.

Chromoendoscopy: A procedure in which a dye is sprayed onto the lining of the esophagus during esophagoscopy. Increased staining of certain areas of the lining may be a sign of early Barrett esophagus.

Fluorescence spectroscopy: A procedure that uses a special light to view tissue in the lining of the esophagus. The light probe is passed through an endoscope and shines on the lining of the esophagus. The light given off by the cells lining the esophagus is then measured. Malignant tissue gives off less light than normal tissue.

407

Risks of Esophageal Cancer Screening

The risks of esophageal cancer screening tests include the following:

Finding esophageal cancer may not improve health or help a person live longer: Screening may not improve your health or help you live longer if you have advanced esophageal cancer or if it has already spread to other places in your body. Some cancers never cause symptoms or become life-threatening, but if found by a screening test, the cancer may be treated. It is not known if treatment of these cancers will help you live longer than if no treatment were given, and treatments for cancer may have serious side effects.

False-negative test results can occur: Screening test results may appear to be normal even though esophageal cancer is present. A person who receives a false-negative test result (one that shows there is no cancer when there really is) may delay seeking medical care even if there are symptoms.

False-positive test results can occur: Screening test results may appear to be abnormal even though no cancer is present. A false-positive test result (one that shows there is cancer when there really isn't) can cause anxiety and is usually followed by more tests (such as biopsy), which also have risks.

Side effects may be caused by the test itself: There are rare but serious side effects that may occur with esophagoscopy and biopsy. These include the following:

- A small hole (puncture) in the esophagus
- Problems with breathing
- Heart attack
- Passage of food, water, stomach acid, or vomit into the airway
- Severe bleeding that may need to be treated in a hospital

Section 41.7

Lung Cancer Screening

Excerpted from PDQ® Cancer Information Summary. National Cancer Institute: Bethesda, MD. "Lung Cancer Screening (PDQ®)–Patient Version." Updated March 2010. Available at http://cancer.gov. Accessed April 1, 2011.

Lung cancer is a disease in which malignant (cancer) cells form in the tissues of the lung. The lungs are a pair of cone-shaped breathing organs inside the chest. The lungs bring oxygen into the body when breathing in and send carbon dioxide out of the body when breathing out. There are two types of lung cancer: small cell lung cancer and non-small cell lung cancer. Lung cancer is the leading cause of cancer death in the United States. Lung cancer is the leading cause of cancer death and the most common nonskin cancer in men and women combined in the United States. Tobacco smoking is the most important risk factor for lung cancer.

Two tests have commonly been used to screen for lung cancer. It has not yet been shown that screening for lung cancer with either of the following tests decreases the chance of dying from lung cancer:

Chest x-ray: A chest x-ray is an x-ray of the organs and bones inside the chest. An x-ray is a type of energy beam that can go through the body and onto film, making a picture of areas inside the body.

Sputum cytology: Sputum cytology is a procedure in which a sample of sputum (mucus that is brought up from the lungs by coughing) is viewed under a microscope to check for cancer cells.

New Test Being Studied in Clinical Trials

Spiral computed tomography (CT) scan: A procedure that makes a series of very detailed pictures of areas inside the body using an x-ray machine that scans the body in a spiral path. The pictures are made by a computer linked to the x-ray machine. This procedure is also called a helical CT scan.

Risks of Lung Cancer Screening

The risks of lung cancer screening tests include the following:

Finding lung cancer may not improve health or help you live longer: Screening may not improve your health or help you live longer if you have advanced lung cancer or if it has already spread to other places in your body. Some cancers never cause symptoms or become life-threatening, but if found by a screening test, the cancer may be treated. It is not known if treatment of these cancers would help you live longer than if no treatment were given, and treatments for cancer may have serious side effects.

False-negative test results can occur: Screening test results may appear to be normal even though lung cancer is present. A person who receives a false-negative test result (one that shows there is no cancer when there really is) may delay seeking medical care even if there are symptoms.

False-positive test results can occur: Screening test results may appear to be abnormal even though no cancer is present. A false-positive test result (one that shows there is cancer when there really isn't) can cause anxiety and is usually followed by more tests (such as biopsy), which also have risks. A biopsy to diagnose lung cancer can cause part of the lung to collapse. Sometimes surgery is needed to reinflate the lung.

Chest x-rays expose the chest to radiation: Radiation exposure from chest x-rays may increase the risk of developing certain cancers, such as breast cancer.

Your doctor can advise you about your risk for lung cancer and your need for screening tests.

Section 41.8

Oral Cancer Screening

Excerpted from PDQ® Cancer Information Summary. National Cancer Institute: Bethesda, MD. "Oral Cancer Screening (PDQ®)–Patient Version." Updated June 2009. Available at http://cancer.gov. Accessed April 1, 2011.

Oral cancer is a disease in which malignant (cancer) cells form in the lips, oral cavity, or oropharynx. Most oral cancers start in squamous cells, the thin, flat cells that line the lips, oral cavity, and oropharynx. Cancer that forms in squamous cells is called squamous cell carcinoma. The number of new cases of oral cancer and the number of deaths from oral cancer have been decreasing slowly. Most oral cancers occur in people older than 45 years, and more often in blacks than in whites. Even though the total number of new cases and deaths from oral cancer has decreased slowly over the past 20 years, the number of new cases of oral cancer (especially of the tongue) has been increasing in adults younger than 40 years. Tobacco and alcohol use can affect the risk of developing oral cancer.

Screening for Oral Cancer

There is no standard or routine screening test for oral cancer. Screening for oral cancer may be done during a routine check-up by a dentist or doctor. The exam will include looking for lesions, including areas of leukoplakia (an abnormal white patch of cells) and erythroplakia (an abnormal red patch of cells). Leukoplakia and erythroplakia lesions on the mucous membranes may become cancerous. Higher-risk areas of the mouth that are checked for cancer include the following:

- Floor of the mouth
- Front and sides of the tongue
- Soft palate

If lesions are seen in the mouth, the following procedures may be used to find abnormal tissue that might develop into oral cancer:

- **Toluidine blue stain:** A procedure in which lesions in the mouth are coated with a blue dye. Areas that stain darker are more likely to be cancer or become cancer.

- **Fluorescence staining:** A procedure in which lesions in the mouth are viewed using a special light. After the patient uses a fluorescent mouth rinse, normal tissue looks different from abnormal tissue when seen under the light.

- **Exfoliative cytology:** A procedure to collect cells from the lip or oral cavity. A piece of cotton, a brush, or a small wooden stick is used to gently scrape cells from the lips, tongue, mouth, or throat. The cells are viewed under a microscope to find out if they are abnormal.

- **Brush biopsy:** The removal of cells using a brush that is designed to collect cells from all layers of a lesion. The cells are viewed under a microscope to find out if they are abnormal.

Early-stage oral cancer can be cured, but most oral cancers have already spread to lymph nodes or other areas by the time they are found. No studies have been done to find out if screening would decrease the risk of dying from this disease.

Risks of Oral Cancer Screening

False-negative test results can occur: Screening test results may appear to be normal even though oral cancer is present. A person who receives a false-negative test result (one that shows there is no cancer when there really is) may delay seeking medical care even if there are symptoms. Exfoliative cytology has a high number of false-negative results.

False-positive test results can occur: Screening test results may appear to be abnormal even though no cancer is present. A false-positive test result (one that shows there is cancer when there really isn't) can cause anxiety and is usually followed by more tests and procedures (such as biopsy) which also have risks. Oral exams have a high number of false-positive results.

Section 41.9

Prostate Cancer Screening

This section begins with an excerpt from "Understanding Prostate Changes: A Health Guide for Men," National Cancer Institute (NCI), October 29, 2010; and concludes with text from "What Comes after PSA?" NCI, October 7, 2008.

Types of Tests to Check the Prostate for Cancer

Health history and current symptoms: This first step lets your doctor hear and understand your prostate concerns. You will be asked whether you have symptoms, how long you have had them, and how much they affect your lifestyle. Your personal medical history also includes any risk factors, pain, fever, or trouble passing urine. You may be asked to give a urine sample for testing.

Digital rectal exam (DRE): DRE is a standard way to check the prostate. With a gloved and lubricated finger, your doctor feels the prostate from the rectum. The test lasts about 10–15 seconds.

This exam checks for:

- the size, firmness, and texture of the prostate;

- any hard areas, lumps, or growth spreading beyond the prostate;

- any pain caused by touching or pressing the prostate.

The DRE allows the doctor to feel only one side of the prostate. A prostate-specific antigen (PSA) blood test is another way to help your doctor check the health of your prostate.

PSA test: The U.S. Food and Drug Administration (FDA) has approved the use of the PSA test along with a DRE to help detect prostate cancer in men age 50 and older. PSA is a protein made by prostate cells. It is normally secreted into ducts in the prostate, where it helps make semen, but sometimes it leaks into the blood. When PSA is in the blood, it can be measured with a blood test called the PSA test.

In prostate cancer, more PSA gets into the blood than is normal. However, a high PSA blood level is not proof of cancer, and many other things can cause a false-positive test result. For example, blood PSA levels are often increased in men with prostatitis or BPH. Even things that disturb the prostate gland—such as riding a bicycle or motorcycle, or having a DRE, an orgasm within the past 24 hours, a prostate biopsy, or prostate surgery—may increase PSA levels.

Also, some prostate glands naturally produce more PSA than others. PSA levels go up with age. African-American men tend to have higher PSA levels in general than men of other races. And some drugs, such as finasteride and dutasteride, can cause a man's PSA level to go down. PSA tests are often used to follow men after prostate cancer treatment to check for signs of cancer recurrence.

It is not yet known for certain whether PSA testing to screen for prostate cancer can reduce a man's risk of dying from the disease. Researchers are working to learn more about:

- the PSA test's ability to help doctors tell the difference between prostate cancer and benign prostate problems;

- the best thing to do if a man has a high PSA level.

For now, men and their doctors use PSA readings over time as a guide to see if more follow-up is needed.

What do PSA results mean?

PSA levels are measured in terms of the amount of PSA per volume of fluid tested. Doctors often use a value of four nanograms (ng) or higher per milliliter of blood as a sign that further tests, such as a prostate biopsy, are needed. Your doctor may monitor your PSA velocity, which means the rate of change in your PSA level over time. Rapid increases in PSA readings may suggest cancer. If you have a mildly elevated PSA level, you and your doctor may choose to do PSA tests on a scheduled basis and watch for any change in the PSA velocity.

Free PSA test: This test is used for men who have higher PSA levels. The standard PSA test measures total PSA, which includes both PSA that is attached, or bound, to other proteins and PSA that is free, or not bound. The free PSA test measures free PSA only. Free PSA is linked to benign prostate conditions, such as benign prostatic hyperplasia (BPH), whereas bound PSA is linked to cancer. The percentage of free PSA can help tell what kind of prostate problem you have.

- If both total PSA and free PSA are higher than normal (high percentage of free PSA), this suggests BPH rather than cancer.

- If total PSA is high but free PSA is not (low percentage of free PSA), cancer is more likely. More testing, such as a biopsy, should be done.

You and your doctor should talk about your personal risk and free PSA results. Then you can decide together whether to have follow-up biopsies and, if so, how often. "There is no magic PSA level below which a man can be assured of having no risk of prostate cancer nor above which a biopsy should automatically be performed. A man's decision to have a prostate biopsy requires a thoughtful discussion with his physician, considering not only the PSA level, but also his other risk factors, his overall health status, and how he perceives the risks and benefits of early detection." (Dr. Howard Parnes, Chief of the Prostate and Urologic Cancer Research Group, Division of Cancer Prevention, National Cancer Institute.)

Prostate Biopsy

If your symptoms or test results suggest prostate cancer, your doctor will refer you to a specialist (a urologist) for a prostate biopsy. A biopsy is usually done in the doctor's office.

For a biopsy, small tissue samples are taken directly from the prostate. Your doctor will take samples from several areas of the prostate gland. This can help lower the chance of missing any areas of the gland that may have cancer cells. Like other cancers, prostate cancer can be diagnosed only by looking at tissue under a microscope.

Most men who have biopsies after prostate cancer screening exams do not have cancer. A second opinion is advisable before getting a biopsy.

If a biopsy is positive: A positive test result after a biopsy means prostate cancer is present. A pathologist will check your biopsy sample for cancer cells and will give it a Gleason score. The Gleason score ranges from 2–10 and describes how likely it is that a tumor will spread. The lower the number, the less aggressive the tumor is and the less likely it will spread. Treatment options depend on the stage (or extent) of the cancer (stages range from 1–4), Gleason score, PSA level, your age, and general health. This information will be available from your doctor and is listed on your pathology report.

What Comes after PSA?

When the U.S. Preventive Services Task Force issued new recommendations advising against routine use of prostate-specific antigen

(PSA) testing to screen men aged 75 or older for prostate cancer, it caused some controversy. But at its core, the recommendation emphasized an important fact: Although the PSA test is one of the most commonly used cancer screening tests—approximately two out of every three men aged 50 to 74 have undergone PSA screening in the preceding two years—there is still no hard evidence that it actually saves lives.

In addition, explains Dr. Howard Parnes, chief of the Prostate and Urologic Cancer Research Group in NCI's Division of Cancer Prevention, the NCI-sponsored Prostate Cancer Prevention Trial has shown that "the true prevalence of prostate cancer is much higher than previously thought, and that the lower we set the PSA threshold for recommending biopsy, the more overdiagnosis there will be." Overdiagnosis refers to the detection of cancers that would never become clinically apparent during a man's lifetime, many of which will be treated, often with surgery, accompanied by potentially serious and lifelong side effects.

The overdiagnosis conundrum has been one of the factors driving the search for a new prostate cancer screening test. Progress on that front has been steady but slow. However, the research that has been done, some investigators caution, suggests that the PSA test will not be going away any time soon. But it may, eventually, be combined with some new tests.

Ideally, many prostate cancer researchers say, a new test will not only detect the disease at its earliest stages, but provide a window into a patient's prognosis: Is it an aggressive cancer that requires immediate treatment, or can it be monitored with active surveillance (or watchful waiting) because it's unlikely to ever become life threatening?

Because of the time and expense involved in such trials, it is hoped that novel approaches or study designs can be developed that have a shorter time course and can move new screening tests for prostate cancer into clinical practice more quickly, particularly for men who are at high risk for the disease.

Section 41.10

Skin Cancer Screening

Excerpted from PDQ® Cancer Information Summary. National Cancer Institute: Bethesda, MD. "Skin Cancer Screening (PDQ®)–Patient Version." Updated June 2010. Available at: http://cancer.gov. Accessed April 1, 2011.

Skin cancer is a disease in which malignant (cancer) cells form in the tissues of the skin. The skin is the body's largest organ. It protects against heat, sunlight, injury, and infection. Skin also helps control body temperature and stores water, fat, and vitamin D. The skin has several layers, but the two main layers are the epidermis (upper or outer layer) and the dermis (lower or inner layer). Skin cancer begins in the epidermis, which is made up of three kinds of cells:

- Squamous cells: Thin, flat cells that form the top layer of the epidermis.

- Basal cells: Round cells under the squamous cells.

- Melanocytes: Found in the lower part of the epidermis, these cells make melanin, the pigment that gives skin its natural color. When skin is exposed to the sun, melanocytes make more pigment, causing the skin to tan, or darken.

Skin cancer is the most common cancer in the United States. The three most common types of skin cancer are basal cell carcinoma, squamous cell carcinoma, and melanoma. Basal cell carcinoma is the most common and melanoma is the least common skin cancer. Most basal cell and squamous cell skin cancers can be cured, but people with these types of cancer have a higher risk for developing other skin cancers. Melanoma causes about three-fourths of skin cancer deaths in the United States. Skin color and exposure to sunlight can affect the risk of developing melanoma.

Skin Cancer Screening

Skin examinations are commonly used to screen for melanoma. Regular examination of the skin by both you and your doctor increases the chance of finding melanoma early. Most melanomas that appear in the skin can be seen by the naked eye. Usually, there is a long period of time when the tumor grows beneath the top layer of skin but does not grow into the deeper skin layers. This period of slow growth allows time for skin cancer to be found early. Skin cancer may be cured if the tumor is found before it spreads deeper. Monthly self-examination of the skin may help find changes that should be reported to a doctor. Regular skin checks by a doctor are important for people who have already had skin cancer.

If an area on the skin looks abnormal, a biopsy is usually done. The doctor will remove as much of the suspicious tissue as possible with a local excision. A pathologist then looks at the tissue under a microscope to check for cancer cells. Because it is sometimes difficult to tell if a skin growth is benign (not cancer) or malignant (cancer), you may want to have the biopsy sample checked by a second pathologist.

Risks of Skin Cancer Screening

The risks of melanoma screening tests include the following:

Finding melanoma may not improve health or help a person live longer: Screening may not improve your health or help you live longer if you have advanced melanoma or if it has already spread to other places in your body. Some cancers never cause symptoms or become life-threatening, but if found by a screening test, the cancer may be treated. It is not known if treatment of these cancers would help you live longer than if no treatment were given, and treatments for cancer may have serious side effects.

False-negative test results can occur: Screening test results may appear to be normal even though melanoma is present. A person who receives a false-negative test result (one that shows there is no cancer when there really is) may delay seeking medical care even if there are symptoms.

False-positive test results can occur: Screening test results may appear to be abnormal even though no cancer is present. A false-positive test result (one that shows there is cancer when there really isn't) can cause anxiety and is usually followed by more tests (such as a biopsy), which also have risks.

A biopsy may cause scarring: When a skin biopsy is done, the doctor will try to leave the smallest scar possible, but there is a risk of scarring and infection.

Your doctor can advise you about your risk for skin cancer and your need for screening tests.

Section 41.11

Testicular Cancer Screening

Excerpted from PDQ® Cancer Information Summary. National Cancer Institute: Bethesda, MD. "Testicular Cancer Screening (PDQ®)–Patient Version." Updated June 2009. Available at http://cancer.gov. Accessed April 1, 2011.

Testicular cancer is very rare, but it is the most common cancer found in men between the ages of 15 and 35. Although there has been an increase in the number of new cases in the last 40 years, the number of deaths caused by testicular cancer has decreased greatly because of better treatments for it. A condition called cryptorchidism (an undescended testicle) is a main risk factor for developing testicular cancer.

Testicular Cancer Screening

There is no standard or routine screening test used for early detection of testicular cancer. Most often, testicular cancer is first found by men themselves, either by chance or during self-exam. Sometimes the cancer is found by a doctor during a routine physical exam. No studies have been done to find out if testicular self-exams or regular exams by a doctor would decrease the risk of dying from this disease.

Routine screening probably would not decrease the risk of dying from testicular cancer, partly because it can usually be cured at any stage. However, finding testicular cancer early may make it easier to treat. Less chemotherapy and surgery may be needed, resulting in fewer side effects.

Men who have already had testicular cancer have a higher risk of developing a tumor in the other testicle or in other parts of the body. There is an increased risk of second cancers for at least 35 years after treatment for testicular cancer. Lifelong follow-up exams are very important for men who have been treated for testicular cancer.

Section 41.12

Tumor Markers

What are they?

Tumor markers are substances, usually proteins, that are produced by the body in response to cancer growth or by the cancer tissue itself and that may be detected in blood, urine, or tissue samples. Some tumor markers are specific for a particular type of cancer, while others are seen in several cancer types. Most of the well-known markers may also be elevated in non-cancerous conditions. Consequently, tumor markers alone are not diagnostic for cancer.

There are only a handful of well-established tumor markers that are routinely used by physicians. Many other potential markers are still being researched. Some markers cause great excitement when they are first discovered but, upon further investigation, prove to be no more useful than markers already in use.

The goal is to be able to screen for and diagnose cancer early, when it is the most treatable and before it has had a chance to grow and spread. So far, the only tumor marker to gain wide acceptance as a screening test is prostate specific antigen (PSA) for prostate cancer in men. Even with PSA there is continued debate among experts and national organizations over the usefulness of this test for screening asymptomatic men. Other markers are either not specific enough (too many false positives, leading to expensive and unnecessary follow-up testing) or they are not elevated early enough in the disease process to be useful for screening.

Some people are at a higher risk for particular cancers because they have inherited a genetic mutation. While not considered tumor makers, there are tests that look for these mutations in order to estimate the risk of developing a particular type of cancer. BRCA1 and BRCA2 are examples of gene mutations related to an inherited risk of breast cancer and ovarian cancer.

Table 41.1. Common Tumor Markers Currently in Use

Tumor markers	Cancers	What else?	When/how used	Usual sample
AFP (alpha-fetoprotein)	Liver, germ cell cancer of ovaries or testes	Also elevated during pregnancy	Help diagnose, monitor treatment, and determine recurrence	Blood
B2M (beta-2 microglobulin)	Multiple myeloma and lymphomas	Present in many other conditions, including Crohn disease and hepatitis; often used to determine cause of renal failure	Determine prognosis	Blood
CA 15-3 (cancer antigen 15-3)	Breast cancer and others, including lung, ovarian	Also elevated in benign breast conditions; doctor can use CA 15-3 or CA 27.29 (two different assays for same marker)	Stage disease, monitor treatment, and determine recurrence	Blood
CA 19-9 (cancer antigen 19-9)	Pancreatic, sometimes colorectal and bile ducts	Also elevated in pancreatitis and inflammatory bowel disease	Stage disease, monitor treatment, and determine recurrence	Blood
CA-125 (cancer antigen 125)	Ovarian	Also elevated with endometriosis, some other benign diseases and conditions; not recommended as a general screen	Help diagnose, monitor treatment, and determine recurrence	Blood
Calcitonin	Thyroid medullary carcinoma	Also elevated in pernicious anemia and thyroiditis	Help diagnose, monitor treatment, and determine recurrence	Blood
CEA (carcinoembryonic antigen)	Colorectal, lung, breast, thyroid, pancreatic, liver, cervix, and bladder	Elevated in other conditions such as hepatitis, COPD, colitis, pancreatitis, and in cigarette smokers	Monitor treatment and determine recurrence	Blood
Chromogranin A (CgA)	Neuroendocrine tumors (carcinoid tumors, neuroblastoma)	May be most sensitive tumor marker for carcinoid tumors	To help diagnose and monitor	Blood
Estrogen receptors	Breast	Increased in hormone-dependent cancer	Determine prognosis and guide treatment	Tissue
hCG (human chorionic gonadotropin)	Testicular and trophoblastic disease	Elevated in pregnancy, testicular failure	Help diagnose, monitor treatment, and determine recurrence	Blood, urine
Her-2/neu	Breast	Oncogene that is present in multiple copies in 20–30% of invasive breast cancer	Determine prognosis and guide treatment	Tissue
Monoclonal immunoglobulins	Multiple myeloma and Waldenström's macroglobulinemia	Overproduction of an immunoglobulin or antibody, usually detected by protein electrophoresis	Help diagnose, monitor treatment, and determine recurrence	Blood, urine
Progesterone receptors	Breast	Increased in hormone-dependent cancer	Determine prognosis and guide treatment	Tissue

421

Table 41.1. *continued*

Tumor markers	Cancers	What else?	When/how used	Usual sample
PSA (prostate specific antigen), total and free	Prostate	Elevated in benign prostatic hyperplasia, prostatitis and with age	Screen for and help diagnose, monitor treatment, and determine recurrence	Blood
Thyroglobulin	Thyroid	Used after thyroid is removed to evaluate treatment	Determine recurrence	Blood
Other Tumor Markers Less Widely Used				
BTA (bladder tumor antigen)	Bladder	Not widely available, but gaining acceptance	Help diagnose and determine recurrence	Urine
CA 72-4 (cancer antigen 72-4)	Ovarian	No evidence that it is better than CA-125 but may be useful when combined with it; still being studied	Help diagnose	Blood
Des-gamma-carboxy prothrombin (DCP)	Hepatocellular carcinoma (HCC)	New test; often used along with an imaging study plus AFP and/or AFP-L3% to evaluate if someone with chronic liver disease has developed HCC	To evaluate risk of developing HCC; to evaluate treatment; to monitor for recurrence	Blood
EGFR (Her-1)	Solid tumors, such as of the lung (non small cell), head and neck, colon, pancreas, or breast	Not available in every laboratory	Guide treatment and determine prognosis	Tissue
NSE (neuron-specific enolase)	Neuroblastoma, small cell lung cancer	May be better than CEA for following this particular kind of lung cancer	Monitor treatment	Blood
NMP22	Bladder	Not widely used	Help diagnose and determine recurrence	Urine
Prostate-specific membrane antigen (PSMA)	Prostate	Not widely used; levels increase normally with age	Help diagnose	Blood
Prostatic acid phosphatase (PAP)	Metastatic prostate cancer, myeloma, lung cancer	Not widely used anymore; elevated in prostatitis and other conditions	Help diagnose	Blood
S-100	Metastatic melanoma	Not widely used	Help diagnose	Blood
Soluble mesothelin-related peptides (SMRP)	Mesothelioma	Often used in conjunction with imaging tests	To monitor progression or recurrence	Blood
TA-90	Metastatic melanoma	Not widely used, being studied	Help diagnose	Blood

Why are they done?

Tumor markers are not diagnostic in themselves. A definitive diagnosis of cancer is made by looking at tissue biopsy specimens under a microscope. However, tumor markers provide information that can be used to do the following:

- **Screen:** Most markers are not suited for general screening, but some may be used in people with a strong family history of a particular cancer. As mentioned, PSA testing may be used to screen for prostate cancer.

- **Diagnose:** In a person who has symptoms, tumor markers may be used to help identify the source of the cancer, such as CA-125 for ovarian cancer, and to help differentiate it from other conditions. Remember that tumor markers cannot diagnose cancer by themselves but aid in this process.

- **Stage:** If a person does have cancer, tumor marker elevations can be used to help determine how far the cancer has spread into other tissues and organs.

- **Determine prognosis:** Some tumor markers can be used to help doctors determine how aggressive a cancer is likely to be.

- **Guide treatment:** A few tumor markers, such as Her2/neu, will give doctors information about what treatments their patients may respond to (for instance, breast cancer patients who are Her2/neu positive are more likely to respond to Herceptin treatment).

- **Monitor treatment:** Tumor markers can be used to monitor the effectiveness of treatment, especially in advanced cancers. If the marker level drops, the treatment is working; if it stays elevated, adjustments are needed. The information must be used with care, however, since other conditions can sometimes cause tumor markers to rise or fall.

- **Determine recurrence:** Currently, one of the most important uses for tumor markers is to monitor for cancer recurrence. If a tumor marker is elevated before treatment, low after treatment, and then begins to rise over time, then it is likely that the cancer is returning. (If it remains elevated after surgery, then chances are that not all of the cancer was removed.)

Chapter 42

Celiac Disease Tests

What is celiac disease?

Celiac disease is a digestive disease that damages the small intestine and interferes with absorption of nutrients from food. People who have celiac disease cannot tolerate gluten, a protein in wheat, rye, and barley. Gluten is found mainly in foods but may also be found in everyday products such as medicines, vitamins, and lip balms.

Celiac disease is both a disease of malabsorption—meaning nutrients are not absorbed properly—and an abnormal immune reaction to gluten. Celiac disease is genetic, meaning it runs in families. Sometimes the disease is triggered—or becomes active for the first time—after surgery, pregnancy, childbirth, viral infection, or severe emotional stress.

Recognizing celiac disease can be difficult because some of its symptoms are similar to those of other diseases. Celiac disease can be confused with irritable bowel syndrome, iron-deficiency anemia caused by menstrual blood loss, inflammatory bowel disease, diverticulitis, intestinal infections, and chronic fatigue syndrome. As a result, celiac disease has long been underdiagnosed or misdiagnosed. As doctors become more aware of the many varied symptoms of the disease and reliable blood tests become more available, diagnosis rates are increasing.

This chapter begins with excerpts from "Celiac Disease," National Institute of Diabetes and Digestive and Kidney Diseases (NIDDK), September 2008; and concludes with "Testing for Celiac Disease," under the heading "Serologic and Genetic Testing for Celiac Disease," NIDDK, April 2009.

425

Intestinal Biopsy

If blood tests and symptoms suggest celiac disease, a biopsy of the small intestine is performed to confirm the diagnosis. During the biopsy, the doctor removes tiny pieces of tissue from the small intestine to check for damage to the villi. To obtain the tissue sample, the doctor eases a long, thin tube called an endoscope through the patient's mouth and stomach into the small intestine. The doctor then takes the samples using instruments passed through the endoscope.

Dermatitis Herpetiformis

Dermatitis herpetiformis (DH) is an intensely itchy, blistering skin rash that affects 15–25% of people with celiac disease. The rash usually occurs on the elbows, knees, and buttocks. Most people with DH have no digestive symptoms of celiac disease.

DH is diagnosed through blood tests and a skin biopsy. If the antibody tests are positive and the skin biopsy has the typical findings of DH, patients do not need to have an intestinal biopsy. Both the skin disease and the intestinal disease respond to a gluten-free diet and recur if gluten is added back into the diet. The rash symptoms can be controlled with antibiotics such as dapsone. Because dapsone does not treat the intestinal condition, people with DH must maintain a gluten-free diet.

Screening

Screening for celiac disease means testing for the presence of autoantibodies in the blood in people without symptoms. Americans are not routinely screened for celiac disease. However, because celiac disease is hereditary, family members of a person with the disease may wish to be tested. Four to 12% of an affected person's first-degree relatives will also have the disease.

Serologic and Genetic Testing for Celiac Disease

Intestinal biopsy is the gold standard for diagnosing celiac disease, but serologic tests provide an effective first step in identifying biopsy candidates. In addition, genetic tests that confirm the presence or absence of specific genes associated with celiac disease may be useful in some circumstances. However, serologic and genetic tests are adjuncts to, not replacements for, biopsies. If serologic or genetic tests indicate the possibility of celiac disease, a biopsy should be done promptly and before initiating any change in the patient's diet.

Serologic Tests

Serologic tests look for three antibodies common in celiac disease: anti-tissue transglutaminase (tTG) antibodies, endomysial antibodies (EMA), and antigliadin antibodies (AGA). The most sensitive antibody tests are of the immunoglobulin A (IgA) class, but immunoglobulin G (IgG) tests may be used in patients with IgA deficiency. Because no one serologic test is ideal, panels are often used. However, the tests included in a celiac panel vary by lab and may include one or more that are unwarranted. The American Gastroenterological Association recommends beginning with tTG in the clinical setting.[1] For accurate diagnostic test results, patients must be on a gluten-containing diet.

Anti-tissue transglutaminase (tTG) antibody: The tTG test is an enzyme-linked immunosorbent assay (ELISA) test. The tTG test has a sensitivity of more than 90%, yielding few false negative results. The test also has a specificity of more than 95%, meaning it yields few false positive results.[1] Point-of-care tTG tests have been developed but are not yet approved for use by clinicians in the United States.

Endomysial antibodies (EMA): The test for EMA is slightly less sensitive than tTG but is highly specific for celiac disease, approaching 100% accuracy.[2] EMA is measured by indirect immunofluorescent assay, a more expensive and time-consuming process than ELISA testing. In addition, the EMA test is subject to operator interpretation, making the results more subjective than those for tTG.

Some studies show the titers, or relative concentrations, of tTG and EMA are correlated with the degree of intestinal damage, making these tests less sensitive among patients with milder celiac disease.[3]

Antigliadin antibodies (AGA): Tests for AGA are not sensitive or specific enough for routine use. However, they may be useful for screening children younger than 18 months old in whom tTG and EMA tests may yield false negative results.[2]

A new generation of tests that use deaminated gliadin peptides (DGP) have sensitivity and specificity that are substantially better than the older gliadin tests.[4] DGP tests are more accurate than tTG and AGA and may be the most reliable tests to detect celiac disease in people with IgA deficiency.

IgA deficiency: Between 2% and 3% of celiac patients have selective IgA deficiency—a rate about ten times higher than in the general population. If IgA, tTG, or IgA EMA are negative but celiac disease is still suspected, total IgA should be measured to identify selective

IgA deficiency. In cases of IgA deficiency, IgG tTG or DGP-IgG should be measured.

Genetic Screening Tests

Nearly all people with celiac disease have gene pairs that encode for at least one of the human leukocyte antigen (HLA) gene variants, or alleles, designated *HLA-DQ2* or *HLA-DQ8*. However, these alleles are common. They are found in about 40% of the general U.S. population, and most people with these alleles do not have celiac disease. Negative findings for *HLA-DQ2* and *HLA-DQ8* can essentially rule out current or future celiac disease in patients for whom other tests, including biopsy, do not provide a clear diagnostic result.

References

1. American Gastroenterological Association. AGA Institute medical position statement on the diagnosis and management of celiac disease. *Gastroenterology*. 2006;131:1977–1980.

2. Green PHR, Cellier C. Medical progress: celiac disease. *The New England Journal of Medicine*. 2007;357:1731–1743.

3. Tursi A, Brandimarte G, Giorgetti GM. Prevalence of anti-tissue transglutaminase antibodies in different degrees of intestinal damage in celiac disease. *Journal of Clinical Gastroenterology*. 2003;36(3):219–221.

4. Rashtak S, Ettore MW, Homburger HA, Murray JA. Combination testing for antibodies in the diagnosis of celiac disease: comparison of multiplex immunoassay and ELISA methods. *Alimentary Pharmacology & Therapeutics*. 2008;28(6):805–813.

Chapter 43

Cystic Fibrosis (CF) Tests

Chapter Contents

Section 43.1

Sputum CF Respiratory Screen

What It Is

Kids with cystic fibrosis (CF) tend to get frequent respiratory infections, sometimes caused by bacteria or fungi. A sputum (mucus) CF respiratory screen or culture helps doctors detect and identify these bacteria or fungi so they can prescribe effective antibiotics.

Why It's Done

A sputum culture can help identify specific causes of infections in the lungs and airways. Such infections can lead to coughing that produces yellow, greenish, or blood-tinged sputum, in addition to fever and difficulty breathing.

Preparation

Before the test, be sure to tell the doctor whether your child has taken antibiotics recently. The best time for testing is usually in the morning, before your child has had anything to eat or drink. Also, make sure your child doesn't use mouthwash before the test because it may contain antibacterial ingredients that could affect results.

The Procedure

Your child will be asked to rinse his or her mouth out with water, then breathe deeply and cough deeply to produce sputum from the airway.

You or the health professional helping your child may need to gently tap on your child's chest to loosen the sputum in the lungs. If your child can't produce a sample, the lab technician may need to use a tongue depressor to stimulate a cough, or your child may need to inhale a mist solution to help produce a cough.

If your child is scheduled for a bronchoscopy (a test done with a small telescope to evaluate the upper airway and bronchi), a sputum screen is likely to be done at this time.

What to Expect

Your child may experience mild discomfort when taking a deep breath or coughing. If your child inhales the mist solution, the urge to cough may be strong. It may take several attempts at coughing to produce the amount of sputum needed for the test.

Getting the Results

The sputum sample is collected into a sterile container and sent to a laboratory. The sample is then placed on a special plate that enables growth of certain bacteria and fungi if an infection is present.

If your child has a bacterial infection, the organisms may need 48 hours to grow. Fungi need a week or longer. These organisms will be identified under a microscope or through chemical tests. If the tests indicate an infection, an additional 1–2 days may be required to determine which antibiotic is best suited to treat it.

Risks

Coughing to produce the sputum specimen may be mildly uncomfortable, but there are no risks associated with this procedure.

Helping Your Child

Explaining the test in terms your child can understand might help ease any fear. Also reassure your child that the procedure doesn't hurt.

If you have questions about the sputum respiratory screen, speak with your doctor.

Section 43.2

Sweat Electrolytes Test

Sweat electrolytes is a test that measures the level of chloride in sweat. Although genetic tests have become important methods for determining whether a child has cystic fibrosis, the sweat chloride test remains important.

How the Test is Performed

In the first part of the test, a colorless, odorless chemical that causes sweating is applied to a small area on an arm or leg. An electrode is then attached to the arm or leg, which allows the technician to apply a weak electrical current to the area to stimulate sweating. People may feel a tingling sensation in the area, or a feeling of warmth. This part of the procedure lasts approximately five minutes.

The next part of the test involves cleaning the stimulated area and collecting the sweat on a piece of filter paper or gauze, or in a plastic coil. After 30 minutes, the collected sweat is sent to a hospital laboratory for analysis. The entire collection procedure takes about one hour.

How to Prepare for the Test

No special preparation is necessary. Make sure the center where the test is being performed is a cystic fibrosis testing center.

How the Test Will Feel

Though the test is not painful, some people describe a tingling sensation at the site of the electrode. In smaller children or infants, the sensation can cause irritability or discomfort.

Why the Test Is Performed

Sweat testing is the standard method for diagnosing cystic fibrosis. People with cystic fibrosis have higher amounts of sodium and chloride in their sweat, which the test can detect. Some people are referred for testing because of symptoms such as poor growth, many respiratory infections, or foul-smelling stools. In some states, newborn screening programs test for cystic fibrosis, and the sweat test is used to confirm these results.

Normal Results

- A sweat chloride test result less than or equal to 39 milliequivalent per liter (mEq/L) in an infant over six months old probably means cystic fibrosis is not present.

- A result between 40–59 mEq/L does not give a clear diagnosis. Further testing is needed.

- If the result is 60 mEq/L or greater, cystic fibrosis is present.

Normal value ranges may vary slightly among different laboratories. Talk to your doctor about the meaning of your specific test results.

Alternative Names

Sweat test, sweat chloride, iontophoretic sweat test

Chapter 44

Diabetes Tests

Chapter Contents

Section 44.1

Screening Tests for Diabetes

This section begins with excerpts from "Diagnosis of Diabetes,"
National Institute of Diabetes and Digestive and Kidney Diseases
(NIDDK), October 2008; and concludes with excerpts from "A1C Test
Recommended for Diagnosis of Diabetes," NIDDK, August 2010.

How are diabetes and pre-diabetes diagnosed?

The following tests are used for diagnosis:

- A fasting plasma glucose (FPG) test measures blood glucose in a
  person who has not eaten anything for at least eight hours. This
  test is used to detect diabetes and pre-diabetes.

- An oral glucose tolerance test (OGTT) measures blood glucose
  after a person fasts at least eight hours and two hours after the
  person drinks a glucose-containing beverage. This test can be
  used to diagnose diabetes and pre-diabetes.

- A random plasma glucose test, also called a casual plasma glucose test, measures blood glucose without regard to when the
  person being tested last ate. This test, along with an assessment of symptoms, is used to diagnose diabetes but not pre-
  diabetes.

Test results indicating that a person has diabetes should be confirmed with a second test on a different day.

Fasting plasma glucose test: The FPG test is the preferred test
for diagnosing diabetes because of its convenience and low cost. However, it will miss some diabetes or pre-diabetes that can be found with
the OGTT. The FPG test is most reliable when done in the morning.

- People with a fasting glucose level of 100 to 125 milligrams
  per deciliter (mg/dL) have a form of pre-diabetes called impaired fasting glucose (IFG). Having IFG means a person has
  an increased risk of developing type 2 diabetes but does not
  have it yet.

- A level of 126 mg/dL or above, confirmed by repeating the test on another day, means a person has diabetes.

Oral glucose tolerance test (OGTT): Research has shown that the OGTT is more sensitive than the FPG test for diagnosing pre-diabetes, but it is less convenient to administer. The OGTT requires fasting for at least eight hours before the test. The plasma glucose level is measured immediately before and two hours after a person drinks a liquid containing 75 grams of glucose dissolved in water.

- If the blood glucose level is between 140 and 199 mg/dL two hours after drinking the liquid, the person has a form of pre-diabetes called impaired glucose tolerance (IGT). Having IGT, like having IFG, means a person has an increased risk of developing type 2 diabetes but does not have it yet.

- A 2-hour glucose level of 200 mg/dL or above, confirmed by repeating the test on another day, means a person has diabetes.

Gestational diabetes is also diagnosed based on plasma glucose values measured during the OGTT, preferably by using 100 grams of glucose in liquid for the test. Blood glucose levels are checked four times during the test. If blood glucose levels are above normal at least twice during the test, the woman has gestational diabetes.

Random plasma glucose test: A random, or casual, blood glucose level of 200 mg/dL or higher, plus the presence of the following symptoms, can mean a person has diabetes:

- increased urination

- increased thirst

- unexplained weight loss

Table 44.1. Gestational Diabetes: Above-Normal Results for the OGTT*

When	Plasma Glucose Result (mg/dL)
Fasting	95 or higher
At 1 hour	180 or higher
At 2 hours	155 or higher
At 3 hours	140 or higher

Note: Some laboratories use other numbers for this test.
*These numbers are for a test using a drink with 100 grams of glucose.

Other symptoms can include fatigue, blurred vision, increased hunger, and sores that do not heal. The doctor will check the person's blood glucose level on another day using the FPG test or the OGTT to confirm the diagnosis.

A1C Test Recommended for Diagnosis of Diabetes

The A1C test, long used as a diabetes management tool, is now recommended by the American Diabetes Association (ADA) for use in the diagnosis of diabetes and pre-diabetes. The test is an alternative to standard glucose testing with the fasting plasma glucose (FPG) test and the oral glucose tolerance test (OGTT). The recommendation was made in the ADA's "Standards of Medical Care in Diabetes–2010," published in the January 2010 issue of *Diabetes Care*.

Also called the hemoglobin A1C test or the glycated hemoglobin test, the A1C test provides an estimate of average blood glucose levels over the preceding 2–3 months. A normal A1C level is around 5%. An A1C level of 6.5% or above indicates diabetes. An A1C level of 5.7% to 6.4% is considered pre-diabetes.

Although the A1C test is not more accurate than the FPG test and the OGTT, it does not require fasting and can be measured at any time of day. Experts hope the convenience of the test will result in more people who are at risk of diabetes or pre-diabetes being tested, thus reducing the number of people with undiagnosed diabetes in the United States.

The ADA recommends that when used for diagnosis, the A1C test should be performed in a laboratory using a method certified by the National Glycohemoglobin Standardization Program (NGSP). A1C tests done in doctors' offices—point of care tests—are useful in guiding therapy but are not sufficiently accurate to be used for diagnosis of diabetes. The A1C test should not be used to diagnose diabetes in people with conditions that shorten red blood cell survival, including certain types of anemia and pregnancy.

Section 44.2

Glucose Meters Monitor Blood Sugar Levels

This section includes excerpts from "Getting Up to Date on Glucose Meters," U.S. Food and Drug Administration (FDA), February 23, 2009; and excerpts from "Home Healthcare Medical Devices: Blood Glucose Meters–Getting the Most Out of Your Meter," FDA, July 16, 2009.

Note: The Food and Drug Administration (FDA) is reminding people with diabetes to use only the test strips that are recommended for use with their glucose meter. FDA is aware of instances where incorrect results were obtained when brands and models of meters and test strips were not used in proper combination.

Using a glucose meter to monitor blood sugar is a daily part of life for millions of Americans. Glucose meters are usually small battery-operated devices, which make it convenient for people to check their glucose levels anywhere. Most work by reading a drop of blood the user has placed on a disposable test strip.

To begin testing, users place the test strip into a slot in the meter, prick a fingertip, and then place a drop of blood onto the strip. Before pricking the skin, the user should clean the selected testing site to ensure it is free of sugar residues. If the site is not clean, the readings may not be accurate.

In a short time, the meter will show a result in its digital display window. Users record their test results and talk with their health care provider to help with overall disease management. Users may also test control materials to ensure that the meter and test strip are working correctly.

FDA reviews all glucose meters and test strips before they can be marketed to the public. The agency also requires that manufacturers demonstrate that their test system provides acceptable accuracy and consistency of results. Recently, we have seen the emergence of advanced glucose meters that include features such as download capabilities that allow the transfer of test results to a home computer. Some meters can now test blood taken not from the fingertips, but from "alternate sites" such as the forearm and palm.

Tips for Proper Use

Read instructions carefully. Glucose meters and test strips must come with instructions for use. Your user manual should also include a toll-free phone number that you can use to contact the manufacturer. How often you use your glucose meter, and the results you should expect, should be based on the recommendations of your health care provider.

Use the test strips that are recommended for your glucose meter. It is important to only use the test strips that are specified for your glucose meter. Otherwise, the device may fail to give results or may generate inaccurate results.

Know that readings taken from "alternate sites" may not always be as accurate as readings from the fingertips. These readings can differ at times when glucose levels are changing rapidly. This is common after a meal, after taking insulin, during exercise, or when you are ill or under stress.

Use blood from a fingertip rather than an alternate site if you think your blood glucose is low, you do not normally have symptoms when your blood glucose is low, or the results from the alternate site does not match how you are feeling.

Know the factors that affect meter accuracy. These may include:

- testing conducted on unclean skin;
- improper storage of test strips;
- the amount of red blood cells (hematocrit) in the blood;
- other substances present in the blood such as uric acid, glutathione, and vitamin C;
- altitude, temperature, and humidity;
- use of test strips developed as a less expensive option than the strips intended for a certain meter;
- test strips that cannot distinguish between glucose and other sugars.

Perform quality-control checks with test control solutions to ensure that the test strips and meter are working properly together. Some meters may also provide electronic test strips that induce a signal to indicate if the meter (and only the meter) is working properly. In addition, perform quality control checks with control solutions regularly to ensure the meter is working properly.

Ask your health care provider to watch you test yourself. He or she can tell you if you are using the meter correctly.

Know when and how to clean your meter. Some meters need regular cleaning. Others do not need regular cleaning, but contain electronic alerts indicating when you should clean them. You should follow the directions given in the manual on how to clean the meter. Only the manufacturer can clean some meters.

Understand what the meter display means. The range of glucose values can be different among meters. Be sure you know how high and low glucose values are displayed on your meter. Sometimes they are displayed as LO or HI when the glucose level is beyond the range than the meter can measure.

Getting the Most Out of Your Meter

It is important to test your blood glucose (sugar) accurately so you can manage your blood glucose levels. Keeping your blood glucose under control helps you feel better and lowers the risk of blindness, kidney disease, and nerve damage.

Preparing to Test

- Read and save all instructions for your meter and test strips.

- Watch and practice with an experienced blood glucose meter user, a diabetes educator, or a health care professional. Do not be afraid to ask questions.

- Wash your hands. Even small amounts of food or sugar on your fingers can affect your results.

- Read the test strip packaging to make sure the strips will work with your meter.

- Do not use test strips from a cracked or damaged bottle.

- Do not use test strips that have passed their expiration dates.

- Make sure you have entered the correct calibration code (if your meter requires one).

Testing Your Blood Glucose

- Use the correct blood drop size. If there is not enough blood on the test strip, the meter may not read the blood glucose level accurately. Repeat the test if you have any doubts.

- Let the blood flow freely from your fingertip; do not squeeze your finger. Squeezing your finger can affect the results.

- Use a whole test strip each time you use your meter.

- Insert the test strip into the meter until you feel it stop against the end of the meter guide.

Maintaining Your Blood Glucose Meter

- Keep your meter clean.

- Test your meter regularly with control solution.

- Keep extra batteries charged and ready.

- Store your meter and supplies properly. Heat and humidity can damage test strips.

- Replace the bottle cap promptly after removing a test strip.

Following Up

- Take your meter with you when you visit your doctor so you can compare it with your laboratory results.

- Talk with your doctor or call the manufacturer's toll-free phone number if you are having problems with your meter.

Blood Glucose Meters Are Not Perfect

Although blood glucose meters are generally reliable and help to manage diabetes, they are not perfect. The technology used in blood glucose meters is not as accurate as testing done in a hospital or a doctor's office.

Your blood glucose meter may give a wrong reading if you are dehydrated, are going into shock, or have a high red blood cell count (hematocrit). Even a very low blood glucose level can cause an incorrect reading.

If you suspect your blood glucose is too low or too high, call your doctor or go to an emergency room immediately—even if your meter shows that everything is fine.

Section 44.3

Continuous Glucose Monitoring

Excerpted from "Continuous Glucose Monitoring," National Institute of
Diabetes and Digestive and Kidney Diseases (NIDDK), October 2008.

What is continuous glucose monitoring?

Continuous glucose monitoring (CGM) systems use a tiny sensor
inserted under the skin to check glucose levels in tissue fluid. The sensor stays in place for several days to a week and then must be replaced.
A transmitter sends information about glucose levels via radio waves
from the sensor to a pager-like wireless monitor. The user must check
blood samples with a glucose meter to program the devices. Because
currently approved CGM devices are not as accurate and reliable as
standard blood glucose meters, users should confirm glucose levels
with a meter before making a change in treatment.

CGM systems are more expensive than conventional glucose monitoring, but they may enable better glucose control. CGM devices produced by Abbott, DexCom, and Medtronic have been approved by the
U.S. Food and Drug Administration (FDA) and are available by prescription. These devices provide real-time measurements of glucose
levels, with glucose levels displayed at five-minute or one-minute intervals. Users can set alarms to alert them when glucose levels are too
low or too high. Special software is available to download data from the
devices to a computer for tracking and analysis of patterns and trends,
and the systems can display trend graphs on the monitor screen.

What are the prospects for an artificial pancreas?

To overcome the limitations of current insulin therapy, researchers
have long sought to link glucose monitoring and insulin delivery by
developing an artificial pancreas. An artificial pancreas is a system
that will mimic, as closely as possible, the way a healthy pancreas
detects changes in blood glucose levels and responds automatically
to secrete appropriate amounts of insulin. Although not a cure, an
artificial pancreas has the potential to significantly improve diabetes

care and management and to reduce the burden of monitoring and managing blood glucose.

The first pairing of a CGM system with an insulin pump—the MiniMed Paradigm REAL-Time System—is not an artificial pancreas, but it does represent the first step in joining glucose monitoring and insulin delivery systems using the most advanced technology available. Additional CGM devices are being developed and tested.

Chapter 45

Hearing Assessments

Difference between Hearing Screening and Hearing Evaluation

The difference between hearing screening and hearing evaluation can sometimes be confusing. A hearing screening is usually a preliminary step in which an individual's hearing is checked to see if further evaluation is required. In other words, hearing screening is a quick and cost-effective way to separate people into two groups: a pass group and a fail group. Those who pass hearing screenings are presumed to have no hearing loss. Those who fail are in need of more detailed hearing evaluation by a qualified audiologist.

It is recommended that all hearing screening programs be conducted under the supervision of an audiologist holding the American Speech-Language-Hearing Association (ASHA) Certificate of Clinical Competence (CCC).

A hearing evaluation is an in-depth assessment of an individual's hearing by an audiologist. The purpose of this evaluation is to determine the nature and degree of the hearing loss and the best treatment options. Audiologists use a number of different tests in this evaluation.

Text in this chapter is reprinted with permission from "Hearing Screening and Testing," available from the website of the American Speech-Language-Hearing Association: http://www.asha.org/public/hearing/testing/assess.htm. © 2011 American Speech-Language-Hearing Association. All rights reserved. For additional information, or to use the American Speech-Language-Hearing Association's professional referral service to locate an audiologist near you, visit www.asha.org.

Hearing Screening

Newborns and Infants

Today, most hospitals screen babies' hearing shortly after they are born. Failing the hearing screening does not necessarily mean that the baby has a hearing loss. Not all babies pass the hearing screening the first time. Infants who do not pass a screening are usually given a second screening to confirm the findings.

If your baby has failed a hearing screening, you will be referred to a pediatric audiologist for a more thorough hearing test. This is called a hearing evaluation. Keep in mind that an audiologic evaluation is much more than just a hearing test.

Infant screening is very important because, without such programs, the average age of detection of significant hearing loss is approximately 14 months. When hearing loss is detected late, language development is delayed, affecting a child's ability to learn and perform in school. Even if your infant passes screening, hearing loss may develop later in life. If you have any concerns about your child's hearing, talk to your doctor and request a hearing evaluation with a certified audiologist.

The Individuals with Disabilities Education Act (IDEA) requires that infants and toddlers with disabilities be identified and provided appropriate screening. You should contact your local school district or your state or local health department to find out how to obtain screenings/evaluations and intervention services through your state's Early Intervention program.

The screening procedures for newborns and infants are simple and painless, and can be done while the infant is resting quietly. The two common screening methods used with infants are otoacoustic emissions (OAEs) and auditory brainstem response (ABR). These tools can detect hearing loss averaging 30 to 40 decibels (dB) or more in the frequency region important for speech recognition (approximately 500–4000 Hertz [Hz]).

Older Children and Adults

In the case of older children and adults, the most commonly used initial screen involves a pure-tone test. School age children should be screened periodically through their school. Adults are often screened at their doctor's office or community health fairs. You should be wary of anyone who offers to screen your hearing over the telephone.

Who Should Be Screened for Hearing Loss?

People of any age can be screened for hearing loss. Newborn infants are now routinely screened before leaving the hospital. Most preschoolers and school-age children are screened periodically at their schools or in their doctors' offices. Adults can receive screenings from their doctor or at health fairs.

Hearing loss increases as a function of age, especially for frequencies of 2000 Hertz (Hz) and above. Sounds above 2000 Hz are the soft consonant sounds such as /s/ in sun and /th/ in thumb. While more than 30% of people over age 65 have some type of hearing loss, 14% of those between 45 and 64 have hearing loss. Close to eight million people between the ages of 18 and 44 have hearing loss. Adults should be screened at least every decade through age 50 and at three-year intervals thereafter.

Certainly, anytime you have a concern about your hearing or your child's hearing, you should ask your doctor about getting a hearing screening. Anyone failing a hearing screening should be referred to a certified audiologist for a more comprehensive audiologic (hearing) evaluation. The follow-up evaluation should be conducted as soon as possible after the failed hearing screening and no more than three months later.

Self-Test for Hearing Loss

You can use this self-administered test as an initial screen for yourself or your child and to find out if an audiologic (hearing) evaluation is needed.

Does my child have a hearing loss that needs to be evaluated by a professional?

If you observe any of the following behaviors or symptoms of hearing loss, you should consider having your child's hearing evaluated further by a certified audiologist:

- Your child is inconsistently responding to sound.

- Language and speech development is delayed.

- Speech is unclear.

- Volume is turned up high on electronic equipment (radio, television, CD player, and so forth).

- Your child does not follow directions.

447

- Your child often says, "Huh?"

- Your child does not respond when called.

Do I have a hearing loss that needs to be evaluated by a professional?

If you answer yes to more than two of the following questions, you should have your hearing evaluated further by a certified audiologist:

- Do you have a problem hearing over the telephone?

- Do you hear better through one ear than the other when you are on the telephone?

- Do you have trouble following the conversation with two or more people talking at the same time?

- Do people complain that you turn the television volume up too high?

- Do you have to strain to understand conversation?

- Do you have trouble hearing in a noisy background?

- Do you have trouble hearing in restaurants?

- Do you have dizziness, pain, or ringing in your ears?

- Do you find yourself asking people to repeat themselves?

- Do family members or coworkers remark about your missing what has been said?

- Do many people you talk to seem to mumble (or not speak clearly)?

- Do you misunderstand what others are saying and respond inappropriately?

- Do you have trouble understanding the speech of women and children?

- Do people get annoyed because you misunderstand what they say?

Audiologic (Hearing) Evaluation

On your first visit to an audiologist, he or she will start by asking you questions about your medical and hearing history. This is called the case history. Next, the audiologist will look into your ears using a light, called an otoscope, and check for anything in the ear canal that might affect the test results or require referral to your doctor. Finally, the audiologist will conduct a test or series of tests to assess the following:

- Whether there is a hearing loss
- The cause of the hearing loss (to the extent possible)
- The degree and configuration (one or both ears?) of hearing loss
- The best treatment options

A variety of tests can be used to identify and diagnose a hearing loss. The method used depends in part on the age of the individual and other factors.

- Pure-tone testing
- Speech testing
- Tests of the middle ear
- Auditory brainstem response (ABR)
- Otoacoustic emissions (OAEs)

Hearing Case History

On your first visit, the audiologist will ask several questions to better understand your (or your child's) medical and hearing background. For example:

- What brought you here today?
- Have you noticed difficulty with your hearing? What have you noticed, and for how long? When do you think the hearing loss began?
- Does your hearing problem affect both ears or just one ear?
- Has your difficulty with hearing been gradual or sudden?
- Do you have ringing (tinnitus) in your ears?
- Do you have a history of ear infections?
- Have you noticed any pain in your ears or any discharge from your ears?
- Do you experience dizziness?
- Is there a family history of hearing loss?
- Do you have greater difficulty hearing women's, men's, or children's voices?
- Do people comment on the volume setting of your television?
- Has someone said that you speak too loudly in conversation?

- Do you frequently have to ask people to repeat?

- Do you hear people speaking but can't understand what is being said?

- Do you have any history of exposure to noise at home, at work, in recreational activities, or in the military?

- Are there situations where it is particularly difficult for you to follow a conversation, such as a noisy restaurant, the theater, in a car, or in large groups?

For children, the questions that are asked will center on the following:

- Speech and language development

- Health history

- Recognition of and response to familiar sounds

- The startle response to loud, unexpected sounds

- The presence of other disabilities

- Any previous hearing screening or testing results

Audiogram

The audiogram is a graph showing the results of the pure-tone hearing tests. It illustrates the type, degree, and configuration of hearing loss. The frequency or pitch of the sound is referred to in Hertz (Hz). The intensity or loudness of the sound is measured in decibels (dB). The responses are recorded on a chart called an audiogram that shows intensity levels for each frequency tested.

Pitch or Frequency

Each vertical line from left to right represents a pitch, or frequency, in Hertz (Hz). The graph starts with the lowest pitches on the left side and moves to the very highest pitches (frequencies) tested on the right side. The range of frequencies tested by the audiologist are 125 Hz, 250 Hz, 500 Hz, 1000 Hz, 2000 Hz, 3000Hz, 4000 Hz, and 8000 Hz.

Examples of sounds in everyday life that would be considered low-frequency are a bass drum, tuba, and vowel sounds such as "oo" in who.

Examples of sounds in everyday life that would be considered high-frequency are a bird chirping, a triangle being played, and the consonant sound "s" as in sun.

Loudness or Intensity

Each horizontal line on the audiogram from top to bottom represents loudness or intensity in units of decibels (dB). Lines at the top of the chart (-10 dB and 0 dB) represent soft sounds. Lines at the bottom of the chart represent very loud sounds.

Examples of sounds in everyday life that would be considered soft are a clock ticking, a voice whispering, and leaves rustling.

Examples of sounds in everyday life that would be considered loud are a lawnmower, a car horn, and a rock concert.

If we were to compare normal conversational loudness level (typically 60 dB) with whispering (typically 30 dB), we'd say that whispering is softer than conversation.

On the audiogram, the pattern of hearing loss (configuration) and degree are recorded. For example, your hearing might be normal in the low pitches while you have hearing loss in high pitches. In this case, you might hear speech, but it would sound muffled and unclear. If you have hearing loss at all pitches, you might have difficulty hearing any speech.

The audiologist uses a red O to indicate the right ear and a blue X to record the left ear. The farther down the audiogram the Xs and Os appear, the worse the hearing.

Table 45.1. Hearing Loss Classification System

Degree of hearing loss	Hearing loss range (dB HL)
Normal	−10 to 15
Slight	16 to 25
Mild	26 to 40
Moderate	41 to 55
Moderately severe	56 to 70
Severe	71 to 90
Profound	91+

Source: Clark, J. G. (1981). *Uses and abuses of hearing loss classification.* ASHA, 23, 493–500.

Types of Hearing Loss

Hearing loss can be categorized by which part of the auditory system is damaged. There are three basic types of hearing loss: conductive hearing loss, sensorineural hearing loss, and mixed hearing loss.

Degree of Hearing Loss

Degree of hearing loss refers to the severity of the loss. Table 45.1 shows one of the more commonly used classification systems. The numbers are representative of the patient's hearing loss range in decibels (dB HL).

Configuration of Hearing Loss

The configuration, or shape, of the hearing loss refers to the degree and pattern of hearing loss across frequencies (tones), as illustrated in a graph called an audiogram. For example, a hearing loss that only affects the high tones would be described as a high-frequency loss. Its configuration would show good hearing in the low tones and poor hearing in the high tones.

On the other hand, if only the low frequencies are affected, the configuration would show poorer hearing for low tones and better hearing for high tones. Some hearing loss configurations are flat, indicating the same amount of hearing loss for low and high tones.

Other descriptors associated with hearing loss are these:

- **Bilateral versus unilateral:** Bilateral means hearing loss in both ears. Unilateral means hearing loss in one ear.

- **Symmetrical versus asymmetrical:** Symmetrical means the degree and configuration of hearing loss are the same in each ear. Asymmetrical means degree and configuration of hearing loss are different in each ear.

- **Progressive versus sudden hearing loss:** Progressive means that hearing loss becomes worse over time. Sudden means hearing loss that happens quickly. Such a hearing loss requires immediate medical attention to determine its cause and treatment.

- **Fluctuating versus stable hearing loss:** Fluctuating means hearing loss that changes over time—sometimes getting better, sometimes getting worse.

Chapter 46

Heart and Vascular Disease Screening and Diagnostic Tests

Chapter Contents

Section 46.1

Cardiomyopathy

Excerpted from "Cardiomyopathy," National Heart, Lung,
and Blood Institute (NHLBI), December 2008.

Cardiomyopathy refers to diseases of the heart muscle. These diseases have many causes, signs and symptoms, and treatments. In cardiomyopathy, the heart muscle becomes enlarged, thick, or rigid. In rare cases, the muscle tissue in the heart is replaced with scar tissue. As cardiomyopathy worsens, the heart becomes weaker. It is less able to pump blood through the body and maintain a normal electrical rhythm. This can lead to heart failure or irregular heartbeats called arrhythmias. In turn, heart failure can cause fluid to build up in the lungs, ankles, feet, legs, or abdomen. The weakening of the heart also can cause other complications, such as heart valve problems.

How Is Cardiomyopathy Diagnosed?

Your doctor will diagnose cardiomyopathy based on your medical and family histories, a physical exam, and the results from tests and procedures. Often, a cardiologist or pediatric cardiologist diagnoses and treats cardiomyopathy. A cardiologist specializes in diagnosing and treating heart diseases. A pediatric cardiologist is a cardiologist who treats children.

Medical and family histories: Your doctor will want to learn about your medical history. He or she will want to know what signs and symptoms you have and how long you have had them. Your doctor also will want to know whether anyone in your family has had cardiomyopathy, heart failure, or sudden cardiac arrest.

Physical exam: Your doctor will use a stethoscope to listen to your heart and lungs for sounds that may suggest cardiomyopathy. These sounds may even suggest a certain type of the disease. For example, the loudness, timing, and location of a heart murmur may suggest obstructive hypertrophic cardiomyopathy. A crackling sound in the lungs may be a sign of heart failure. (Heart failure often develops in the later stages of cardiomyopathy.) Physical signs also help your doctor diagnose cardiomyopathy. Swelling of the ankles, feet, legs, abdomen, or veins in your neck suggests fluid buildup, a sign of heart failure. Your doctor may notice signs and symptoms of cardiomyopathy during a routine exam. For example, he or she may hear a heart murmur, or you may have abnormal test results.

Diagnostic Tests

Your doctor may recommend one or more of the following tests to diagnose cardiomyopathy.

Blood tests: During a blood test, a small amount of blood is taken from your body. It is often drawn from a vein in your arm using a needle. Blood tests give your doctor information about your heart and help rule out other conditions.

Chest x-ray: A chest x-ray takes pictures of the organs and structures inside your chest, such as your heart, lungs, and blood vessels. This test can show whether your heart is enlarged. A chest x-ray also can show whether fluid is building up in your lungs.

EKG (electrocardiogram): An EKG is a simple test that records the heart's electrical activity. The test shows how fast the heart is beating and its rhythm (steady or irregular). An EKG also records the strength and timing of electrical signals as they pass through each part of the heart. This test is used to detect and study many heart problems, such as heart attacks, arrhythmias (irregular heartbeats), and heart failure. EKG results also can suggest other disorders that affect heart function. A standard EKG only records the heartbeat for a few seconds. It will not detect problems that do not happen during the test. To diagnose heart problems that come and go, your doctor may have you wear a portable EKG monitor. The two most common types of portable EKGs are Holter and event monitors.

Holter and event monitors: Holter and event monitors are small, portable devices. They record your heart's electrical activity while you do your normal daily activities. A Holter monitor records the heart's electrical activity for a full 24- or 48-hour period. An event monitor records your heart's electrical activity only at certain times while you are wearing it. For many event monitors, you push a button to start the monitor when you feel symptoms. Other event monitors start automatically when they sense abnormal heart rhythms.

Echocardiography: A test that uses sound waves to create a moving picture of your heart. The picture shows how well your heart is working and its size and shape. There are several types of echo, including stress echo. This test is done as part of a stress test. Stress echo can show whether you have decreased blood flow to your heart, a sign of coronary heart disease. Another type of echo is transesophageal echo, or TEE. TEE provides a view of the back of the heart. For this test, a sound wave wand is put on the end of a special tube. The tube is gently passed down your throat and into your esophagus (the passage leading from your mouth to your stomach). Because this passage is right behind the heart, TEE can create detailed pictures of the heart's structures. Before TEE, you are given medicine to help you relax, and your throat is sprayed with numbing medicine.

Stress test: Some heart problems are easier to diagnose when your heart is working hard and beating fast. During stress testing, you exercise (or are given medicine if you are unable to exercise) to make your heart work hard and beat fast while heart tests are done. These tests may include nuclear heart scanning, echo, and positron emission tomography (PET) scanning of the heart.

Diagnostic Procedures

You may have one or more medical procedures to confirm a diagnosis or to prepare for surgery (if surgery is planned). These procedures may include cardiac catheterization, coronary angiography, or myocardial biopsy.

Cardiac catheterization: This procedure checks the pressure and blood flow in your heart's chambers. The procedure also allows your doctor to collect blood samples and look at your heart's arteries using x-ray imaging. During cardiac catheterization, a long, thin, flexible tube called a catheter is put into a blood vessel in your arm, groin (upper thigh), or neck and threaded to your heart. This allows your doctor to study the inside of your arteries for blockages.

Coronary angiography: This procedure often is done with cardiac catheterization. During the procedure, dye that can be seen on an x-ray is injected into your coronary arteries. The dye lets your doctor study blood flow through your heart and blood vessels. Dye also may be injected into your heart chambers. This allows your doctor to study the pumping function of your heart.

Myocardial biopsy: For this procedure, your doctor removes a piece of your heart muscle. This can be done during cardiac catheterization.

The heart muscle is studied under a microscope to see whether changes in cells have occurred. These changes may suggest cardiomyopathy.

Genetic testing: Some types of cardiomyopathy run in families. Thus, your doctor may suggest genetic testing to look for the disease in your parents, brothers and sisters, or other family members.

Section 46.2

Carotid Artery Disease Assessments

Excerpted from "Carotid Artery Disease," National Heart,
Lung, and Blood Institute (NHLBI), March 2008.

Carotid artery disease is a disease in which a waxy substance called plaque builds up inside the carotid arteries. You have two common carotid arteries, one on each side of your neck. They each divide into internal and external carotid arteries. The internal carotid arteries supply oxygen-rich blood to your brain. The external carotid arteries supply oxygen-rich blood to your face, scalp, and neck. Carotid artery disease is serious because it can cause a stroke, also called a brain attack. A stroke occurs if blood flow to your brain is cut off.

How Is Carotid Artery Disease Diagnosed?

Your doctor will diagnose carotid artery disease based on your medical history, a physical exam, and test results.

Medical history: Your doctor will find out whether you have any of the major risk factors for carotid artery disease. He or she also will ask whether you've had any signs or symptoms of a mini-stroke or stroke.

Physical exam: To check your carotid arteries, your doctor will listen to them with a stethoscope. He or she will listen for a whooshing sound called a bruit. This sound may indicate changed or reduced blood flow due to plaque buildup. To find out more, your doctor may recommend tests.

Diagnostic Tests

The following tests are common for diagnosing carotid artery disease. If you have symptoms of a mini-stroke or stroke, your doctor may use other tests as well.

Carotid ultrasound (also called sonography): The most common test for diagnosing carotid artery disease. It is a painless, harmless test that uses sound waves to create pictures of the insides of your carotid arteries. This test can show whether plaque has narrowed your carotid arteries and how narrow they are. A standard carotid ultrasound shows the structure of your carotid arteries. A Doppler carotid ultrasound shows how blood moves through your carotid arteries.

Carotid angiography: A special type of x-ray. This test may be used if the ultrasound results are unclear or do not give your doctor enough information. For this test, your doctor will inject a substance (called contrast dye) into a vein, most often in your leg. The dye travels to your carotid arteries and highlights them on x-ray pictures.

Magnetic resonance angiography (MRA): Uses a large magnet and radio waves to take pictures of your carotid arteries. Your doctor can see these pictures on a computer screen. For this test, your doctor may give you contrast dye to highlight your carotid arteries on the pictures.

Computed tomography (CT) angiography: Takes x-ray pictures of the body from many angles. A computer combines the pictures into two- and three-dimensional images. For this test, your doctor may give you contrast dye to highlight your carotid arteries on the pictures.

Section 46.3

Congenital Heart Defects Tests

Excerpted from "Congenital Heart Defects," National
Heart, Lung, and Blood Institute (NHLBI), August 2009.

Congenital heart defects are problems with the heart's structure
that are present at birth. These defects can involve the interior walls
of the heart, the valves inside the heart, or the arteries and veins that
carry blood to the heart or out to the body. Congenital heart defects
change the normal flow of blood through the heart.

There are many types of congenital heart defects. They range from
simple defects with no symptoms to complex defects with severe, life-
threatening symptoms. Congenital heart defects are the most common
type of birth defect. They affect eight of every 1,000 newborns.

How Are Congenital Heart Defects Diagnosed?

Severe congenital heart defects are generally found during pregnancy or soon after birth. Less severe defects are not diagnosed until
children are older. Minor defects often have no signs or symptoms and
are diagnosed based on results from a physical exam and tests done
for another reason.

Physical exam: During a physical exam, the doctor will:

- listen to your child's heart and lungs with a stethoscope; and

- look for signs of a heart defect, such as cyanosis (a bluish tint to
the skin, lips, or fingernails), shortness of breath, rapid breathing, delayed growth, or signs of heart failure.

Diagnostic Tests

Echocardiography (echo): A painless test that uses sound waves
to create a moving picture of the heart. During the test, the sound
waves (called ultrasound) bounce off the structures of the heart. A
computer converts the sound waves into pictures on a screen. Echo

allows the doctor to clearly see any problem with the way the heart is formed or the way it is working.

Echo is an important test for both diagnosing a heart problem and following the problem over time. In children who have congenital heart defects, echo can show problems with the heart's structure and how the heart is reacting to these problems. Echo will help your child's cardiologist decide if and when treatment is needed.

During pregnancy, if your doctor suspects that your baby has a congenital heart defect, a fetal echo can be done. This test uses sound waves to create a picture of the baby's heart while the baby is still in the womb. The fetal echo usually is done at about 18 to 22 weeks of pregnancy. If your child is diagnosed with a congenital heart defect before birth, your doctor can plan treatment before the baby is born.

EKG (electrocardiogram): An EKG is a simple, painless test that records the heart's electrical activity. The test shows how fast the heart is beating and its rhythm (steady or irregular). It also records the strength and timing of electrical signals as they pass through each part of the heart. An EKG can detect if one of the heart's chambers is enlarged, which can help diagnose a heart problem.

Chest x-ray: A chest x-ray is a painless test that creates pictures of the structures in the chest, such as the heart and lungs. This test can show whether the heart is enlarged or whether the lungs have extra blood flow or extra fluid, a sign of heart failure.

Pulse oximetry: Shows how much oxygen is in the blood. For this test, a small sensor is attached to a finger or toe (like an adhesive bandage). The sensor gives an estimate of how much oxygen is in the blood.

Cardiac catheterization: During cardiac catheterization, a thin, flexible tube called a catheter is put into a vein in the arm, groin (upper thigh), or neck and threaded to the heart. Special dye is injected through the catheter into a blood vessel or a chamber of the heart. The dye allows the doctor to see the flow of blood through the heart and blood vessels on an x-ray image.

The doctor also can use cardiac catheterization to measure the pressure and oxygen level inside the heart chambers and blood vessels. This can help the doctor determine whether blood is mixing between the two sides of the heart. Cardiac catheterization also is used to repair some heart defects.

Section 46.4

Peripheral Arterial Disease (PAD) Assessments

Excerpted from "Peripheral Arterial Disease," National Heart, Lung, and Blood Institute (NHLBI), September 2008.

Peripheral arterial disease (PAD) occurs when plaque builds up in the arteries that carry blood to your head, organs, and limbs. Plaque is made up of fat, cholesterol, calcium, fibrous tissue, and other substances in the blood. When plaque builds up in arteries, the condition is called atherosclerosis. Over time, plaque can harden and narrow the arteries. This limits the flow of oxygen-rich blood to your organs and other parts of your body. PAD usually affects the legs, but also can affect the arteries that carry blood from your heart to your head, arms, kidneys, and stomach.

How Is Peripheral Arterial Disease Diagnosed?

Peripheral arterial disease (PAD) is diagnosed based on your medical and family histories, a physical exam, and results from tests. PAD often is diagnosed after symptoms are reported. An accurate diagnosis is important, because people who have PAD are at increased risk for coronary artery disease (CAD), heart attack, stroke, and transient ischemic attack (mini-stroke). A cardiologist may be involved in treating people who have PAD. Cardiologists treat heart problems, such as CAD and heart attack, which often affect people who have PAD.

Medical and family histories: To learn about your medical and family histories, your doctor may ask:

- whether you have any risk factors for PAD;

- about your symptoms, including any symptoms that occur when walking, exercising, sitting, standing, or climbing;

- about your diet;

- about any medicines you take, including prescription and over-the-counter medicines;

- whether anyone in your family has a history of cardiovascular disease.

Physical exam: During the physical exam, your doctor will look for signs and symptoms of PAD. He or she may check the blood flow in your legs or feet to see whether you have weak or absent pulses. Your doctor also may check the pulses in your leg arteries for an abnormal whooshing sound called a bruit. He or she can hear this sound with a stethoscope. A bruit may be a warning sign of a narrowed or blocked section of artery. During the physical exam, your doctor may compare blood pressure between your limbs to see whether the pressure is lower in the affected limb. He or she also may check for poor wound healing or any changes in your hair, skin, or nails that may be signs of PAD.

Diagnostic Tests

Ankle-brachial index (ABI): A simple test that is often used to diagnose PAD. The ABI compares blood pressure in your ankle to blood pressure in your arm. This test shows how well blood is flowing in your limbs. ABI can show whether PAD is affecting your limbs, but it will not show which blood vessels are narrowed or blocked. A normal ABI result is 1.0 or greater (with a range of 0.90 to 1.30). The test takes about 10–15 minutes to measure both arms and both ankles. This test may be done yearly to see whether PAD is getting worse.

Doppler ultrasound: A test that uses sound waves to show whether a blood vessel is blocked. This test uses a blood pressure cuff and special device to measure blood flow in the veins and arteries of the limbs.

Treadmill test: This test can show how severe your symptoms are and what level of exercise brings them on. For this test, you walk on a treadmill. This shows whether you have any problems during normal walking. You may have an ABI test done before and after the treadmill test. This will help compare blood flow in your arms and legs before and after exercise.

Magnetic resonance angiogram (MRA): MRA uses magnetic and radio wave energy to take pictures of blood vessels inside your body. An MRA is a type of magnetic resonance imaging (MRI). An MRA can find the location of a blocked blood vessel and show how severe the blockage is.

Arteriogram: An arteriogram provides a road map of the arteries. It is used to find the exact location of a blocked artery. For this test, dye is injected through a needle or catheter (tube) into an artery. After the dye is injected, an x-ray is taken that can show the location, type, and extent of the blockage in the artery. Some hospitals use a newer method of arteriogram that uses tiny ultrasound cameras that take pictures of the insides of the blood vessels. This method is called intravascular ultrasound.

Blood tests: Your doctor may recommend blood tests to check for PAD risk factors. For example, you may get a blood test to check for diabetes, or to check your cholesterol levels.

Chapter 47

Infectious Disease Testing

Chapter Contents

Section 47.1

Diagnosis and Screening of Infectious Diseases

This section includes an excerpt from "Understanding Microbes in Sickness and in Health," National Institute of Allergy and Infectious Diseases (NIAID), September 2009.

Infectious Diseases Are Diagnosed in Many Ways

Sometimes your health care provider can diagnose an infectious disease by listening to your medical history and doing a physical exam. For example, listening to you describe what happened and any symptoms you have noticed plays an important part in helping your doctor find out what's wrong.

Blood and urine tests are other ways to diagnose an infection. A laboratory expert can sometimes see the offending microbe in a sample of blood or urine viewed under a microscope. One or both of these tests may be the only way to determine what caused the infection, or they may be used to confirm a diagnosis.

In another type of test, your health care provider will take a sample of blood or other body fluid, such as vaginal secretion, and then put it into a special container called a Petri dish to see whether any microbe grows. This test is called a culture. Lab workers usually can identify certain bacteria, such as chlamydia, and viruses, such as herpes simplex, using this method.

X-rays, scans, and biopsies (taking a tiny sample of tissue from the infected area and inspecting it under a microscope) are among other tools your health care provider can use to make an accurate diagnosis.

All of these procedures are relatively safe, and some can be done in your health care provider's office or a clinic. Others pose a higher risk to you because they involve procedures that go inside your body. One such invasive procedure is taking a biopsy from an internal organ. For example, one way a doctor can diagnose *Pneumocystis carinii* pneumonia, a lung disease caused by a fungus, is by doing a biopsy on lung tissue and then examining the sample under a microscope.

Section 47.2

Human Immunodeficiency Virus (HIV) and Sexually Transmitted Disease Testing

Excerpted from "National HIV and STD Testing Resources: Frequently Asked Questions," Centers for Disease Control and Prevention (CDC).

Should I get a human immunodeficiency virus (HIV) test?

The following are behaviors that increase your chances of getting human immunodeficiency virus (HIV). If you answer yes to any of them, you should definitely get an HIV test. If you continue with any of these behaviors, you should be tested every year. Talk to a health care provider about an HIV testing schedule that is right for you.

- Have you injected drugs or steroids or shared equipment (such as needles, syringes, works) with others?

- Have you had unprotected vaginal, anal, or oral sex with men who have sex with men, multiple partners, or anonymous partners?

- Have you exchanged sex for drugs or money?

- Have you been diagnosed with or treated for hepatitis, tuberculosis (TB), or a sexually transmitted disease (STD), like syphilis?

- Have you had unprotected sex with someone who could answer yes to any of the above questions?

If you have had sex with someone whose history of sex partners and/or drug use is unknown to you, or if you or your partner has had many sex partners, then you have more of a chance of being infected with HIV. Both you and your new partner should get tested for HIV, and learn the results, before having sex for the first time.

For women who plan to become pregnant, testing is even more important. If a woman is infected with HIV, medical care and certain drugs given during pregnancy can lower the chance of passing HIV to her baby. All women who are pregnant should be tested during each pregnancy.

How long after a possible exposure should I wait to get tested for HIV?

Most HIV tests are antibody tests that measure the antibodies your body makes against HIV. It can take some time for the immune system to produce enough antibodies for the antibody test to detect and this time period can vary from person to person. This time period is commonly referred to as the window period. Most people will develop detectable antibodies within 2–8 weeks (the average is 25 days). Even so, there is a chance that some individuals will take longer to develop detectable antibodies. Therefore, if the initial negative HIV test was conducted within the first three months after possible exposure, repeat testing should be considered three months after the exposure occurred to account for the possibility of a false-negative result. Ninety-seven percent will develop antibodies in the first three months following the time of their infection. In very rare cases, it can take up to six months to develop antibodies to HIV.

Another type of test is an ribonucleic acid (RNA) test, which detects the HIV virus directly. The time between HIV infection and RNA detection is 9–11 days. These tests, which are more costly and used less often than antibody tests, are used in some parts of the United States.

How do HIV tests work?

The most common HIV tests use blood to detect HIV infection. Tests using saliva or urine are also available. Some tests take a few days for results, but rapid HIV tests can give results in about 20 minutes. All positive HIV tests must be followed up by another test to confirm the positive result. Results of this confirmatory test can take a few days to a few weeks.

What are the different HIV screening tests available in the United States?

In most cases the EIA (enzyme immunoassay), used on blood drawn from a vein, is the most common screening test used to look for antibodies to HIV. A positive (reactive) EIA must be used with a follow-up (confirmatory) test such as the Western blot to make a positive diagnosis. There are EIA tests that use other body fluids to look for antibodies to HIV. These include:

- **Oral fluid tests** use oral fluid (not saliva) that is collected from the mouth using a special collection device. This is an EIA

468

antibody test similar to the standard blood EIA test. A follow-up confirmatory Western Blot uses the same oral fluid sample.

- **Urine tests** use urine instead of blood. The sensitivity and specificity (accuracy) are somewhat less than that of the blood and oral fluid tests. This is also an EIA antibody test similar to blood EIA tests and requires a follow-up confirmatory Western blot using the same urine sample.

Rapid tests: A screening test that produces very quick results, in approximately 20 minutes. Rapid tests use blood from a vein or from a finger stick, or oral fluid to look for the presence of antibodies to HIV. As is true for all screening tests, a reactive rapid HIV test result must be confirmed with a follow-up confirmatory test before a final diagnosis of infection can be made. These tests have similar accuracy rates as traditional EIA screening tests.

Home testing kits: Consumer-controlled test kits (popularly known as home testing kits) were first licensed in 1997. Although home HIV tests are sometimes advertised through the internet, currently only the Home Access HIV-1 Test System is approved by the Food and Drug Administration. (The accuracy of other home test kits cannot be verified). The Home Access HIV-1 Test System can be found at most local drug stores. It is not a true home test, but a home collection kit. The testing procedure involves pricking a finger with a special device, placing drops of blood on a specially treated card, and then mailing the card in to be tested at a licensed laboratory. Customers are given an identification number to use when phoning in for the results. Callers may speak to a counselor before taking the test, while waiting for the test result, and when the results are given. All individuals receiving a positive test result are provided referrals for a follow-up confirmatory test, as well as information and resources on treatment and support services.

RNA tests: Look for genetic material of the virus and can be used in screening the blood supply and for detection of very early infection rare cases when antibody tests are unable to detect antibodies to HIV.

Section 47.3

Tuberculosis (TB) Test

Excerpted from "Diagnosis of Tuberculosis Disease," Centers
for Disease Control and Prevention (CDC), July 1, 2010.

A complete medical evaluation for tuberculosis (TB) includes the
following:

Medical history: Clinicians should ask about the patient's history
of TB exposure, infection, or disease. It is also important to consider
demographic factors (such as country of origin, age, ethnic or racial
group, occupation) that may increase the patient's risk for exposure to
TB or to drug-resistant TB. Also, clinicians should determine whether
the patient has medical conditions, especially HIV infection, that increase the risk of latent TB infection progressing to TB disease.

Physical examination: A physical exam can provide valuable
information about the patient's overall condition and other factors
that may affect how TB is treated, such as HIV infection or other
illnesses.

Test for TB infection: The Mantoux tuberculin skin test (TST) or
the special TB blood test can be used to test for *M. tuberculosis* infection. Additional tests are required to confirm TB disease. The Mantoux
tuberculin skin test is performed by injecting a small amount of fluid
called tuberculin into the skin in the lower part of the arm. The test
is read within 48 to 72 hours by a trained health care worker, who
looks for a reaction (induration) on the arm. The special TB blood test
measures the patient's immune system reaction to *M. tuberculosis*.

Chest radiograph: A posterior-anterior chest radiograph is used to
detect chest abnormalities. Lesions may appear anywhere in the lungs
and may differ in size, shape, density, and cavitation. These abnormalities may suggest TB, but cannot be used to definitively diagnose TB.
However, a chest radiograph may be used to rule out the possibility of
pulmonary TB in a person who has had a positive reaction to a TST
or special TB blood test and no symptoms of disease.

Diagnostic microbiology: The presence of acid-fast-bacilli (AFB) on a sputum smear or other specimen often indicates TB disease. Acid-fast microscopy is easy and quick, but it does not confirm a diagnosis of TB because some acid-fast-bacilli are not *M. tuberculosis*. Therefore, a culture is done on all initial samples to confirm the diagnosis. (However, a positive culture is not always necessary to begin or continue treatment for TB.) A positive culture for *M. tuberculosis* confirms the diagnosis of TB disease. Culture examinations should be completed on all specimens, regardless of AFB smear results. Laboratories should report positive results on smears and cultures within 24 hours by telephone or fax to the primary health care provider and to the state or local TB control program, as required by law.

Drug resistance: For all patients, the initial *M. tuberculosis* isolate should be tested for drug resistance. It is crucial to identify drug resistance as early as possible to ensure effective treatment. Drug susceptibility patterns should be repeated for patients who do not respond adequately to treatment or who have positive culture results despite three months of therapy. Susceptibility results from laboratories should be promptly reported to the primary health care provider and the state or local TB control program.

Chapter 48

Lung Disease Tests

Lung function tests, also called pulmonary function tests, measure how well your lungs work. These tests are used to look for the cause of breathing problems, such as shortness of breath. Lung function tests measure:

- How much air you can take into your lungs. This amount is compared to that of other people your age, height, and sex. This allows your doctor to see whether you're in the normal range.

- How much air you can blow out of your lungs and how fast you can do it.

- How well your lungs deliver oxygen to your blood.

- The strength of your breathing muscles.

Doctors use lung function tests to help diagnose conditions such as asthma, pulmonary fibrosis (scarring of the lung tissue), and COPD (chronic obstructive pulmonary disease). Lung function tests also are used to check the extent of damage caused by conditions such as pulmonary fibrosis and sarcoidosis. Also, these tests may be used to check how well treatments, such as asthma medicines, are working.

Excerpted from "Lung Function Tests," National Heart, Lung, and Blood Institute (NHLBI), August 2010.

Types of Lung Function Tests

Spirometry measures how much air you breathe in and out and how fast you blow it out. This is measured two ways: peak expiratory flow rate (PEFR) and forced expiratory volume in one second (FEV1). PEFR refers to the amount of air you can blow out as quickly as possible. FEV1 refers to the amount of air you can blow out in one second.

Lung volume measurement: This test measures the size of your lungs and how much air you can breathe in and out is measured to test how much air your lungs can hold.

Lung diffusion capacity: This test measures how well oxygen passes from your lungs to your bloodstream.

Tests to measure oxygen level: Pulse oximetry and arterial blood gas tests show how much oxygen is in your blood.

Testing in Infants and Young Children

Spirometry and other measures of lung function usually can be done in children older than six years, if they can follow directions well. Spirometry may be tried in children as young as five years. However, technicians who have special training with young children may need to do the testing.

Instead of spirometry, a growing number of medical centers measure respiratory system resistance. This is another way to test lung function in young children. The child wears nose clips and has his or her cheeks supported with an adult's hands. The child breathes in and out quietly on a mouthpiece, while the technician measures changes in pressure at the mouth. During these lung function tests, parents can help comfort their children and encourage them to cooperate.

Very young children (younger than two years) may need an infant lung function test. This requires special equipment and medical staff. This type of test is available only at a few medical centers. The doctor gives the child medicine to help him or her sleep through the test. A technician places a mask over the child's nose and mouth and a vest around the child's chest. The mask and vest are attached to a lung function machine. The machine gently pushes air into the child's lungs through the mask. As the child exhales, the vest slightly squeezes his or her chest. This helps push more air out of the lungs. The exhaled air is then measured.

In children younger than five years, doctors likely will use signs and symptoms, medical history, and a physical exam to diagnose lung problems. Pulse oximetry and arterial blood gas tests can be used for children of all ages.

Diagnosing Lung Conditions

Your doctor will diagnose a lung condition based on your medical and family histories, a physical exam, and test results.

Medical and family histories: Your doctor will ask you questions, such as these:

- Do you ever feel like you cannot get enough air?

- Does your chest feel tight sometimes?

- Do you have periods of coughing or wheezing (a whistling sound when you breathe)?

- Do you ever have chest pain?

- Can you walk or run as fast as other people your age?

Your doctor also will ask whether you or anyone in your family has ever:

- had asthma and/or allergies,

- had heart disease,

- smoked,

- traveled to places where they may have been exposed to tuberculosis,

- had a job that exposed them to dust, fumes, or particles (like asbestos).

Physical exam: Your doctor will check your heart rate, breathing rate, and blood pressure. He or she also will listen to your heart and lungs with a stethoscope and feel your abdomen and limbs. Your doctor will look for signs of heart or lung disease, or another disease that may be causing your symptoms.

Lung and heart tests: Based on your medical history and physical exam, your doctor will recommend tests. A chest x-ray usually is the first test done to find the cause of a breathing problem. This test takes pictures of the organs and structures inside your chest. Your doctor may do lung function tests to find out even more about how well your lungs work.

Your doctor also may do tests to check your heart, such as an EKG (electrocardiogram) or a stress test. An EKG detects and records your heart's electrical activity. A stress test shows how well your heart works during physical activity.

What to Expect before Lung Function Tests

If you take breathing medicines, your doctor may ask you to stop them for a short time before spirometry, lung volume measurement, or lung diffusion capacity tests. No special preparation is needed before pulse oximetry and arterial blood gas tests. If you are getting oxygen therapy, your doctor may ask you to stop using it for a short time before the tests. This allows your doctor to check your blood oxygen level without the added oxygen.

What to Expect during Lung Function Tests

Breathing Tests

Spirometry may be done in your doctor's office or in a special lung function laboratory (lab). Lung volume measurement and lung diffusion capacity tests are done in a special lab or clinic. For these tests, you sit in a chair next to a machine that measures your breathing. For spirometry, you sit or stand next to the machine.

Before the tests, a technician places soft clips on your nose. This allows you to breathe only through a tube that's attached to the testing machine. The technician will tell you how to breathe into the tube. For example, you may be asked to breathe normally, slowly, or rapidly. The deep breathing done in some of the tests may make you feel short of breath, dizzy, or light-headed, or it may make you cough.

Spirometry: For this test, you take a deep breath and then exhale as fast and as hard as you can into the tube. With spirometry, your doctor may give you a medicine that helps open your airways. Your doctor will want to see whether the medicine changes or improves the test results.

Lung volume measurement: For this test, you sit in a clear glass booth and breathe through the tube attached to the testing machine. The changes in pressure inside the booth are measured to show how much air you can breathe into your lungs. Sometimes you breathe in nitrogen or helium gas and then exhale. The gas that you breathe out is measured.

Lung diffusion capacity: During this test, you breathe in gas through the tube, hold your breath for ten seconds, and then rapidly blow it out. The gas contains a small amount of carbon monoxide, which won't harm you.

Tests to Measure Oxygen Level

Pulse oximetry is done in a doctor's office or hospital. An arterial blood gas test is done in a lab or hospital.

Pulse oximetry: For this test, a small sensor is attached to your finger or ear using a clip or flexible tape. The sensor is then attached to a cable that leads to a small machine called an oximeter. The oximeter shows the amount of oxygen in your blood. This test is painless and no needles are used.

Arterial blood gas: During this test, your doctor or technician inserts a needle into an artery, usually in your wrist, and takes a sample of blood. You may feel some discomfort when the needle is inserted. The sample is then sent to a lab where its oxygen level is measured. After the needle is removed, you may feel mild pressure or throbbing at the needle site. Applying pressure to the area for 5–10 minutes should stop the bleeding.

What Lung Function Tests Show

Spirometry can show whether you have the following:

- A blockage (obstruction) in your airways. This may be a sign of asthma, COPD (chronic obstructive pulmonary disease), or another obstructive lung disorder.

- Smaller than normal lungs (restriction). This may be a sign of heart failure, pulmonary fibrosis (scarring of the lung tissue), or another restrictive lung disorder.

Lung volume measurement: This test shows the size of your lungs. Abnormal test results may show that you have pulmonary fibrosis or a stiff and/or weak chest wall.

Lung diffusion capacity: This test can show a problem with oxygen moving from your lungs into your bloodstream. This may be a sign of loss of lung tissue, emphysema (a type of COPD), or problems with blood flow through the body's arteries.

Pulse oximetry and arterial blood gas tests measure the oxygen level in your blood. These tests show how well your lungs are taking in oxygen and moving it into the bloodstream. A low level of oxygen in the blood may be a sign of a lung or heart disorder.

Chapter 49

Neurological Diagnostic Tests

Diagnostic tests and procedures are vital tools that help physicians confirm or rule out the presence of a neurological disorder or other medical condition. Researchers and physicians use a variety of diagnostic imaging techniques and chemical and metabolic analyses to detect, manage, and treat neurological disease. Some procedures are performed in specialized settings, conducted to determine the presence of a particular disorder or abnormality. Many tests that were previously conducted in a hospital are now performed in a physician's office or at an outpatient testing facility, with little if any risk to the patient. Depending on the type of procedure, results are either immediate or may take several hours to process.

What are some of the more common screening tests?

Laboratory screening tests of blood, urine, or other substances are used to help diagnose disease, better understand the disease process, and monitor levels of therapeutic drugs. Certain tests, ordered by the physician as part of a regular check-up, provide general information, while others are used to identify specific health concerns. For example, blood and blood product tests can detect brain and/or spinal cord infection, bone marrow disease, hemorrhage, blood vessel damage, toxins that affect the nervous system, and the presence of antibodies that signal the presence of an autoimmune disease. Blood tests are

"Neurological Diagnostic Tests," National Institute of Neurological Disorders and Stroke (NINDS), December 18, 2009.

also used to monitor levels of therapeutic drugs used to treat epilepsy and other neurological disorders. Genetic testing of deoxyribonucleic acid (DNA) extracted from white cells in the blood can help diagnose Huntington disease and other congenital diseases. Analysis of the fluid that surrounds the brain and spinal cord can detect meningitis, acute and chronic inflammation, rare infections, and some cases of multiple sclerosis. Chemical and metabolic testing of the blood can indicate protein disorders, some forms of muscular dystrophy and other muscle disorders, and diabetes. Urinalysis can reveal abnormal substances in the urine or the presence or absence of certain proteins that cause diseases including the mucopolysaccharidoses.

Genetic testing or counseling can help parents who have a family history of a neurological disease determine if they are carrying one of the known genes that cause the disorder or find out if their child is affected. Genetic testing can identify many neurological disorders, including spina bifida, in utero (while the child is inside the mother's womb). Genetic tests include amniocentesis, chorionic villus sampling, and uterine ultrasound.

What is a neurological examination?

A neurological examination assesses motor and sensory skills, the functioning of one or more cranial nerves, hearing and speech, vision, coordination and balance, mental status, and changes in mood or behavior, among other abilities. Items including a tuning fork, flashlight, reflex hammer, ophthalmoscope, and needles are used to help diagnose brain tumors, infections such as encephalitis and meningitis, and diseases such as Parkinson disease, Huntington disease, amyotrophic lateral sclerosis (ALS), and epilepsy. Some tests require the services of a specialist to perform and analyze results.

X-rays of the patient's chest and skull are often taken as part of a neurological work-up. Fluoroscopy is a type of x-ray that uses a continuous or pulsed beam of low-dose radiation to produce continuous images of a body part in motion. The fluoroscope (x-ray tube) is focused on the area of interest and pictures are either videotaped or sent to a monitor for viewing. A contrast medium may be used to highlight the images. Fluoroscopy can be used to evaluate the flow of blood through arteries.

What are some diagnostic tests used to diagnose neurological disorders?

Based on the result of a neurological exam, physical exam, patient history, x-rays of the patient's chest and skull, and any previous screening or testing, physicians may order one or more of the following diagnostic tests to determine the specific nature of a suspected neurological disorder or injury. These diagnostics generally involve either nuclear medicine imaging, in which very small amounts of radioactive materials are used to study organ function and structure, or diagnostic imaging, which uses magnets and electrical charges to study human anatomy.

The following list of available procedures—in alphabetical rather than sequential order—includes some of the more common tests used to help diagnose a neurological condition.

Angiography is a test used to detect blockages of the arteries or veins. A cerebral angiogram can detect the degree of narrowing or obstruction of an artery or blood vessel in the brain, head, or neck. It is used to diagnose stroke and to determine the location and size of a brain tumor, aneurysm, or vascular malformation.

Biopsy involves the removal and examination of a small piece of tissue from the body. Muscle or nerve biopsies are used to diagnose neuromuscular disorders and may also reveal if a person is a carrier of a defective gene that could be passed on to children.

Brain scans are imaging techniques used to diagnose tumors, blood vessel malformations, or hemorrhage in the brain. These scans are used to study organ function or injury or disease to tissue or muscle.

Cerebrospinal fluid analysis involves the removal of a small amount of the fluid that protects the brain and spinal cord. The fluid is tested to detect any bleeding or brain hemorrhage, diagnose infection to the brain and/or spinal cord, identify some cases of multiple sclerosis and other neurological conditions, and measure intracranial pressure.

Computed tomography, also known as a CT scan, is a noninvasive, painless process used to produce rapid, clear two-dimensional images of organs, bones, and tissues. Neurological CT scans are used to view the brain and spine.

Discography is often suggested for patients who are considering lumbar surgery or whose lower back pain has not responded to conventional treatments. This outpatient procedure is usually performed at a testing facility or a hospital. The patient is asked to put on a metal-free hospital gown and lie on an imaging table. The physician numbs the skin with anesthetic and inserts a thin needle, using x-ray guidance, into the spinal disc. Once the needle is in place, a small amount of contrast dye is injected and CT scans are taken. The contrast dye outlines any damaged areas. More than one disc may be imaged at the same time. Patient recovery usually takes about an hour. Pain medicine may be prescribed for any resulting discomfort.

An intrathecal contrast-enhanced CT scan (also called cisternography) is used to detect problems with the spine and spinal nerve roots. This test is most often performed at an imaging center.

Electroencephalography, or EEG, monitors brain activity through the skull. EEG is used to help diagnose certain seizure disorders, brain tumors, brain damage from head injuries, inflammation of the brain and/or spinal cord, alcoholism, certain psychiatric disorders, and metabolic and degenerative disorders that affect the brain. EEGs are also used to evaluate sleep disorders, monitor brain activity when a patient has been fully anesthetized or loses consciousness, and confirm brain death.

Electromyography, or EMG, is used to diagnose nerve and muscle dysfunction and spinal cord disease. It records the electrical activity from the brain and/or spinal cord to a peripheral nerve root (found in the arms and legs) that controls muscles during contraction and at rest. An EMG is usually done in conjunction with a nerve conduction velocity (NCV) test, which measures electrical energy by assessing the nerve's ability to send a signal. This two-part test is conducted most often in a hospital.

Electronystagmography (ENG) describes a group of tests used to diagnose involuntary eye movement, dizziness, and balance disorders, and to evaluate some brain functions.

Evoked potentials (also called evoked response) measure the electrical signals to the brain generated by hearing, touch, or sight. These tests are used to assess sensory nerve problems and confirm neurological conditions including multiple sclerosis, brain tumor, acoustic neuroma (small tumors of the inner ear), and spinal cord injury. Evoked potentials are also used to test sight and hearing (especially in infants and young children), monitor brain activity among coma patients, and confirm brain death.

Magnetic resonance imaging (MRI) uses computer-generated radio waves and a powerful magnetic field to produce detailed images of body structures including tissues, organs, bones, and nerves. Neurological uses include the diagnosis of brain and spinal cord tumors, eye disease, inflammation, infection, and vascular irregularities that may lead to stroke. MRI can also detect and monitor degenerative disorders such as multiple sclerosis and can document brain injury from trauma.

Functional MRI (fMRI) uses the blood's magnetic properties to produce real-time images of blood flow to particular areas of the brain. An fMRI can pinpoint areas of the brain that become active and note how long they stay active. It can also tell if brain activity within a region occurs simultaneously or sequentially. This imaging process is used to assess brain damage from head injury or degenerative disorders such as Alzheimer disease and to identify and monitor other neurological disorders, including multiple sclerosis, stroke, and brain tumors.

Myelography involves the injection of a water- or oil-based contrast dye into the spinal canal to enhance x-ray imaging of the spine. Myelograms are used to diagnose spinal nerve injury, herniated discs, fractures, back or leg pain, and spinal tumors.

Positron emission tomography (PET) scans provide two- and three-dimensional pictures of brain activity by measuring radioactive isotopes that are injected into the bloodstream. PET scans of the brain are used to detect or highlight tumors and diseased tissue, measure cellular and/or tissue metabolism, show blood flow, evaluate patients who have seizure disorders that do not respond to medical therapy and patients with certain memory disorders, and determine brain changes following injury or drug abuse, among other uses.

A polysomnogram measures brain and body activity during sleep. It is performed over one or more nights at a sleep center.

Single photon emission computed tomography (SPECT), a nuclear imaging test involving blood flow to tissue, is used to evaluate certain brain functions. The test may be ordered as a follow-up to an MRI to diagnose tumors, infections, degenerative spinal disease, and stress fractures.

Thermography uses infrared sensing devices to measure small temperature changes between the two sides of the body or within a specific organ. Also known as digital infrared thermal imaging, thermography may be used to detect vascular disease of the head and neck, soft tissue injury, various neuromusculoskeletal disorders, and the presence or absence of nerve root compression.

Ultrasound imaging, also called ultrasound scanning or sonography, uses high-frequency sound waves to obtain images inside the body. Neurosonography (ultrasound of the brain and spinal column) analyzes blood flow in the brain and can diagnose stroke, brain tumors, hydrocephalus (build-up of cerebrospinal fluid in the brain), and vascular problems. It can also identify or rule out inflammatory processes causing pain. Transcranial Doppler ultrasound is used to view arteries and blood vessels in the neck and determine blood flow and risk of stroke.

Chapter 50

Osteoporosis Diagnosis

Osteoporosis is a condition of low bone density that can progress silently over a long period of time. If diagnosed early, the fractures associated with the disease can often be prevented. An examination to diagnose osteoporosis can involve several steps that predict your chances of future fracture, diagnose osteoporosis, or both. It might include a physical exam, x-rays, laboratory tests, and a bone density test.

Before performing any tests, your doctor will record information about your medical history and lifestyle and will ask questions related to your:

- risk factors, including information about any fractures you have had;

- family history of disease, including osteoporosis;

- medication history;

- general intake of calcium and vitamin D;

- exercise pattern;

- menstrual history (for women).

Excerpted from "Osteoporosis: The Diagnosis," Osteoporosis and Related Bone Diseases National Resource Center (ORBD-NRC) of the National Institutes of Health (NIH), May 2009.

X-Ray Tests

If you have back pain or have experienced a loss of height or a change in posture, your doctor may order an x-ray of your spine. However, because an x-ray can detect bone loss only after 30% of the skeleton has been depleted, the presence of osteoporosis may be missed.

Bone Mineral Density Tests

A bone mineral density (BMD) test is the best way to determine your bone health. BMD tests can identify osteoporosis, determine your risk for fractures, and measure your response to osteoporosis treatment. The most widely recognized BMD test is called a dual-energy x-ray absorptiometry, or DXA test. The BMD test is painless, a bit like having an x-ray, but with much less exposure to radiation. It measures bone density at your hip and spine.

During a BMD test, an extremely low energy source is passed over part or all of the body. A computer program evaluates the information and allows the doctor to see how much bone mass you have. Because bone mass serves as an approximate measure of bone strength, this information also helps the doctor to detect low bone mass accurately, make a definitive diagnosis of osteoporosis, and determine your risk of future fractures.

BMD tests provide doctors with a measurement called a T-score, a number value that results from comparing your bone density to optimal bone density. When a T-score appears as a negative number (such as −1, −2 or −2.5), it indicates low bone mass. The greater the negative the number, the greater is the risk of fracture.

Although no bone density test is 100% accurate, this type of test is the single most important predictor of whether a person will have a fracture in the future.

Bone Scans

For some people, the doctor may order a bone scan. A bone scan is different from the BMD test, although the term "bone scan" often is used incorrectly to describe a bone density test. A bone scan involves injecting the patient with a dye that allows a scanner to identify differences in the conditions of various areas of bone tissue. A bone scan can show the doctor changes in bone tissue that may indicate cancer, bone lesions, inflammation, or new fractures.

Lab Tests

A number of lab tests may be performed on blood and urine samples. The results of these tests can help your doctor identify conditions that may be contributing to your bone loss.

The most common blood tests evaluate:

- blood calcium levels,

- blood vitamin D levels,

- thyroid function,

- parathyroid hormone levels,

- estradiol levels to measure estrogen (in women),

- follicle stimulating hormone (FSH) test to establish menopause status,

- testosterone levels (in men),

- osteocalcin levels to measure bone formation.

The most common urine tests are:

- 24-hour urine collection to measure calcium metabolism, and

- tests to measure the rate at which a person is breaking down or resorbing bone.

Chapter 51

Prenatal and Infertility Tests

Chapter Contents

Section 51.1

Prenatal Tests

Text in this section is excerpted from "Healthy Pregnancy:
Prenatal Care and Tests," U.S. Department of Health and
Human Services (HHS), September 27, 2010.

Tests are used during pregnancy to check your and your baby's
health. At your fist prenatal visit, your doctor will use tests to check
for a number of things, such as the following:

• Your blood type and Rh factor

• Anemia

• Infections, such as toxoplasmosis and sexually transmitted infections (STIs), including hepatitis B, syphilis, chlamydia, and human immunodeficiency virus (HIV)

• Signs that you are immune to rubella (German measles) and
chicken pox

Throughout your pregnancy, your doctor or midwife may suggest
a number of other tests, too. Some tests are suggested for all women,
such as screenings for gestational diabetes, Down syndrome, and HIV.
Other tests might be offered based on your:

• age,

• personal or family health history,

• ethnic background, or

• results of routine tests.

Some tests are screening tests. They detect risks for or signs of
possible health problems in you or your baby. Based on screening test
results, your doctor might suggest diagnostic tests. Diagnostic tests
confirm or rule out health problems in you or your baby.

Descriptions of Some of the Most Common Prenatal Tests

Amniocentesis: This test can diagnosis certain birth defects, including Down syndrome, Cystic fibrosis, and spina bifida. It is performed at 14–20 weeks. It may be suggested for couples at higher risk for genetic disorders. It also provides deoxyribonucleic acid (DNA) for paternity testing. For this test, a thin needle is used to draw out a small amount of amniotic fluid and cells from the sac surrounding the fetus. The sample is sent to a lab for testing.

Biophysical profile (BPP): This test is used in the third trimester to monitor the overall health of the baby and to help decide if the baby should be delivered early. BPP involves an ultrasound exam along with a nonstress test. The BPP looks at the baby's breathing, movement, muscle tone, heart rate, and the amount of amniotic fluid.

Chorionic villus sampling (CVS): A test done at 10–13 weeks to diagnose certain birth defects, including chromosomal disorders, Down syndrome and other genetic disorders, such as cystic fibrosis. CVS may be suggested for couples at higher risk for genetic disorders. It also provides DNA for paternity testing. This test involves having a needle remove a small sample of cells from the placenta to be tested.

First trimester screen: A screening test done at 11–14 weeks to detect higher risk of chromosomal disorders, including Down syndrome and trisomy 18, and other problems such as heart defects. It also can reveal multiple births. Based on test results, your doctor may suggest other tests to diagnose a disorder. This test involves both a blood test and an ultrasound exam called nuchal translucency screening. The blood test measures the levels of certain substances in the mother's blood. The ultrasound exam measures the thickness at the back of the baby's neck. This information, combined with the mother's age, help doctors determine risk to the fetus.

Glucose challenge screening: A screening test done at 26–28 weeks to determine the mother's risk of gestational diabetes. Based on test results, your doctor may suggest a glucose tolerance test. For this test, you consume a special sugary drink from your doctor. A blood sample is taken one hour later to look for high blood sugar levels.

Glucose tolerance test: This test is done at 26–28 weeks to diagnose gestational diabetes. Your doctor will tell you what to eat a few days before the test. Then, you cannot eat or drink anything but sips of water for 14 hours before the test. Your blood is drawn to test your fasting blood glucose level. Then, you will consume a sugary drink. Your blood will be tested every hour for three hours to see how well your body processes sugar.

Group B streptococcus infection: This test is done at 36–37 weeks to look for bacteria that can cause pneumonia or serious infection in newborn. To do this test, a swab is used to take cells from your vagina and rectum to be tested.

Maternal serum screen (also called quad screen, triple test, triple screen, multiple marker screen, or AFP): A screening test done at 15–20 weeks to detect higher risk of chromosomal disorders, including Down syndrome and trisomy 18, and neural tube defects such as spina bifida. Based on test results, your doctor may suggest other tests to diagnose a disorder. The test draws blood to measure the levels of certain substances in the mother's blood.

Nonstress test (NST): This test is performed after 28 weeks to monitor your baby's health. It can show signs of fetal distress, such as your baby not getting enough oxygen. A belt is placed around the mother's belly to measure the baby's heart rate in response to its own movements.

Ultrasound exam: An ultrasound exam can be performed at any point during the pregnancy. Ultrasound exams are not routine. But it is not uncommon for women to have a standard ultrasound exam between 18 and 20 weeks to look for signs of problems with the baby's organs and body systems and confirm the age of the fetus and proper growth. It also might be able to tell the sex of your baby.

Ultrasound exam is also used as part of the first trimester screen and biophysical profile (BPP). Based on exam results, your doctor may suggest other tests or other types of ultrasound to help detect a problem. Ultrasound uses sound waves to create a picture of your baby on a monitor. With a standard ultrasound, a gel is spread on your abdomen. A special tool is moved over your abdomen, which allows your doctor and you to view the baby on a monitor.

Urine test: A urine sample can look for signs of health problems, such as urinary tract infection, diabetes, and preeclampsia. If your doctor suspects a problem, the sample might be sent to a lab for more in-depth testing. For this test, you will collect a small sample of clean, midstream urine in a sterile plastic cup. Testing strips that look for certain substances in your urine are dipped in the sample. The sample also can be looked at under a microscope.

Understanding Prenatal Tests and Test Results

If your doctor suggests certain prenatal tests, do not be afraid to ask lots of questions. Learning about the test, why your doctor is suggesting it for you, and what the test results could mean can help you cope with any worries or fears you might have. Keep in mind that screening tests do not diagnose problems. They evaluate risk. So if a screening test comes back abnormal, this does not mean there is a problem with your baby. More information is needed. Your doctor can explain what test results mean and possible next steps.

Avoid Keepsake Ultrasounds

You might think a keepsake ultrasound is a must-have for your scrapbook. But, doctors advise against ultrasound when there is no medical need to do so. Some companies sell keepsake ultrasound videos and images. Although ultrasound is considered safe for medical purposes, exposure to ultrasound energy for a keepsake video or image may put a mother and her unborn baby at risk. Don't take that chance.

Section 51.2

Infertility Tests

Excerpted from "Infertility: FAQs," U.S. Department of
Health and Human Services (HHS), July 1, 2009.

How will doctors find out if a woman and her partner have fertility problems?

Doctors will do an infertility checkup. This involves a physical exam. The doctor will also ask for both partners' health and sexual histories. Sometimes this can find the problem. However, most of the time, the doctor will need to do more tests.

In men, doctors usually begin by testing the semen. They look at the number, shape, and movement of the sperm. Sometimes doctors also suggest testing the level of a man's hormones.

In women, the first step is to find out if she is ovulating each month. There are a few ways to do this. A woman can track her ovulation at home by:

- writing down changes in her morning body temperature for several months,

- writing down how her cervical mucus looks for several months, or

- using a home ovulation test kit (available at drug or grocery stores).

Doctors can also check ovulation with blood tests. Or they can do an ultrasound of the ovaries. If ovulation is normal, there are other fertility tests available.

Some common tests of fertility in women include:

- **Hysterosalpingography:** This is an x-ray of the uterus and fallopian tubes. Doctors inject a special dye into the uterus through the vagina. This dye shows up in the x-ray. Doctors can then watch to see if the dye moves freely through the uterus and fallopian tubes. This can help them find physical blocks that may be causing infertility. Blocks in the system can keep the egg from moving from the fallopian tube to the uterus. A block could also keep the sperm from reaching the egg.

- **Laparoscopy:** A minor surgery to see inside the abdomen. The doctor does this with a small tool with a light called a laparoscope. She or he makes a small cut in the lower abdomen and inserts the laparoscope. With the laparoscope, the doctor can check the ovaries, fallopian tubes, and uterus for disease and physical problems. Doctors can usually find scarring and endometriosis by laparoscopy.

Finding the cause of infertility can be a long and emotional process. It may take time to complete all the needed tests. So do not worry if the problem is not found right away.

Chapter 52

Sleep Disorder Tests

What are sleep studies?

Sleep studies allow doctors to measure how much and how well you sleep. They also help show whether you have sleep problems and how severe they are. Sleep studies are important because untreated sleep disorders can increase your risk of high blood pressure, heart attack, stroke, and other medical conditions. Sleep disorders also have been linked to an increased risk of injury due to falls and car accidents.

Doctors can diagnose and treat sleep disorders. Talk with your doctor if you snore regularly or feel very tired while at work or school most days of the week. You also may want to talk with your doctor if you often have trouble falling or staying asleep, or if you wake up too early and are not able to go back to sleep. These are common signs of a sleep disorder.

Before a Sleep Study

Before a sleep study, your doctor may ask you about your sleep habits and whether you feel well rested and alert during the day. You may be asked to keep a sleep diary or sleep log. You'll record information such as when you went to bed, when you woke up, how many times you woke up during the night, and more.

This chapter begins with text excerpted from "Sleep Studies," National Heart, Lung, and Blood Institute (NHLBI), December 2009; and concludes with an excerpt from "Monitoring Sleep One Z at a Time: June 27, 2008," National Institute of Biomedical Imaging and Bioengineering (NIBIB), July 14, 2009.

You may need to stop or limit the use of tobacco, caffeine and other stimulants, and some medicines before having a sleep study. Your doctor may ask you about alcohol, medicines, or other substances that you take. Make sure you tell your doctor about all of the medicines you take, including over-the-counter products. Your doctor also may ask about any allergies you have. Talk with your doctor before the sleep study and never stop taking your medicines unless the doctor who prescribed them tells you to do so.

You should try to sleep well the night before you have a maintenance of wakefulness test (MWT) because you will have to try to stay awake during the test. If you are being tested as a requirement for a transportation- or safety-related job, you may be asked to take a drug-screening test. You also should try to sleep well for a night or two before you have a multiple sleep latency test (MSLT) because the results will be more accurate.

If you are going to have a home-based sleep test with a portable monitor, you'll need to visit a sleep center or your doctor's office to pick up the equipment. Your doctor or a technician will tell you how to use the equipment.

Sleep Study

Sleep studies are painless. The polysomnogram (PSG), multiple sleep latency test (MSLT), and maintenance of wakefulness test (MWT) usually are done at a sleep center. The room the sleep study is done in may look like a hotel room. A technician makes the room comfortable for you and sets the temperature to your liking. Most of your contact at the sleep center will be with nurses or technicians. You can ask them questions about the sleep study. They can answer questions about the test itself, but they usually cannot give you the test results.

Sticky patches and sensors called electrodes are placed on your scalp, face, chest, limbs, and a finger. While you sleep, these sensors record your brain activity, eye movements, heart rate and rhythm, blood pressure, and the amount of oxygen in your blood.

Elastic belts are placed around your chest and abdomen. They measure chest movements and the strength and duration of inhaled and exhaled breaths. Wires attached to the sensors transmit the data to a computer in the next room. The wires are very thin and flexible and are bundled together so they don't restrict movement, disrupt your sleep, or cause other discomfort.

If you have signs of sleep apnea, you may have a split-night sleep study. During the first half of the night, the technician records your sleep patterns. At the start of the second half of the night, he or she wakes you to fit a CPAP (continuous positive airway pressure) mask over your nose and/or mouth. The mask is connected to a small machine that gently blows air through the mask. This creates mild pressure that keeps your airway open while you sleep. The technician checks how you sleep with the CPAP machine. He or she adjusts the flow of air through the mask to find the setting that's right for you.

At the end of the PSG, the technician removes the sensors. If you are having a daytime sleep study, such as an MSLT, some of the sensors may be left on for that test. Parents usually are required to spend the night with their child during the child's PSG.

During a Multiple Sleep Latency Test (MSLT)

The MSLT is a daytime sleep study that's usually done after a PSG. Sensors on your scalp, face, and chin usually are used for this test. These sensors record brain activity. They show various stages of sleep and how long it takes you to fall asleep. Sometimes your breathing also is checked during an MSLT. A technician in another room watches these recordings as you sleep. He or she fixes any problems with the recordings that occur.

About 1.5–3 hours after you wake from the PSG, you are asked to relax in a quiet room for about 30 minutes. The test is repeated four or five times throughout the day. This is because your ability to fall asleep changes throughout the day. You get two-hour breaks between tests. You need to stay awake during the breaks.

The MSLT records whether you fall asleep during the test and what types and stages of sleep you have. Sleep has two basic types: rapid eye movement (REM) and non-REM. Non-REM sleep has three distinct stages. REM sleep and the three stages of non-REM sleep occur in patterns throughout the night. The types and stages of sleep you have during the day can help your doctor diagnose sleep disorders such as narcolepsy and idiopathic hypersomnia.

During a Maintenance of Wakefulness Test

This sleep study occurs during the day. It is usually done after a PSG and takes most of the day. Sensors on your scalp, face, and chin are used to measure when you are awake or asleep. You sit quietly on a bed in a comfortable position and look straight ahead. Then you simply try to stay awake for a period of time.

An MWT typically includes four trials lasting about 40 minutes each. If you fall asleep, the technician will wake you after about 90 seconds. There usually are two-hour breaks between trials. During these breaks, you can read, watch television, and so forth. If you are being tested as a requirement for a transportation- or safety-related job, you may need a drug-screening test before a MWT.

During a Home-Based Portable Monitor Test

If you're having a home-based portable monitor test, you'll need to set up the equipment at home before you go to sleep. When you pick up the equipment at the sleep center or your doctor's office, someone will tell you how to use it.

During Actigraphy

You do not have to go to a sleep center for this test. An Actigraph is a small device that is usually worn like a wristwatch. You can go about your normal routine while you wear it. You remove it while bathing or swimming. The Actigraph measures your sleep-wake behavior over 3–7 days and nights. Results give your doctor a better idea about your sleep habits, such as when you sleep or nap and whether the lights are on while you sleep. You may be asked to keep a sleep diary while you wear an Actigraph.

What to Expect after a Sleep Study

Once the sensors are removed after a polysomnogram (PSG), multiple sleep latency test, or maintenance of wakefulness test, you can go home. If you used an Actigraph or a home-based portable monitor, you will return the equipment to a sleep center or your doctor's office.

You will not receive a diagnosis right away. Your primary care doctor or sleep specialist will review the results of your sleep study or sleep studies. He or she will use your medical history, your sleep history, and the test results to make a diagnosis.

New Technology for Monitoring Sleep

Assessing individuals who suffer from poor sleep may get easier as a new device based on technology developed by researchers at the Beth Israel Deaconess Medical Center in Boston finds its way to sleep labs and doctors' offices. The new device, designed by Embla Systems, a Denver-based sleep diagnostic equipment firm, may also help cardiologists more precisely track heart failure and track therapies that reduce its impact since heart failure is often associated with poor-quality sleep.

Because of the device's small size and portability, it may also permit at-home monitoring of sleep quality.

The new device has been delivered to sleep labs, sleep physicians, and primary care physicians in the U.S. The device, currently about the size of a cell phone, would include data storage so that information taken through the night could be transmitted to a doctor's office. This would be of particular use for the 13 million U.S. patients who must wear masks attached to continuous positive airway pressure machines that blow air down the patient's airway. Weight gain or loss over time can alter pressure needs. The new device would allow clinicians to remotely monitor the sleep quality of those patients and change their pressures as needed rather than requiring patients to return to a sleep lab for assessment. Baker anticipates medical insurance reimbursement for the device for in-home use. He also sees an opportunity for the device in sports. Teams could track how well the team or key players sleep, and then manage their schedules for optimal performance.

Chapter 53

Thyroid and Other Endocrine Tests

Chapter Contents

Section 53.1

Recognizing Endocrine System Dysfunction

"Endocrine System and Syndromes: Overview, Summary Table, Tests, and Treatments," © 2011 American Association for Clinical Chemistry. Reprinted with permission. For additional information about clinical lab testing, visit the Lab Tests Online website at www.labtestsonline.org.

What Is the Endocrine System?

The endocrine system is made up of various glands located throughout the body. Together with the nervous system, it controls and regulates all bodily functions. While the nervous system uses nerve impulses as a means of control, the endocrine system uses chemical messenger molecules called hormones. These hormones are released by the endocrine glands into the blood stream, where they have an effect on specific target tissues. The targets have specific receptors for the hormones, like fitting a key to a lock. Sometimes the target tissue of a hormone is another gland. The hormone stimulates the receptor gland to produce and release another hormone into the blood, which in turn can affect different target tissues. An example of this is the hypothalamus gland that releases thyrotropin-releasing hormone (TRH). This hormone stimulates the pituitary gland to release thyrotropin (more commonly called TSH or thyroid-stimulating hormone). TSH in turn stimulates the thyroid gland to produce thyroid hormones thyroxine (T_4) and triiodothyronine (T_3), which help to regulate the rate of metabolism throughout the body.

All of the endocrine glands are carefully controlled with the use of feedback systems. For example, the amount of thyroid hormone in the bloodstream acts as a regulating factor on the hypothalamus and pituitary, stimulating them to release more TRH and TSH respectively when thyroid hormone concentrations in the blood decrease. In some cases, such as thyroid hormone, the body strives to keep a relatively constant amount in the blood.

Some hormones have a daily or monthly pattern of release. For example, concentrations of the adrenal hormone cortisol are high in the morning and lower late in the evening, while levels of the pituitary hormones follicle-stimulating hormone (FSH) and luteinizing hormone (LH) increase and decrease in regular patterns to regulate a woman's monthly menstrual cycle. Other hormones are generally present in very small quantities in the blood and are released in specific situations, such as the release of epinephrine (adrenaline) from the adrenal glands in response to stress.

Table 53.1 includes a listing of endocrine glands, the hormones they produce, and the diseases and conditions associated with their improper function.

Tests

The goals of endocrine testing are to identify the hormone(s) that are being over- or under-produced, to determine which gland(s) are involved, and to determine the cause of the hormone imbalance. This may involve measuring hormone levels and their metabolites in the blood and/or urine. Stimulation or suppression testing may be utilized to evaluate hormone production and/or gland interaction with other glands and hormones. If a tumor is suspected, then imaging scans may be used to help locate the tumor. If symptoms are suspected to be due to an inherited condition, then genetic testing may be recommended. Patients often see an endocrinologist (an endocrine gland specialist) to help them determine the appropriate testing and treatment.

Treatments

Treatment of endocrine gland-related conditions depends on the cause. If the problem is due to a drug therapy, then the patient may be switched to another medication. It is important that patients do not abruptly stop taking a medication without consulting their doctor. This can cause additional, sometimes serious, complications. If the condition is due to hyperplasia, then the action of the hormone may be able to be blocked. If the condition is due to a tumor, then the tumor may be able to be surgically removed. Often this will resolve the problem or decrease the disorder to the point that it can be controlled.

In some cases, after a gland has been removed, the patient may need to take replacement medications, such as taking thyroid hormone after the thyroid gland has been removed. Replacement is also often used when a patient's gland has been damaged or is otherwise not capable of producing a sufficient quantity of one or more hormones. When patients have a gene mutation associated with MEN-1 or MEN-2, careful lifetime monitoring may be necessary. Treatment of all endocrine-related conditions will be tailored to the individual. Patients should work with their doctor to determine the right course of action for them.

Table 53.1. Table of Endocrine Glands

Endocrine Gland	Location/ Description	Hormones Gland Produces	Gland/ Hormone Function	Examples of Disorders Associated with Improper Function
Hypothalamus	Lower middle of the brain	Growth hormone-releasing hormone (GHRH)	Communicates with both nervous and endocrine systems;	Precocious puberty (early GnRH production)
		Thyrotropin-releasing hormone (TRH)	Stimulates (GHRH, TRH, CRH, GnRH) or inhibits (PIF) hormone production in the pituitary	Kallmann syndrome (inadequate GnRH production)
		Corticotropin-releasing hormone (CRH)		Thyroid diseases
		Gonadotropin-releasing hormone (GnRH)		
		Prolactin Inhibitory Factor (PIF, dopamine)		
		Oxytocin	Uterine contraction during labor	Diabetes insipidus (inadequate AVP production)
		Arginine vasopressin (AVP), also called antidiuretic hormone (ADH)	Water balance	
Pituitary	Below hypothalamus, behind sinus cavity	Prolactin	Milk production	Hypopituitarism
		Growth Hormone (GH)	Bone growth	Empty Sella Syndrome
		ACTH	Stimulates cortisol	Galactorrhea (milk production not during pregnancy due to high prolactin)
		TSH	Stimulates thyroid hormone	Acromegaly or Gigantism (excess GH)
		LH, FSH	Regulation of testosterone and estrogen, fertility	Growth Hormone Deficiency (GHD)
				Cushing disease (excess ACTH)
				Hyper/hypothyroidism
				Loss of menstrual period
				Loss of sex drive
				Infertility

Gland	Location	Hormones	Function	Related Conditions
Thyroid	Butterfly-shaped; lies flat against windpipe in the throat	T_4 (thyroxine) T_3 (triiodothyronine) Calcitonin	Helps regulate the rate of metabolism Helps regulate bone status, blood calcium	Thyroid diseases (including hypo and hyperthyroidism)
Parathyroid	4 tiny glands located behind, next to, or below the thyroid	Parathyroid hormone (PTH)	Regulates blood calcium	Hyperparathyroidism Hypoparathyroidism MEN1
Adrenal	2 triangular organs, on top of each kidney	Epinephrine (adrenaline) norepinephrine Aldosterone Cortisol DHEA-S	Blood pressure regulation, stress reaction Salt, water balance Stress reaction Body hair development at puberty	Pheochromocytoma (MEN2) Conn Syndrome Cushing Syndrome Addison Disease Cancer Adrenal Hyperplasia
Ovaries (females only)	2, located in the pelvis	Estrogen Progesterone	Female sexual characteristics	Polycystic ovary syndrome (PCOS)
Testes (males only)	2, located in the groin	Testosterone	Male sexual characteristics	Hypogonadism
Pancreas	Large, gourd-shaped gland, located behind the stomach	Insulin Glucagon Somatostatin	Glucose regulation	Diabetes mellitus MEN1 Zollinger-Ellison syndrome
Pineal	Lower side of the brain	Melatonin	Not well understood; Helps control sleep patterns, affects reproduction	

Section 53.2

Thyroid Function Tests

This section is excerpted from "Thyroid Function Tests," National Institute of Diabetes and Digestive and Kidney Diseases (NIDDK), January 2010.

Why Are Thyroid Function Tests Performed?

Thyroid function tests are used to evaluate the thyroid's functioning and to diagnose and help determine the cause of thyroid diseases. Sometimes the body produces too much or too little thyroid hormone. Too much thyroid hormone in the bloodstream causes hyperthyroidism, which results in increased metabolic rate, weight loss, sweating, rapid heart rate, and high blood pressure, among other symptoms. Too little thyroid hormone causes hypothyroidism, which slows down bodily functions and leads to fatigue, weight gain, cold intolerance, and related symptoms.

Hyperthyroidism and hypothyroidism are most often caused by autoimmune diseases. Normally, the immune system produces antibodies that defend the body against foreign substances such as bacteria. In autoimmune diseases, however, the immune system produces autoantibodies that attack the body's own healthy cells and tissues—in this case, the thyroid. Graves disease is the most common cause of autoimmune hyperthyroidism. Hashimoto disease is the most common cause of autoimmune hypothyroidism. Both Graves disease and Hashimoto disease are due to an immune attack on the thyroid. In Graves disease, the attacking antibodies stimulate thyroid hormone production.

Blood tests assess thyroid function by measuring TSH and thyroid hormone levels and detecting certain autoantibodies present in autoimmune thyroid disease. Radiologic tests either assess thyroid function or detect abnormalities in the thyroid gland.

What Blood Tests Are Used to Assess Thyroid Function?

Usually the first blood test performed is the TSH test. TSH is the key hormone for diagnosing hyperthyroidism and hypothyroidism. If results of the TSH test are abnormal, one or more additional tests are needed to help determine the cause of the problem.

TSH Test

This blood test is the most sensitive test of thyroid function available. The TSH test can detect TSH blood levels as low as 0.01 milli-international units per liter (mIU/L). The normal range for TSH is between 0.3 and 4.0 mIU/L, although the range varies from one laboratory to another.

The TSH test is based on the way TSH and thyroid hormones work together. Normally, the pituitary boosts TSH production when thyroid hormone levels in the blood are low. The thyroid responds by making more hormone. Then, when the body has enough thyroid hormone circulating in the blood, TSH output drops. The cycle repeats continuously to maintain a healthy level of thyroid hormone in the body. The TSH test measures the amount of TSH being secreted by the pituitary.

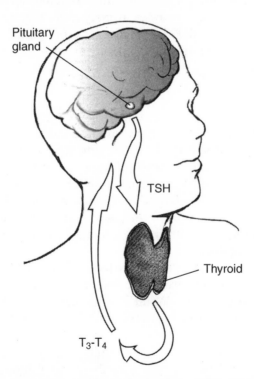

Figure 53.1. The thyroid gland's production of thyroid hormones (T_3 and T_4) is regulated by thyroid-stimulating hormone (TSH), which is made by the pituitary gland.

In people whose thyroid produces too much thyroid hormone, the pituitary shuts down TSH production, leading to low or even undetectable TSH levels in the blood. An abnormally low TSH level suggests hyperthyroidism.

In people whose thyroid is not functioning normally and produces too little thyroid hormone, the thyroid cannot respond normally to TSH by producing thyroid hormone. As a result, the pituitary keeps making TSH, trying to get the thyroid to respond. An abnormally high TSH level suggests hypothyroidism.

Occasionally, however, a low TSH level can indicate a type of hypothyroidism called secondary hypothyroidism. Instead of a problem with the thyroid gland, this type of hypothyroidism is caused by an abnormality in the pituitary that prevents it from making enough TSH to stimulate thyroid hormone production.

Very rarely, hyperthyroidism can result from a problem with the pituitary rather than the thyroid. Noncancerous, or benign, pituitary tumors may overproduce TSH and cause thyroid hormone levels to rise. However, such tumors are extremely rare. The usual cause of a high TSH level is an under-functioning thyroid gland or inadequate dosage of thyroid hormone medication in patients taking replacement hormone.

T_4 Tests

T_4 is the principal thyroid hormone and exists in two forms—T_4 that is bound to proteins in the blood and kept in reserve until the body needs it, and a small amount of unbound or free T_4 (FT_4), which is the active form of the hormone and is available to body tissues. The normal range for total T_4—bound and free together—is usually about 4.5 to 12.6 micrograms per deciliter (µg/dL), although the range varies from one laboratory to another. The normal FT_4 range is about 0.7 to 1.8 nanograms per deciliter (ng/dL).

Elevated total T_4 or FT_4 suggests hyperthyroidism, and low total T_4 or FT_4 suggests hypothyroidism. Sometimes total T_4 levels are abnormal because the protein-bound T_4 is abnormally high or low due to elevated or low concentrations of the protein that binds T_4. Therefore, FT_4 must be calculated separately.

Measuring FT_4 directly requires complicated laboratory procedures, so FT_4 is usually estimated based on the ratio of binding protein to total T_4. Normal FT_4 levels, when the total T_4 is high or low, indicate the issue is the binding protein, not the thyroid. For example, pregnancy or the use of oral contraceptives increases levels of binding protein in the blood. In this case, the total T_4 will be high due to the binding protein but the person does not have hyperthyroidism. Severe illness or the use of corticosteroids—a class of medications that treat asthma, arthritis, and skin conditions, among other health problems—can decrease binding protein levels. The total T_4 measurement will be low as a consequence, but the person does not have hypothyroidism. In either case—having high binding protein or having low binding protein—the FT_4 will be normal and the person has normal thyroid function—also called euthyroid.

T_3 *Test*

Only about 20% of the T_3 circulating in the blood comes from the thyroid gland, while all of the circulating T_4 comes from the thyroid. The remaining 80% of circulating T_3 comes from various cells all over the body where T_4 is converted to T_3. T_3 is far more active than T_4 and, like T_4, exists in both bound and free states. In some cases of hyperthyroidism, FT_4 is normal but free T_3 (FT_3) is elevated, so measuring both forms is useful if hyperthyroidism is suspected. The normal FT_3 range is about 0.2 to 0.5 ng/dL. The T_3 test is not useful in diagnosing hypothyroidism because levels are not reduced until the hypothyroidism is severe.

Thyroid-Stimulating Immunoglobulin (TSI) Test

TSI is an autoantibody present in Graves disease, the most common cause of hyperthyroidism. TSI mimics TSH by stimulating the thyroid cells, causing the thyroid gland to secrete excess hormone. The TSI test detects TSI circulating in the blood and is usually measured in specific instances in people with Graves disease—when the diagnosis is obscure, during pregnancy, and to determine if remission has occurred.

Antithyroid Antibody Test

Antithyroid antibodies are present in Hashimoto disease, the most common cause of hypothyroidism. Antithyroid antibodies are markers in the blood, and their presence is extremely helpful in diagnosing Hashimoto disease. Two principal types of antithyroid antibodies are anti-TG antibodies, which attack a protein in the thyroid called thyroglobulin; and anti-thyroperoxidase, or anti-TPO, antibodies, which attack an enzyme in thyroid cells called thyroperoxidase.

What Radiologic Tests Are Used to Assess Thyroid Function?

Two radiologic tests—the radioactive iodine uptake (RAIU) test and a thyroid scan—may be used to aid diagnosis and treatment.

RAIU Test

The thyroid uses iodine from food to make thyroid hormone. The RAIU test measures the amount of iodine the thyroid collects from the bloodstream. The test helps doctors evaluate how the thyroid is functioning and determine the cause of hyperthyroidism. The RAIU is not used to assess hypothyroidism.

For this test, the patient swallows a small amount of radioactive iodine in liquid or capsule form. After 4–6 hours and again at 24 hours, the patient returns to the testing center, where the doctor measures the amount of radioactive iodine taken up by the thyroid. The measurement is taken with a small device called a gamma probe, which resembles a microphone. The gamma probe is positioned near the patient's neck over the thyroid gland. Measurement takes only a few minutes and is painless.

In the diagnosis of hyperthyroidism, a high RAIU reading usually indicates an overactive thyroid that produces too much thyroid hormone, as seen in Graves disease or toxic nodular goiter, an enlargement of the thyroid gland. A low RAIU reading suggests the thyroid is not overactive.

Thyroiditis may cause leakage of thyroid hormone and iodine out of the thyroid gland into the bloodstream, which can lead to high T_4 levels. Because the thyroid is inflamed, it does not take up the radioactive iodine given as part of the RAIU test. Hyperthyroidism seen in Graves disease would be marked by high blood T_4 and a high RAIU. In thyroiditis, temporary hyperthyroidism may exist because of the release of T_4 into the blood, but the RAIU is low because of the inflammation. Temporary hyperthyroidism in thyroiditis is often followed by a period of hypothyroidism before the thyroid heals.

The radioactive compound used in the RAIU test is safe to ingest in the small amount given. Pregnant and nursing women should not undergo this test, however, because the radioactive material can travel across the placenta to the baby's bloodstream or be transmitted to the baby via breast milk.

Thyroid Scan

A thyroid scan does not test thyroid function per se, but instead uses radioactive material to create a picture of the thyroid. The scan shows the size and shape of the thyroid and provides images of irregularities such as nodules. Nodules are tumors in the thyroid that can either be benign or cancerous and can sometimes produce excess thyroid hormone. The scan does not identify whether the nodules are benign or cancerous.

For the scan, radioactive iodine or radioactive technetium is either injected into the patient's vein or swallowed in liquid or capsule form. The scan takes place 30 minutes after an injection or 6–24 hours after the radioactive substance is swallowed. The patient lies on an examining table for the scan, which takes about 30 minutes. A device called a gamma camera is suspended over the table or may be located within a large, doughnut-shaped machine that resembles a computerized tomography (CT) scanner.

The gamma camera detects the radioactive material and sends images to a computer that show how and where the radioactive substance has been distributed in the thyroid. Nodules that produce excess thyroid hormone—so-called hot, or toxic, nodules—show up clearly because they absorb more radioactive material than normal thyroid tissue. Graves disease shows up as a diffuse, overall increase in radioactivity rather than a localized spot.

Table 53.2. Typical thyroid function test results: Hyperthyroidism

		Test		
Cause:	TSH	T_3/T_4	TSI	RAIU
Graves Disease	↓	↑	+	↑
Thyroiditis (early state)	↓	↑	–	↑
Thyroid nodules (hot, or toxic)	↓	↑	–	↑ or N

Key: N = Normal; ↑ = Above normal; ↓ = Below normal; + = Positive; – = Negative

Table 53.3. Typical thyroid function test results: Hypothyroidism

		Test	
Cause:	TSH	T_3/T_4	Antithyroid Antibody
Hashimoto disease (thyroiditis)	↑	↓ or N	+
Hashimoto disease (thyroiditis) later stage	↑	↓	+
Pituitary abnormality	↓	↓	–

Key: N = Normal; ↑ = Above normal; ↓ = Below normal; + = Positive; – = Negative

What Do Thyroid Function Test Results Tell Doctors?

The pattern of test results in people with hyperthyroidism or hypothyroidism can help doctors determine the underlying cause of the condition. Because many complex factors affect thyroid function and hormone levels, doctors must take the patient's full medical history into account when interpreting thyroid function tests.

Chapter 54

Vision Tests

Chapter Contents

Section 54.1

Routine Eye Exam

"Why does my eye care professional ask me to read the
letters on an eye chart?" by Catherine Cukras, MD, PhD,
National Eye Institute (NEI), July 2010.

Why Does My Eye Care Professional Ask Me to Read the Letters on an Eye Chart?

"An eye chart helps your eye care professional assess the sharpness
of your vision, or visual acuity," says National Eye Institute (NEI)
ophthalmologist Catherine Cukras, MD, PhD. Visual acuity is a basic
measure of visual function. The measurement that is typically associated with normal vision is 20/20. This number means that when you
are 20 feet away from an object, you can see details that most people
with normal vision can see at that distance. If your vision is 20/40, it
means that when you are 20 feet away from an object, you can only
see what most people see clearly from 40 feet away.

Snellen Chart

There are many different types of eye charts that your eye care
professional may use to measure your visual acuity. The eye chart with
a large "E" at the top and rows of smaller letters below, which was created in the mid-19th century, is known as a Snellen chart. The chart is
named after the Dutch ophthalmologist who developed it.

When clinical research studies became important in vision science
beginning in the 1970s, researchers needed a standardized way to
measure visual acuity. Therefore, a group of NEI scientists developed
a new chart that measures vision consistently, regardless of the exam
environment. It is called an ETDRS chart because it was developed as
part of the Early Treatment for Diabetic Retinopathy Study. This chart
is illuminated from behind in a light box so the lighting is uniform,
and it has the same number of letters on each line that decrease in
size, based on a mathematical formula.

ETDRS Chart

"The ETDRS chart is an important tool to accurately measure visual acuity, especially for multi-center clinical trials where the participants are located around the country," Dr. Cukras says.

Using either chart, eye care professionals can determine if your eye is functioning properly. If your visual acuity is worse than 20/20, your visual system may not be working properly. You may have a refractive error such as nearsightedness that could be corrected with glasses, or you could have a more serious problem such as a cataract, retinal disease, or glaucoma.

"Based on your eye chart measurement, your eye care professional can conduct additional tests to properly diagnose a more serious visual condition," Dr. Cukras says.

Section 54.2

Comprehensive Dilated Eye Exam

Excerpted from "Healthy Eyes Bulletin,"
National Eye Institute (NEI), 2010.

Healthy Eyes Start with a Dilated Eye Exam

Getting a comprehensive dilated eye exam is one of the best things you can do to keep your eyes healthy. In this painless procedure, an eye care professional examines your eyes to look for common vision problems and eye diseases, many of which have no early warning signs. Different from the basic eye exam one has to get glasses or contact lenses, comprehensive dilated eye exams can help protect your sight by making sure you are seeing your best and detecting eye diseases in their early stages, before vision loss has occurred.

A comprehensive dilated eye exam includes the following:

- **Dilation:** Drops are placed in your eyes to dilate, or widen, the pupils. Your eye care professional uses a special magnifying lens to examine your retina to look for signs of damage and other eye problems, such as diabetic retinopathy or age-related macular degeneration. A dilated eye exam also allows your doctor to check for damage to the optic nerve that occurs when a person has glaucoma. After the examination, your close-up vision may remain blurred for several hours.

- **Tonometry:** This test helps to detect glaucoma by measuring eye pressure. Your eye care professional may direct a quick puff of air onto the eye, or gently apply a pressure-sensitive tip near or against the eye. Numbing drops may be applied to your eye for this test. Elevated pressure is a possible sign of glaucoma.

- **Visual field test:** This test measures your side (peripheral) vision. It helps your eye care professional find out if you have lost side vision, a sign of glaucoma.

- **Visual acuity test:** This eye chart test measures how well you see at various distances.

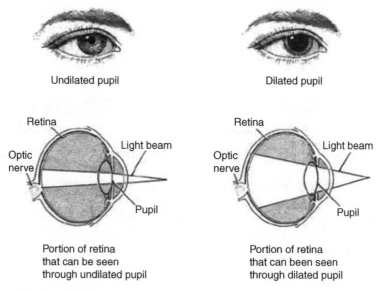

Undilated pupil   Dilated pupil

Figure 54.1. Before and After the Pupil Is Dilated (image courtesy National Eye Institute).

Section 54.3

Common Tests for Glaucoma

Diagnostic Tests

Early detection, through regular and complete eye exams, is the key to protecting your vision from damage caused by glaucoma. It is important to have your eyes examined regularly.

Your eyes should be tested:

• before age 40, every two to four years;

• from age 40 to age 54, every one to three years;

• from age 55 to 64, every one to two years; and

• after age 65, every six to 12 months.

Anyone with high risk factors, should be tested every year or two after age 35.

Four Common Tests for Glaucoma

Regular glaucoma check-ups include two routine eye tests: tonometry and ophthalmoscopy.

Tonometry: The tonometry test measures the inner pressure of the eye. Usually drops are used to numb the eye. Then the doctor or technician will use a special device that measures the eye's pressure.

Ophthalmoscopy: Used to examine the inside of the eye, especially the optic nerve. In a darkened room, the doctor will magnify your eye by using an ophthalmoscope (an instrument with a small light on the end). This helps the doctor look at the shape and color of the optic nerve.

If the pressure in the eye is not in the normal range, or if the optic nerve looks unusual, then one or two special glaucoma tests will be done. These two tests are called perimetry and gonioscopy.

Perimetry: The perimetry test is also called a visual field test. During this test, you will be asked to look straight ahead and then indicate when a moving light passes your peripheral (or side) vision. This helps draw a map of your vision.

Gonioscopy: A painless eye test that checks if the angle where the iris meets the cornea is open or closed, showing if either open-angle or closed-angle glaucoma is present.

Optic Nerve Computer Imaging

In recent years three new techniques of optic nerve imaging have become widely available. These are scanning laser polarimetry (GDx), confocal laser ophthalmoscopy (Heidelberg Retinal Tomography or HRT), and optical coherence tomography (OCT).

The GDx machine does not actually image the optic nerve but rather it measures the thickness of the nerve fiber layer on the retinal surface just before the fibers pass over the optic nerve margin to form the optic nerve. The HRT scans the retinal surface and optic nerve with a laser. It then constructs a topographic (3-D) image of the optic nerve including a contour outline of the optic cup. The nerve fiber layer thickness is also measured. The OCT instrument utilizes a technique called optical coherence tomography which creates images by use of special beams of light. The OCT machine can create a contour map of the optic nerve, optic cup, and measure the retinal nerve fiber thickness. Over time, all three of these machines can detect loss of optic nerve fibers.

Your intraocular eye pressure (IOP) is important to determining your risk for glaucoma. If you have high IOP, careful management of your eye pressure with medications can help prevent vision loss. Recent discoveries about the cornea, the clear part of the eye's protective covering, are showing that corneal thickness is an important factor in accurately diagnosing eye pressure. In response to these findings, the Glaucoma Research Foundation has put together this brief guide to help you understand how your corneal thickness affects your risk for glaucoma, and what you can do to make sure your diagnosis is accurate.

Corneal Thickness

In 2002, the five-year report of the Ocular Hypertension Study (OHTS) was released. The study's goal was to determine if early intervention with pressure lowering medications could reduce the number of ocular hypertensive (OHT) patients that develop glaucoma. During the study, a critical discovery was made regarding corneal thickness and its role in intraocular eye pressure and glaucoma development.

Why Is Corneal Thickness Important?

Corneal thickness is important because it can mask an accurate reading of eye pressure, causing doctors to treat you for a condition that may not really exist or to treat you unnecessarily when readings are normal. Actual IOP may be underestimated in patients with thinner CCT, and overestimated in patients with thicker CCT. This may be important to your diagnosis; some people originally diagnosed with normal tension glaucoma may in fact be more accurately treated as having regular glaucoma; others diagnosed with ocular hypertension may be better treated as normal based on accurate CCT measurement. In light of this discovery, it is important to have your eyes checked regularly and to make sure your doctor takes your CCT into account for diagnosis.

A Thin Cornea—The Danger of Misreading Eye Pressure

Many times, patients with thin corneas (less than 555 micrometers [μm]) show artificially low IOP readings. This is dangerous because if your actual IOP is higher than your reading shows, you may be at risk for developing glaucoma and your doctor may not know it. Left untreated, high IOP can lead to glaucoma and vision loss. It is important that your doctor have an accurate IOP reading to diagnose your risk and decide upon a treatment plan.

A Thicker Cornea May Mean Less Reason to Worry about Glaucoma

Those patients with thicker CCT may show a higher reading of IOP than actually exists. This means their eye pressure is lower than thought, a lower IOP means that risk for developing glaucoma is lowered. However, it is still important to have regular eye exams to monitor eye pressure and stay aware of changes.

Pachymetry—A Simple Test to Determine Corneal Thickness

A pachymetry test is a simple, quick, painless test to measure the thickness of your cornea. With this measurement, your doctor can better understand your IOP reading, and develop a treatment plan that is right for your condition. The procedure takes only about a minute to measure both eyes.

Chapter 55

Vestibular (Balance)
Problem Tests

What is a balance disorder?

A balance disorder is a condition that makes you feel unsteady or dizzy, as if you are moving, spinning, or floating, even though you are standing still or lying down. Balance disorders can be caused by certain health conditions, medications, or a problem in the inner ear or the brain.

Our sense of balance is primarily controlled by a maze-like structure in our inner ear called the labyrinth, which is made of bone and soft tissue. At one end of the labyrinth is an intricate system of loops and pouches called the semicircular canals and the otolithic organs, which help us maintain our balance. At the other end is a snail-shaped organ called the cochlea, which enables us to hear. The medical term for all of the parts of the inner ear involved with balance is the vestibular system (see Figure 55.1).

Our visual system works with our vestibular system to keep objects from blurring when our head moves and to keep us aware of our position when we walk or when we ride in a vehicle. Sensory receptors in our joints and muscles also help us maintain our balance when we stand still or walk. The brain receives, interprets, and processes the information from these systems to control our balance.

Excerpted from "Balance Disorders," National Institute on Deafness an Other Communication Disorders (NIDCD), December 2009.

What are some types of balance disorders?

There are more than a dozen different balance disorders. Some of the most common are:

- **Benign paroxysmal positional vertigo (BPPV) or positional vertigo** is a brief, intense episode of vertigo that occurs because of a specific change in the position of the head. If you have BPPV, you might feel as if you are spinning when you look for an object on a high or low shelf or turn your head to look over your shoulder (such as when you back up your car).

- **Labyrinthitis** is an infection or inflammation of the inner ear that causes dizziness and loss of balance. It frequently is associated with an upper respiratory infection such as the flu.

- **Ménière disease** is associated with a change in fluid volume within parts of the labyrinth. Ménière disease causes episodes of vertigo, irregular hearing loss, tinnitus (a ringing or buzzing in the ear), and a feeling of fullness in the ear. The cause of this disease is unknown.

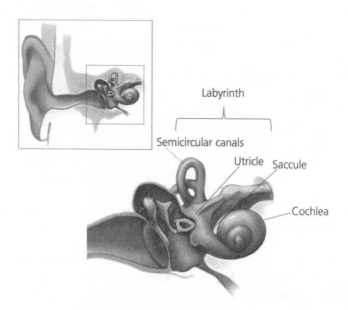

Figure 55.1. *The vestibular system in relation to the ear. (Source: NIH Medical Arts)*

- **Vestibular neuronitis** is an inflammation of the vestibular nerve and may be caused by a virus. Its primary symptom is vertigo.

- **Perilymph fistula** is a leakage of inner ear fluid into the middle ear. It can occur after a head injury, drastic changes in atmospheric pressure (such as when scuba diving), physical exertion, ear surgery, or chronic ear infections. Its most notable symptom, besides dizziness and nausea, is unsteadiness when walking or standing that increases with activity and decreases with rest. Some babies may be born with perilymph fistula, usually in association with hearing loss that is present at birth.

- **Mal de debarquement syndrome (MdDS)** is a balance disorder in which you feel as if you are continuously rocking or bobbing. It generally happens after an ocean cruise or other sea travel. Usually, the symptoms will go away in a matter of hours or days after you reach land. However, severe cases can last months or even years.

How is a balance disorder diagnosed?

Diagnosis of a balance disorder is difficult. There are many potential causes—including medical conditions and medications. To help evaluate a balance problem, your doctor may suggest you see an otolaryngologist. An otolaryngologist is a physician and surgeon who specializes in the ear, nose, and throat. An otolaryngologist may request tests to assess the cause and extent of the balance problem depending on your symptoms and health status.

The otolaryngologist may request a hearing examination, blood tests, an electronystagmogram (which measures eye movements and the muscles that control them), or imaging studies of your head and brain. Another possible test is called posturography. For this test, you stand on a special movable platform in front of a patterned screen. The doctor measures how your body moves in response to movement of the platform, the patterned screen, or both.

How do I know if I have a balance disorder?

Everyone has a dizzy spell now and then, but the term dizziness may mean something different to different people. For some people, dizziness might be a fleeting sensation of spinning, while for others it is intense and lasts a long time. Experts believe that more than four out of ten Americans will experience an episode of dizziness significant enough to send them to a doctor.

To help you decide whether or not you should seek medical help for a dizzy spell, ask yourself the following questions. If you answer yes to any of these questions, talk to your doctor.

- Do I feel unsteady?

- Do I feel as if the room is spinning around me?

- Do I feel as if I'm moving when I know I'm sitting or standing still?

- Do I lose my balance and fall?

- Do I feel as if I'm falling?

- Do I feel lightheaded or as if I might faint?

- Do I have blurred vision?

- Do I ever feel disoriented, such as losing my sense of time or where I am?

How can I help my doctor make a diagnosis?

You can help your doctor make a diagnosis and determine a treatment plan by answering the following questions. Be prepared to discuss this information during your appointment.

1. The best way I can describe my dizziness or balance problem is:

2. How often do I feel dizzy or have trouble keeping my balance?

3. Have I ever fallen? If yes, include the following: When did I fall? Where did I fall? Under what conditions did I fall? How often have I fallen?

4. These are the medicines I take: Include the name of prescription and over-the-counter medicine, amount in milligrams, how often it is taken, and the condition for which the medicine is taken.

Part Six

Home and Self-Ordered Tests

Chapter 56

An Introduction to Home-Use Medical Tests

Chapter Contents

Section 56.1

Convenient, Timely, Not Necessarily Perfect

This section includes "With Home Testing, Consumers Take Charge of Their Health: Introduction, Types of Tests, and Avoiding Errors," © 2011 American Association for Clinical Chemistry. Reprinted with permission. For additional information about clinical lab testing, visit the Lab Tests Online website at www.labtestsonline.org.

You can reap the benefits of home testing—convenience, privacy, control—as long as you educate yourself about the potential tradeoffs.

If you've been to the drugstore lately, you may have noticed an increase in the number of medical tests you can use in the privacy of your own home. Advances in testing technology—and changing attitudes towards patients' responsibility for their own health care—have made home testing a worldwide, billion-dollar-and-growing market. In fact, the word patient itself is gradually disappearing—people like you, who used to think of themselves as patients, are now hearing themselves called consumers who are taking charge of their own health care.

"People today aren't satisfied with just being told everything's fine," says James H. Nichols, PhD. "They want to know the exact number [on a test result] and what it means." Nichols directs the Clinical Chemistry Laboratory and Point-of-Care Testing at Baystate Medical Center in Springfield, Massachusetts. He says that recent market surveys indicate at least 25% of all medical tests are conducted outside the hospital laboratory. But, he adds, you should be cautious when purchasing over-the-counter tests—sometimes there are tradeoffs between convenience and quality. "Tests you buy in your local supermarket can be of similar quality to what we perform in the hospital at the bedside," Nichols says, "but not necessarily equivalent to the quality of testing performed in a laboratory."

Nurses, emergency medical technicians (EMTs), and laboratorians must be trained and certified in the testing procedure, the instrumentation used to perform the test, and quality control practices. There is no such requirement for consumers who purchase home tests, even the ones prescribed or recommended by their doctors.

530

Yet these tests, especially those designed to monitor diseases like diabetes, are important to your quality of life if you live with chronic illness. Home glucose testing, for example, allows you to monitor your blood sugar level and adjust diet or medication accordingly, without having to make frequent lab visits or risking precarious highs and lows in sugar levels.

Home testing offers many benefits, to be sure. But it's also important to recognize the potential tradeoffs between quality and convenience and take steps to protect yourself against bogus tests, the possibility of false results, and your own lack of training.

Tests Available for Home Use

Home tests can be used to screen for, diagnose, or monitor disease. Although a few home tests (for example, those that monitor blood-thinning medication) must be prescribed by your doctor, most are available over the counter (OTC) in local supermarkets or pharmacies or directly from manufacturers by internet, phone, or mail order. Categories of tests cleared by the Food and Drug Administration (FDA) for home use include those that measure:

- cholesterol, for assessing risk of heart disease;

- hemoglobin, for anemia;

- glucose for monitoring diabetes;

- alcohol and the presence of illegal drugs or drugs of abuse;

- nicotine metabolites, urine test to assess smoking status;

- human chorionic gonadotrophin (hCG), to screen for pregnancy;

- prothrombin time, for monitoring blood thinning and clotting;

- fecal occult blood, to screen for colorectal cancer;

- luteinizing hormone, salivary test to predict ovulation;

- sperm counts, to assess infertility;

- follicle stimulating hormone, to screen for menopause;

- urine dipsticks, for determining urinary tract infection.

Some home tests, like those for pregnancy, produce immediate results. Others are sold as collection devices—you use the device to collect a specimen (for example, urine or stool) and then mail the device containing the sample to the laboratory for evaluation. For example, if you want to know if you've contracted human immunodeficiency (HIV), the virus that causes acquired immunodeficiency syndrome (AIDS), you collect a small blood sample by pricking your finger at home and collecting a drop of blood on special filter paper that is then sent to a laboratory for analysis. Home collection kits that are mailed to a laboratory for analysis include the following tests:

- allergy testing for ten common home allergens
- antioxidant levels (urine lipid peroxide)
- male and female hormone testing
- high sensitivity C reactive protein (CRP), to screen for heart disease
- hepatitis C, to determine hepatitis infection
- HIV-1 antibody, for determining HIV infection
- microalbumin, to screen for kidney disease
- hair, urine, and salivary drugs of abuse testing
- hair, to assess mineral and toxic element levels
- performance and stress hormone levels of testosterone, dehydroepiandrosterone (DHEA), and cortisol
- prostate specific antigen, to screen for prostate cancer
- melatonin levels, to assess sleep
- thyroid stimulating hormone (TSH) for thyroid function
- antibodies involved in Celiac disease
- paternity testing
- blood typing

Test results are generally available within a week or two of mailing the specimen to the analyzing laboratory.

To search for information on a particular OTC test (by test name, manufacturer, or test type), visit the FDA's Office of In Vitro Diagnostic Device Evaluation and Safety online at http://www.fda.gov/medical devices/productsandmedicalprocedures/invitrodiagnostics/default.htm. Another FDA website, Currently Waived Analytes, (http://www.access data.fda.gov/scripts/cdrh/cfdocs/cfClia/analyteswaived.cfm) provides links to a broad range of tests kits and devices, including those that have been cleared by the FDA for home use.

Avoiding Errors

Although home tests offer convenience, privacy, and "real-time" results, those results are for your personal information. They do not qualify as official test results that could be recorded in your medical record or be acted on by a physician. Results that are used for medical decision making, and recorded as part of your medical history, must be performed by a laboratory or medical professional. Therefore, your doctor is likely to repeat the test that you've already done at home before acting on the result.

Errors can arise with any type of home test because of a number of possible mistakes. These range from using an expired test kit to storing the kit inappropriately to how you perform the test. Mistakes in the testing procedure often involve how you collect the sample, the time of day you collect it, or how precisely you time the test (not waiting long enough or waiting too long before noting the result). Even the impact of medications you may be taking may interfere with the results and may be a source of error to be considered.

With the possibility of these various errors, your doctor will most likely want to confirm the result of a home test to ensure its validity before proceeding with any course of action or treatment. While some follow-up procedures from erroneous home test results can be viewed simply as inconvenient, others may be costly or have serious implications. That's why your doctor will often choose to repeat even a seemingly straight-forward home pregnancy test.

"Many times, results from pregnancy tests may be invalid," Nichols says. "This is usually because people make mistakes in performing the test." In a study of pregnancy home use tests sold in France, for example, though nearly all of the negative specimens were interpreted correctly, 53% of urine specimens with pregnancy hormone concentrations at the minimal detection limit were considered negative. And 39% of specimens with twice the detection limit were considered negative. Investigators said that the main problem seemed to be the consumer's difficulty in interpreting instructions on the package insert and in following those instructions explicitly.

Regarding home testing for blood-thinning medications, Nichols says that clinicians get nervous about tests that monitor medications like Coumadin because of the consequences of acting on a wrong result. If the number is erroneously low, inadequate treatment could allow blood to clot. If the number is erroneously high, treatment could cause bruising or internal bleeding.

The importance of repeated (and continuous) monitoring was underscored in a report from a 1999 workshop on the standardization of blood coagulation devices. Alan Jacobson, MD, a panelist at the workshop, said that testing frequency, as much or more than testing accuracy, was responsible for most adverse treatment effects. "The average Medicare patient on Coumadin gets tested only four times per year," he said. "Cheap testing, but high price in adverse outcomes." In contrast, at Jacobson's institution, patients perform a test that is then verified by additional, separate tests performed by a clinician and a nurse to ensure that the patient can competently perform the test.

Section 56.2

How to Get the Best Results

This section includes "With Home Testing, Consumers Take Charge of Their Health: Buyer Beware," © 2011 American Association for Clinical Chemistry. Reprinted with permission. For additional information about clinical lab testing, visit the Lab Tests Online website at www.labtestsonline.org.

Caveat Emptor (Let the Buyer Beware)

Home testing offers a way for you to test for medical conditions in the privacy of your own home and to monitor chronic health conditions. If you use home tests, however, protect yourself against the possibility of bogus tests, false results, and your own lack of training by following these guidelines.

Make sure that the test you are purchasing is FDA approved: The Food and Drug Administration (FDA) requires manufacturers to meet stringent controls for quality, precision, and accuracy. Approved home tests must also meet FDA labeling requirements.

Check the expiration date: Do not buy tests if they have expired. The chemicals in the test may have lost their effectiveness, and the results may not be valid.

Follow the package directions on where and how to store the test kit: Do not leave temperature-sensitive kits in places with extreme temperatures, such as the trunk of a car or near a radiator or heater. Some tests may be sensitive to moisture and should not be left in places with high humidity, such as a bathroom.

Note and follow any special precautions before performing the test: For example, check to see when the test is to be performed (morning, evening) or under what conditions (fasting, no physical exertion, and so forth).

Perform the test exactly as instructed: If you have questions or are at all unsure about how to use the test, consider talking to your doctor or health care provider. If you have privacy or security concerns, call the 800 help number listed on the package insert.

Make sure you understand the meaning of the test results and what to do about them: If you do not, call the help number provided by the manufacturer or call your health care provider. The FDA encourages manufacturers to provide professional counseling and referral services through an 800 number.

If you have any questions or concerns about the legitimacy of the product or about whether there have been any adverse effects associated with the device, contact the Manufacturer and User Facility Device Experience Database (MAUDE) (http://www.accessdata.fda.gov/scripts/cdrh/cfdocs/cfmaude/search.cfm) to do an online search. You can search the Center for Devices and Radiological Health's database on medical devices that may have malfunctioned or caused death or serious injury at (http://www.fda.gov/MedicalDevices/DeviceRegulation andGuidance/Databases/default.htm).

Consult the following agencies for additional consumer information: These are general links that will require additional searching for relevant information.

Food and Drug Administration

Website: http://www.fda.gov

National Library of Medicine

Website: http://www.nlm.nih.gov

Center for Devices and Radiological Health (CDRH)

Website: http://www.fda.gov/MedicalDevices/default.htm

Centers for Disease Control and Prevention (CDC)

Website: http://www.cdc.gov

Section 56.3

Buying Diagnostic Tests Online

Excerpted from "Buying Diagnostic Tests from the Internet:
Buyer Beware," U.S. Food and Drug Administration
(FDA), July 16, 2009.

Tests called in vitro diagnostic (IVD for short) tests use a sample of blood, urine, or other specimen taken from the human body. A doctor uses IVD tests along with a physical examination and a medical history to get a picture of a patient's health status. Rarely does one IVD test provide a diagnosis.

Although many quality IVD tests are being sold over the internet, other tests sold online may not work or be harmful. Some tests are illegal, that is, being sold without clearance or approval by the Food and Drug Administration (FDA). Examples of some types of IVD tests available from the internet include pregnancy, hepatitis, fertility, cholesterol, drugs of abuse, blood sugar, human immunodeficiency virus (HIV), and antibodies to silicone. While some of these tests are approved or cleared for sale directly to the consumer (called over-the-counter or OTC), most IVD tests are not. FDA has cleared or approved many tests for use in a doctor's office or for professional use only, but internet marketers are selling them OTC or for unapproved uses.

Misleading advertising is another problem. Ads promise in-home results, but most IVD tests should be followed with a second, more sophisticated laboratory test to confirm the results. For example, tests to detect prostate cancer, called PSA (prostate surface antigen) test, are for screening only and should be used in conjunction with a rectal exam performed by a doctor. Elevated PSA test results often are further evaluated using additional tests such free PSAs or complexed PSA.

Internet sources also heavily advertise tests for detecting the presence of drugs such as marijuana, nicotine, amphetamine, and methamphetamine in children and employees. Again, to be sure of their accuracy, the positive results for these tests must be confirmed by additional laboratory tests. Another example of false advertising is claiming that disposable supplies, such as test strips for blood glucose monitors, will work in "any meter."

So what precautions can a consumer take? If you think that you have a medical condition or disease, see your doctor or health care professional. Don't try to diagnose yourself with questionable products obtained over the internet. If you still want to buy an IVD test over the internet, how can you tell if it is a legitimate product? First, ask if FDA has cleared or approved the product for use at home. Second, be wary if you see that the test:

- claims to diagnose more than one illness, (for example: cancer, arthritis, and anemia);

- is made in a country other than the United States (if so, check to see if FDA has cleared or approved the test for use at home); or

- is made by only one laboratory and sold directly to the public.

Although FDA's resources are limited, the agency is taking action against internet websites with misleading marketing or unsafe products. FDA has sent warning letters that demand the owners of these websites stop selling medical devices until they can prove FDA has cleared or approved the devices for sale. FDA is working with the Federal Trade Commission (FTC) whose laws allow it to quickly regulate practices that are unfair and deceptive. FDA also sends information about deceptive companies to the National Consumer League's Fraud Information Center.

If you have questions or complaints about a particular medical device or website, you can call FDA at 888-INFO-FDA (463-6332) or your local FDA district office. They will be able to tell you if FDA has cleared or approved the medical device in question. Finally, if you want to purchase an IVD test promising a diagnosis for treatment of a serious illness, talk to your healthcare provider before using it to find out if additional tests will be needed.

Report False Claims

Consumer Response Center
Federal Trade Commission (FTC)
Washington, DC 20850
Toll-Free: 877-FTC-HELP (382-4357)
Toll-Free TTY: 866-653-4261
Website: http://www.ftc.gov/complaint

FDA MedWatch
Toll-Free:800-FDA-1088
Website: http://www.fda.gov/
Safety/MedWatch

Chapter 57

Cholesterol Home Use Test

What this test does: This is a home-use test kit to measure total cholesterol.

What cholesterol is: Cholesterol is a fat (lipid) in your blood. High-density lipoprotein (HDL) (good cholesterol) helps protect your heart, but low-density lipoprotein (LDL) (bad cholesterol) can clog the arteries of your heart. Some cholesterol tests also measure triglycerides, another type of fat in the blood.

What type of test this is: This is a quantitative test—you find out the amount of total cholesterol present in your sample.

Why you should do this test: You should do this test to find out if you have high total cholesterol. High cholesterol increases your risk of heart disease. When the blood vessels of your heart become clogged by cholesterol, your heart does not receive enough oxygen. This can cause heart disease.

How often you should do this test: If you are more than 20 years old, you should test your cholesterol about every five years. If your doctor has you on a special diet or drugs to control your cholesterol, you may need to check your cholesterol more frequently. Follow your doctor's recommendations about how often you test your cholesterol.

"Home Use Tests: Cholesterol," U. S. Food and Drug Administration (FDA), March 17, 2010.

What you cholesterol levels should be: Your total cholesterol level should be 200 milligrams per deciliter (mg/dL) or less, according to recommendations in the National Cholesterol Education Program (NCEP) Third Adult Treatment Panel (ATP III). You should try to keep your LDL values less than 100 mg/dL, your HDL values greater or equal to 40 mg/dL, and your triglyceride values less than 150 mg/dL.

How accurate this test is: This test is about as accurate as the test your doctor uses, but you must follow the directions carefully. Total cholesterol tests vary in accuracy from brand to brand. Information about the test's accuracy is printed on its package. Tests that say they are traceable to a program of the Centers for Disease Control and Prevention (CDC) may be more accurate than others.

What to do you if your test shows high cholesterol: Talk to your doctor if your test shows that your cholesterol is higher than 200 mg/dL. Many things can cause high cholesterol levels including diet, exercise, and other factors. Your doctor may want you to test your cholesterol again.

How you do this test: You prick your finger with a lancet to get a drop of blood. Then put the drop of blood on a piece paper that contains special chemicals. The paper will change color depending on how much cholesterol is in your blood. Some testing kits use a small machine to tell you how much cholesterol there is in the sample.

Chapter 58

Drugs of Abuse Home Tests

Chapter Contents

Section 58.1

First Check 12 Drug Test

"Home-Use Tests: Drugs of Abuse (First Check 12 Drug Test),"
U.S. Food and Drug Administration (FDA), March 17, 2010.

What does this test do? The *First Check 12 Drug Test* indicates
if one or more prescription or illegal drugs are present in urine. It is
currently the only over-the-counter test available designed to detect
prescription drugs that are being abused. The test detects the presence of 12 prescription and illegal drugs: marijuana, cocaine, opiates,
methamphetamine, amphetamines, PCP, benzodiazepine, barbiturates,
methadone, tricyclic antidepressants, ecstasy, and oxycodone.

This test is done in two steps. First, you do a quick at-home test.
Second, if the test suggests that drugs may be present, you send the
sample to a laboratory for additional testing.

What are prescription drugs of abuse? Prescription drugs of
abuse are medicines (for example, Oxycodone or Valium) that are obtained legally with a doctor's prescription, but are being taken for a
non-medical purpose. Non-medical purposes include taking the medication for longer than your doctor prescribed it for or for a purpose other
than what the doctor prescribed it for. Medications are not drugs of
abuse if they are taken according to your doctor's instructions.

What type of test is this? This is a qualitative test—you find out
if a particular drug may be in the urine, not how much is present.

When should you do this test? You should use this test when
you think someone you care about might be abusing prescription or
illegal drugs. If you are worried about a specific drug, make sure to
check the label to confirm that this test is designed to detect the drug
you are looking for.

How accurate is this test? The at-home testing part of this test is
fairly sensitive to the presence of drugs in the urine. This means that if
drugs are present, you will usually get a preliminary (or presumptive)
positive test result. If you get a preliminary positive result, you should
send the urine sample to the laboratory for a second test.

It is very important to send the urine sample to the laboratory to confirm a positive at-home result because certain foods, food supplements, beverages, or medicines can affect the results of at-home tests. Laboratory tests are the most reliable way to confirm drugs of abuse.

Note that all amphetamine results should be considered carefully, even those from the laboratory. Some over-the-counter medications cannot be distinguished from illegally-abused amphetamines.

Many things can affect the accuracy of this test, including (but not limited to):

- the way you did the test,

- the way you stored the test or urine,

- what the person ate or drank before taking the test, and

- any other prescription or over-the-counter drugs the person may have taken before the test.

Does a positive test mean that you found drugs of abuse? No. Take no serious actions until you get the laboratory's result. Remember that many factors may cause a false positive result in the home test.

Remember that a positive test for a prescription drug does not mean that a person is abusing the drug, because there is no way for the test to indicate acceptable levels compared to abusive levels of prescribed drugs.

If the test results are negative, can you be sure that the person you tested did not abuse drugs? No. There are several factors that can make the test results negative even though the person is abusing drugs. First, you may have tested for the wrong drugs. Or, you may not have tested the urine when it contained drugs. It takes time for drugs to appear in the urine after a person takes them, and they do not stay in the urine indefinitely; you may have collected the urine too late or too soon. It is also possible that the chemicals in the test went bad because they were stored incorrectly or they passed their expiration date.

If you get a negative test result, but still suspect that someone is abusing drugs, you can test again at a later time. Talk to your doctor if you need more help deciding what steps to take next.

How soon after a person takes drugs, will they show up in a drug test? And how long after a person takes drugs, will they continue to show up in a drug test? The drug clearance rate tells how soon a person may have a positive test after taking a particular drug. It also tells how long the person may continue to test positive after the last time he or she took the drug. Clearance rates for common drugs of abuse are given in Table 58.1. These are only guidelines, however, and the times can vary significantly from these estimates based on how long the person has been taking the drug, the amount of drug they use, or the person's metabolism.

How You Do the Two-Step Test

The kit contains a urine collection cup, a plastic lid containing 12 test strips and an instruction booklet. It also includes a numbered sticker for confidential confirmation testing and packaging for sending samples to the laboratory for confirmation.

You collect a urine sample in the collection cup, and secure the lid onto the cup. The test strips in the lid contain chemicals that react with each possible drug and show a visible result for each drug they detect. Read and follow the directions carefully and exactly. If the test indicates the presence of one or more drugs, you should send the urine sample to the laboratory for confirmation.

Table 58.1. Clearance Rates for Common Drugs

Drug	How soon after taking drug will there be a positive drug test?	How long after taking drug will there continue to be a positive drug test?
Marijuana/pot	1–3 hours	1–7 days
Crack (cocaine)	2–6 hours	2–3 days
Heroin (opiates)	2–6 hours	1–3 days
Speed/uppers (amphetamine, methamphetamine)	4–6 hours	2–3 days
Angel dust/PCP	4-6 hours	7–14 days
Ecstasy	2–7 hours	2–4 days
Benzodiazepine	2– hours	1–4 days
Barbiturates	2–4 hours	1–3 weeks
Methadone	3–8 hours	1–3 days
Tricyclic antidepressants	8–12 hours	2–7 days
Oxycodone	1–3 hours	1–2 days

Section 58.2

Collection Kit

Excerpted from "Home-Use Tests: Drugs of Abuse (Collection Kit),"
U.S. Food and Drug Administration (FDA), March 17, 2010.

What does this test do? This is a home collection kit for drugs of abuse. You collect a sample of urine, hair, saliva, or other human material, and send it to a laboratory for analysis. The laboratory does a quick screening test for drugs, then, if the test suggests that one or more drugs may be present, it performs additional testing.

What are drugs of abuse? Examples of drugs of abuse include marijuana, cocaine, opiates (including heroin), amphetamines (including Ecstasy or MDMA), and PCP (angel dust). Prescription drugs, such as codeine or other painkillers, also may be abused.

What type of test is this? This is a qualitative test—you find out whether or not the person tested took drugs of abuse, not how much is present.

When should you use this test? You should use this test when you think someone you care about might be using drugs of abuse.

How accurate is this test? Laboratories use a very reliable test, with very few errors, to determine whether or not your sample contains drugs of abuse. Note that all amphetamine results should be considered carefully, even those from the laboratory. Some over-the-counter medications contain amphetamines that cannot be distinguished from illegally-abused amphetamines.

If the test results are negative, can you be sure that the person you tested did not take drugs? No. You may not have taken a sample when it contained drugs. It takes time for drugs to appear in urine, hair, saliva, or other human materials, and they do not stay in the materials indefinitely; you may have gotten the sample too soon or too late. If you get a negative test result, but still suspect that someone is abusing drugs, you can test again at a later time. Talk to your doctor if you need more help deciding what steps to take next.

How do you do this test? You do not do the testing yourself. You simply collect a sample of urine, hair, saliva, or other human material and send it to a laboratory for analysis. The laboratory does a preliminary analysis to see if the sample might contain drugs of abuse. If the result is positive, they will do a more complete analysis of the sample and report the results to you. These collection kits contain the sample containers, instructions, and shipping containers. The price you pay for the kit usually pays for the analysis.

Chapter 59

Fecal Occult Blood Home Test

What does this test do? This is a home-use test kit to measure the presence of hidden (occult) blood in your stool (feces).

What is fecal occult blood? Fecal occult blood is blood in your feces that you cannot see in your stool or on your toilet paper after you use the toilet.

What type of test is this? This is a qualitative test—you find out whether or not you have occult blood in your feces, not how much is present.

Why should you do this test? You should do this test, because blood in your feces may be an early sign of a digestive condition, for example abnormal growths (polyps) or cancer in your colon.

How often should you test for fecal occult blood? The American Cancer Society recommends that you test for fecal occult blood every year after you turn 50. Some doctors suggest that you start testing at age 40, if your family is thought to be at increased risk. Follow your doctor's recommendations about how often you test for fecal occult blood.

How accurate is this test? This test is about as accurate as the test your doctor uses, but you must follow the directions carefully. For accurate results, you must prepare properly for the test and get a good stool sample.

This chapter includes "Home Use Tests: Fecal Occult Blood," U.S. Food and Drug Administration (FDA), March 17, 2010.

Does a positive test mean you have hidden blood in your stool? A positive result means that the test has detected blood. This does not mean you have tested positive for cancer or any other illness. False positive results may be caused by diet or medications. Further testing and examinations should be performed by the physician to determine the exact cause and source of the occult blood in the stool.

If the test results are negative, can you be sure that you do not have a bowel condition? No. You could still have bowel condition that you should know about. You should use this test again in a year.

How do you do this test? There are several different methods for detecting hidden blood in the stool. In one method, you collect stool samples and smear them onto paper cards in a holder. You then either send these cards to a laboratory for testing or test them at home. If you test them at home, you add a special solution from your test kit to the paper cards to see if they change color. If the paper cards change color, it means there was blood in the stool.

In another method, you put special paper in the toilet after a bowel movement. If the special paper changes color, it indicates there was blood in the toilet.

You will need to test your feces from three separate bowel movements. These bowel movements should be three in a row, closely spaced in time to minimize the time you need to be on the special diet. This is necessary because if you have polyps, they may not bleed all the time. You improve your chances of catching any bleeding if you sample three different bowel movements.

- Unless you use the method where you put a test solution into the toilet, it is best to catch your feces before it enters the toilet. You can do this by holding a piece of toilet paper in your hand. After you catch it, cut it apart in two places with the little wooden stick you get in the kit. Take a little bit of the feces from each place where you cut it apart and put these bits on one place in the cardboard in the kit. You use the second and third spots on the cardboard for other bowel movements.

What interferes with this test? To get good results with this test, you have to follow the instructions. You may find it difficult because you need to do things you do not ordinarily do. Because the test is for blood, any source of blood will give a positive test. Blood from another source, like bleeding hemorrhoids or your menstrual period, will interfere with the test, so you will not be able to tell what made the test positive.

Pay attention to your diet before the test:

- Eat a high fiber diet, such as one that has cereals and breads with bran.

- Cook your fruits and vegetables well.

- Do not eat raw turnips, radishes, broccoli, or horseradish. These foods can make it look like you have hidden blood when you do not.

- Do not eat red meat. (You may eat poultry or fish). Red meat in your diet can make it look like you have hidden blood when you don't.

Avoid the following drugs for the seven days before the test—they can make it look like you have hidden blood when you don't:

- Aspirin

- Anti-inflammatory drugs, such as Motrin

Do not take vitamin C supplements for the seven days before the test. They can prevent the test from detecting your hidden blood.

Chapter 60

Direct-to-Consumer Genetic Testing

Overview of Food and Drug Administration (FDA) Regulation of Genetic Tests

The purpose of genetic tests includes predicting risk of disease, screening newborns, directing clinical management, identifying carriers, and establishing prenatal or clinical diagnoses or prognoses in individuals, families, or populations.

A genetic test is only subject to FDA oversight if it is a medical device; that is, if it is intended for use in the diagnosis of disease or other conditions, or in the cure, mitigation, treatment, or prevention of disease. For example, a test to determine a person's risk of developing heart disease is a device, whereas a test to determine ancestry is not a device. The type of genetic testing has changed over the past two decades. Whereas early tests tended to identify a single genetic mutation and a patient's risk for developing a disease, some newer tests evaluate thousands of genes or the entire genome and report out risk for a disease based on the combination of dozens of genetic variations.

There currently are two paths to market for a genetic test used in clinical management of patients, as is the case for other in vitro diagnostics (IVD). One is through development of a commercial test kit by an IVD device manufacturer for distribution to multiple laboratories. The FDA has exercised its regulatory authority over these products and has approved several tests for specific genetic factors.

Excerpted from "Direct-to-Consumer Genetic Testing and the Consequences to the Public," U.S. Food and Drug Administration (FDA), July 22, 2010.

The second pathway is through the development of a test by a laboratory for use only by that laboratory; these are commonly called laboratory-developed tests (LDTs). Conservative estimates are that there are between 2,500–5,000 LDTs, including genetic tests that are developed and offered by hundreds of different laboratories. FDA has the authority to regulate LDTs as it does all IVDs. Most genetic tests being offered today are LDTs.

The nature of laboratory-developed tests has changed over the last 30 years, but most dramatically in the last few years. Today, LDTs are increasingly used to assess high-risk but relatively common diseases and conditions, often are used to provide critical information for patient treatment decisions, rely on novel (sometimes preliminary) scientific findings to support their usefulness, often require complex software and may incorporate automated interpretation in lieu of expert interpretation, often are used when there are alternative tests available that have been cleared or approved by FDA, and are performed in commercial laboratory settings that are geographically separate from the patient's primary health care professional and health care setting. In addition, some entities marketed their tests without prior FDA review, claiming that they are LDTs, when they are not. Furthermore, the ability of laboratories to market tests without any regulatory oversight creates a disincentive for traditional manufacturers to develop new tests, thereby stifling innovation.

FDA has observed the following problems with some LDTs in recent years:

- Faulty data analysis
- Exaggerated clinical claims
- Fraudulent data
- Lack of traceability/change control
- Poor clinical study design
- Unacceptable clinical performance

FDA believes that a test used for patient care should have the same assurances of safety and effectiveness whether it is manufactured for distribution to multiple laboratories or created for use in only one laboratory.

Genetic Tests Being Sold Directly to Consumers

An emerging market segment for the laboratory testing industry is direct-to-consumer (DTC) testing. A few companies have sought to popularize genetic testing through advertisements and social media. FDA has been aware of these companies marketing to consumers for several years. At the time of the 2006 Government Accountability Office (GAO) investigation of DTC testing, most of these diagnostics were "nutritional genetic" tests—tests to assess what kinds of foods individual consumers should eat and dietary supplements they should take. FDA followed up with the companies and FDA, Centers for Disease Control and Prevention (CDC), and the Federal Trade Commission (FTC) published a cautionary statement on DTC genetic tests.

New DTC genetic tests subsequently came on the market. FDA met with some of these companies starting in 2007. FDA's Center for Devices and Radiological Health, which is responsible for the oversight of these tests, never informed these companies that they could lawfully market their tests without FDA oversight. Instead, the Center met with these companies to have a better understanding of what the companies were in fact doing or planning to do. Initially their business models were not clear and the tests were being marketed for such purposes as antiquity determinations. However, since then we have seen changes in the number and types of claims being made. For example, one company provided test reports for 17 diseases, conditions, or traits in 2008 but provided over 100 types of results by 2010. In particular, some companies are making claims about high-risk medical indications, such as determining the risk for cancer or the likelihood of responding to a specific drug. Moreover, in many cases the link between the genetic results and the risk of developing a disease or responding/ not responding to a drug has not been well-established.

Marketing genetic tests directly to consumers can increase the risk of a test because a patient may make a decision that adversely affects their health, such as stopping or changing the dose of a medication or continuing an unhealthy lifestyle, without the intervention of a learned intermediary. The risk points up the importance of ensuring that consumers are also provided accurate, complete, and understandable information about the limitations of test results they are obtaining.

Recently, we have seen companies more aggressively market directly to consumers. For example, Pathway Genomics Corporation (PGC) was poised to offer their Pathway Genomics Genetic Health Report, a home use saliva collection kit, directly to consumers through more than 6,000 Walgreen stores. 23andMe is marketing directly to consumers on Amazon.com.

Although FDA has cleared a number of genetic tests since 2003, none of the genetic tests now offered directly to consumers has undergone premarket review by FDA to ensure that the test results being provided to patients are accurate, reliable, and clinically meaningful.

Because of the escalation in risk and aggressive marketing, FDA notified PGC on May 10, 2010, that their offering appeared to meet the definition of a medical device as that term is defined under the Food, Drug, and Cosmetic Act, and clearance or approval by the Agency was necessary in order for them to market their product. The test is intended to report the presence or risk of more than 70 health conditions, including pharmacogenetics (prescription medication response), propensity for complex disease, carrier status, and other information from which one could modify one's lifestyle and health regime, supposedly to live a healthier, longer life. These tests have not been proven safe, effective, or accurate, and patients could be put at risk by making medical decisions based on data that has not received independent premarket review. Following receipt of FDA's letter, PGC stopped marketing directly to consumers.

On June 10, 2010, FDA sent similar letters to four other diagnostic test manufacturing firms that were offering their tests directly to consumers (Knome, Inc.; Navigenics; deCODE Genetics; and 23andMe). FDA considers all of these products to meet the statutory definition of a medical device on the basis of the manufacturers' claims about the test results. For example, the tests claimed to describe the genetic basis of specific disease traits or conditions on which consumers may base medical decisions; provide personalized information on which medications are more likely to work given a person's genetic makeup; and provide genetic predispositions for important health conditions and medication sensitivities.

Chapter 61

Gynecological Concerns Home Tests

Chapter Contents

Section 61.1

Ovulation (Saliva Test)

Text in this section is from "Home Use Tests: Ovulation (Saliva Test),"
U.S. Food and Drug Administration (FDA), March 17, 2010.

What does this test do? This is a home-use test kit to predict ovulation by looking at patterns formed by your saliva. When your estrogen increases near your time of ovulation, your dried saliva may form a fern-shaped pattern.

What type of test is this? This is a qualitative test—you find out whether or not you may be near your ovulation time, not if you will definitely become pregnant.

Why should you do this test? You should do this test if you want to know when you expect to ovulate and be in the most fertile part of your menstrual cycle. This test can be used to help you plan to become pregnant. You should not use this test to help prevent pregnancy, because it is not reliable for that purpose.

How accurate is this test? This test may not work well for you. Some of the reasons are:

- not all women fern;
- you may not be able to see the fern;
- women who fern on some days of their fertile period, don't necessarily fern on all of their fertile days;
- ferning may be disrupted by smoking, eating, drinking, brushing your teeth, how you put your saliva on the slide, or where you were when you did the test.

How do you do this test? In this test, you get a small microscope with built-in or removable slides. You put some of your saliva on a glass slide, allow it to dry, and look at the pattern it makes. You will see dots and circles, a fern (full or partial), or a combination depending on where you are in your monthly cycle.

You will get your best results when you use the test within the five-day period around your expected ovulation. This period includes the two days before and the two days after your expected day of ovulation. The test is not perfect, though, and you might fern outside of this time period or when you are pregnant. Even some men will fern.

Is this test similar to the one my doctor uses? The fertility tests your doctor uses are automated, and they may give more consistent results. Your doctor may use other tests that are not yet available for home use (for example, blood and urine laboratory tests) and information about your history to get a better view of your fertility status.

Does a positive test mean you are ovulating? A positive test indicates that you may be near ovulation. It does not mean that you will definitely become pregnant.

Do negative test results mean that you are not ovulating? No, there may be many reasons why you did not detect your time of ovulation. You should not use this test to help prevent pregnancy, because it is not reliable for that purpose.

Section 61.2

Ovulation (Urine Test)

Text in this section is from "Home Use Tests:
Ovulation (Urine Test)," U.S. Food and Drug
Administration (FDA), March 17, 2010.

What does this test do? This is a home-use test kit to measure
luteinizing hormone (LH) in your urine. This helps detect the LH surge
that happens in the middle of your menstrual cycle, about 1–1½ days
before ovulation. Some tests also measure another hormone—estrone-
3-glucuronide (E3G).

What is LH? Luteinizing hormone (LH) is a hormone produced
by your pituitary gland. Your body always makes a small amount of
LH, but just before you ovulate, you make much more LH. This test
can detect this LH surge, which usually happens 1–1½ days before
you ovulate.

What is E3G? E3G is produced when estrogen breaks down in your
body. It accumulates in your urine around the time of ovulation and
causes your cervical mucus to become thin and slippery. Sperm may
swim more easily in your thin and slippery cervical mucus, increasing
your chances of getting pregnant.

What type of test is this? This is a qualitative test—you find out
whether or not you have elevated LH or E3G levels, not if you will
definitely become pregnant.

Why should you do this test? You should do this test if you want
to know when you expect to ovulate and be in the most fertile part of
your menstrual cycle. This test can be used to help you plan to become
pregnant. You should not use this test to help prevent pregnancy, because it is not reliable for that purpose.

How accurate is this test? How well this test will predict your
fertile period depends on how well you follow the instructions. These
tests can detect LH and E3G reliably about nine times out of ten, but
you must do the test carefully.

How do you do this test? You add a few drops of your urine to the test, hold the tip of the test in your urine stream, or dip the test in a cup of your urine. You either read the test by looking for colored lines on the test or you put the test device into a monitor. You can get results in about five minutes. The details of what the color looks like, or how to use the monitor vary among the different brands.

Most kits come with multiple tests to allow you to take measurements over several days. This can help you find your most fertile period, the time during your cycle when you can expect to ovulate based on your hormone levels. Follow the instructions carefully to get good results. You will need to start your testing at the proper time during your cycle, otherwise the test will be unreliable, and you will not find your hormonal surges or your fertile period.

Is this test similar to the one my doctor uses? The fertility tests your doctor uses are automated, and they may give more consistent results. Your doctor may use other tests that are not yet available for home use (such as blood and urine laboratory tests) and information about your history to get a better view of your fertility status.

Section 61.3

Pregnancy Home Tests

Excerpted from "Pregnancy Tests: FAQs," U.S. Department of
Health and Human Services (HHS), March 20, 2009.

How do pregnancy tests work?

All pregnancy tests work by detecting a certain hormone in the
urine or blood that is only there when a woman is pregnant. This hormone is called human chorionic gonadotropin, or hCG. It is also called
the pregnancy hormone. hCG is made when a fertilized egg implants
in the uterus. This usually happens about six days after the egg and
sperm merge. But studies show that in up to 10% of women, implantation does not occur until much later, after the first day of the missed
period. The amount of hCG rapidly builds up in your body with each
passing day you are pregnant.

Are there different types of pregnancy tests?

Yes. There are two types of pregnancy tests. One tests the blood
for the pregnancy hormone, hCG. You need to see a doctor to have a
blood test. The other checks the urine for the hCG hormone. You can
do a urine test at a doctor's office or at home with a home pregnancy
test (HPT).

These days, many women first use an HPT to find out if they are
pregnant. HPTs are inexpensive, private, and easy to use. HPTs
also are highly accurate if used correctly and at the right time.
HPTs will be able to tell if you are pregnant about one week after
a missed period.

How do you do a home pregnancy test?

There are many different types of home pregnancy tests (HPTs).
Most drugstores sell HPTs over the counter. They are inexpensive. But
the cost depends on the brand and how many tests come in the box.

Most HPTs work in a similar way. Many instruct the user to hold
a stick in the urine stream. Others involve collecting urine in a cup

and then dipping the stick into it. At least one brand tells the woman to collect urine in a cup and then use a dropper to put a few drops of the urine into a special container. Then the woman needs to wait a few minutes. Different brands instruct the woman to wait different amounts of time. Once the time has passed, the user should inspect the result window. If a line or plus symbol appears, you are pregnant. It does not matter how faint the line is. A line, whether bold or faint, means the result is positive. New digital tests show the words pregnant or not pregnant.

Most tests also have a control indicator in the result window. This line or symbol shows whether the test is working properly. If the control indicator does not appear, the test is not working properly. You should not rely on any results from a HPT that may be faulty.

Most brands tell users to repeat the test in a few days, no matter what the results. One negative result (especially soon after a missed period) does not always mean you are not pregnant. All HPTs come with written instructions. Most tests also have toll-free phone numbers to call in case of questions about use or results.

How accurate are home pregnancy tests?

Home pregnancy tests (HPTs) can be quite accurate. But the accuracy depends on:

- **How you use them:** Be sure to check the expiration date and follow the instructions. Wait ten minutes after taking the test to check the results window to get the most accurate result.

- **When you use them:** The amount of hCG or pregnancy hormone in your urine increases with time. So, the earlier after a missed period you take the test, the harder it is to spot the hCG. Many HPTs claim to be 99% accurate on the first day of your missed period. But research suggests that most HPTs do not always detect the low levels of hCG usually present this early in pregnancy. And when they do, the results are often very faint. Most HPTs can accurately detect pregnancy one week after a missed period. Also, testing your urine first thing in the morning may boost the accuracy.

- **Who uses them:** Each woman ovulates at a different time in her menstrual cycle. Plus, the fertilized egg can implant in a woman's uterus at different times. hCG only is produced once implantation occurs. In up to 10% of women, implantation does not occur until after the first day of a missed period.

My home pregnancy test says I am pregnant. What should I do next?

If a home pregnancy test is positive and shows that you are pregnant, you should call your doctor right away. Your doctor can use a more sensitive test along with a pelvic exam to tell for sure if you are pregnant. Seeing your doctor early on in your pregnancy will help you and your baby stay healthy.

My home pregnancy test says that I am not pregnant. Might I still be pregnant?

Yes. So, most home pregnancy tests (HPTs) suggest women take the test again in a few days or a week if the result is negative. Each woman ovulates at a different time in her menstrual cycle. Plus, the fertilized egg can implant in a woman's uterus at different times. So, the accuracy of HPT results varies from woman to woman. Other things can also affect the accuracy. Sometimes women get false negative results when they test too early in the pregnancy. This means that the test says you are not pregnant when you are. Other times, problems with the pregnancy can affect the amount of hCG in the urine.

If your HPT is negative, test yourself again in a few days or one week. If you keep getting a negative result but think you are pregnant, talk with your doctor right away.

Can anything affect home pregnancy test results?

Most medicines should not affect the results of a home pregnancy test (HPT). This includes over-the-counter and prescription medicines, including birth control pills and antibiotics. Only medicines that have the pregnancy hormone hCG in them can give a false positive test result. A false positive is when a test says you are pregnant when you are not. Sometimes medicines containing hCG are used to treat infertility (not being able to get pregnant).

Alcohol and illegal drugs do not affect HPT results. But do not use these substances if you are trying to become pregnant or are sexually active and could become pregnant.

Section 61.4

Vaginal pH

Text in this section is from "Home Use Tests: Vaginal pH,"
U.S. Food and Drug Administration (FDA), March 17, 2010.

What does this test do? This is a home-use test kit to measure the pH of your vaginal secretions.

What is pH? pH is a way to describe how acidic a substance is. It is given by a number on a scale of 1–14. The lower the number, the more acidic the substance.

What type of test is this? This is a quantitative test—you find out how acidic your vaginal secretions are.

Why should you do this test? You should do this test to help evaluate if your vaginal symptoms (such as itching, burning, unpleasant odor, or unusual discharge) are likely caused by an infection that needs medical treatment. The test is not intended for human immunodeficiency virus (HIV), chlamydia, herpes, gonorrhea, syphilis, or group B streptococcus.

How accurate is this test? Home vaginal pH tests showed good agreement with a doctor's diagnosis. However, just because you find changes in your vaginal pH, does not always mean that you have a vaginal infection. pH changes also do not help or differentiate one type of infection from another. Your doctor diagnoses a vaginal infection by using a combination of: pH, microscopic examination of the vaginal discharge, amine (fishy) odor, culture, wet preparation, and Gram stain.

Does a positive test mean you have a vaginal infection? No, a positive test (elevated pH) could occur for other reasons. If you detect elevated pH, you should see your doctor for further testing and treatment. There are no over-the-counter medications for treatment of an elevated vaginal pH.

If test results are negative, can you be sure that you do not have a vaginal infection? No, you may have an infection that does not show up in these tests. If you have no symptoms, your negative test could suggest the possibility of chemical, allergic, or other noninfectious irritation of the vagina. Or, a negative test could indicate the possibility of a yeast infection. You should see your doctor if you find changes in your vaginal pH or if you continue to have symptoms.

How do you do this test? You hold a piece of pH paper against the wall of your vagina for a few seconds, then compare the color of the pH paper to the color on the chart provided with the test kit. The number on the chart for the color that best matches the color on the pH paper is the vaginal pH number.

Is the home test similar to your doctor's test? Yes. The home vaginal pH tests are practically identical to the ones sold to doctors. But your doctor can provide a more thorough assessment of your vaginal status through your history, physical exam, and other laboratory tests than you can using a single pH test in your home.

Chapter 62

Menopause Home Test

What does this test do? This is a home-use test kit to measure follicle stimulating hormone (FSH) in your urine. This may help indicate if you are in menopause or perimenopause.

What is menopause? Menopause is the stage in your life when menstruation stops for at least 12 months. The time before this is called perimenopause and could last for several years. You may reach menopause in your early 40s or as late as your 60s.

What is FSH? Follicle stimulating hormone (FSH) is a hormone produced by your pituitary gland. FSH levels increase temporarily each month to stimulate your ovaries to produce eggs. When you enter menopause and your ovaries stop working, your FSH levels also increase.

What type of test is this? This is a qualitative test—you find out whether or not you have elevated FSH levels, not if you definitely are in menopause or perimenopause.

Why should you do this test? You should use this test if you want to know if your symptoms, such as irregular periods, hot flashes, vaginal dryness, or sleep problems are part of menopause. While many women may have little or no trouble when going through the stages of menopause, others may have moderate to severe discomfort and may want

Text in this chapter is from "Home Use Tests: Menopause," U.S. Food and Drug Administration (FDA), March 17, 2010.

treatment to alleviate their symptoms. This test may help you be better informed about your current condition when you see your doctor.

How accurate is this test? These tests will accurately detect FSH about nine out of ten times. This test does not detect menopause or perimenopause. As you grow older, your FSH levels may rise and fall during your menstrual cycle. While your hormone levels are changing, your ovaries continue to release eggs and you can still become pregnant.

Your test will depend on whether you:

• used your first morning urine;

• drank large amounts of water before the test;

• use, or recently stopped using, oral or patch contraceptives, hormone replacement therapy, or estrogen supplements.

How do you do this test? In this test, you put a few drops of your urine on a test device, put the end of the testing device in your urine stream, or dip the test device into a cup of urine. Chemicals in the test device react with FSH and produce a color. Read the instructions with the test you buy to learn exactly what to look for in this test.

Are the home menopause tests similar to the ones my doctor uses? Some home menopause tests are identical to the one your doctor uses. However, doctors would not use this test by itself. Your doctor would use your medical history, physical exam, and other laboratory tests to get a more thorough assessment of your condition.

Does a positive test mean you are in menopause? A positive test indicates that you may be in a stage of menopause. If you have a positive test, or if you have any symptoms of menopause, you should see your doctor. Do not stop taking contraceptives based on the results of these tests because they are not foolproof and you could become pregnant.

Do negative test results indicate that you are not in menopause? If you have a negative test result, but you have symptoms of menopause, you may be in perimenopause or menopause. You should not assume that a negative test means you have not reached menopause, there could be other reasons for the negative result. You should always discuss your symptoms and your test results with your doctor. Do not use these tests to determine if you are fertile or can become pregnant. These tests will not give you a reliable answer on your ability to become pregnant.

Chapter 63

Hepatitis C Home Test

What does this test do? This is a home-use collection kit to determine if you may have a hepatitis C infection now or had one in the past. You collect a blood sample and send it to a testing laboratory for analysis.

What is hepatitis C infection? Hepatitis C infection is caused by the hepatitis C virus (HCV). Untreated, hepatitis C can cause liver disease.

What type of test is this? This is a qualitative test—you find out whether or not you may have this infection, not how advanced your disease is.

Why should you do this test? You should do this test if you think you may have been infected with HCV. If you are infected with HCV, you should take steps to avoid spreading the disease to others. At least eight out of ten people with acute hepatitis C develop chronic liver infection, and 2–3 out of ten develop cirrhosis. A small number of people may also develop liver cancer. Hepatitis C infection is the number one cause for liver transplantation in the United States.

When should you do this test? The Centers for Disease Control and Prevention(CDC) recommend that you do this test if you:

- have ever injected illegal drugs;
- received clotting factor concentrates produced before 1987;

Text in this chapter is from "Home Use Tests: Hepatitis C," U. S. Food and Drug Administration (FDA), March 17, 2010.

- were ever on long-term dialysis;

- received a blood transfusion before July 1992;

- received an organ transplant before July 1992; or

- are a health care, emergency medicine, or public safety worker who contacted HCV-positive blood through needlesticks, sharps, or mucosal exposure.

How accurate is this test? This test is about as accurate as the test your doctor uses, but you must carefully follow the directions about getting the sample and sending it the testing laboratory. Proper sample collection is important for obtaining accurate results. Researchers found that about 90 of 100 home users were able to obtain acceptable samples to send to the laboratory. After the laboratory got these 90 samples, it could get results for about 81 of them. Of these 81 samples, the laboratory got correct results in 77 and incorrect results in four.

Does a positive test mean you have HCV? If you have a positive test, you either are infected with HCV now or you have been infected with HCV in the past. You need to see your doctor to find out if you have an active infection and what therapy you should have. Some people who become infected with HCV develop antibodies and then are no longer infected.

If your test results are negative, can you be sure that you do not have HCV infection? A negative test does not guarantee that you do not have HCV infection since it takes some time for you to develop antibodies after you are infected with this virus. If you think you were exposed to the virus and might be infected, you should see your doctor for a more accurate laboratory test.

How do you do this test? The test kit comes with a small piece of filter paper, a lancet, and instructions for obtaining a blood sample and placing it on the filter paper. You first prick your finger with the lancet to get a drop of blood. Then, you put your drop of blood on a piece of filter paper and send it in a special container to the testing laboratory. You get the results of your test by phone from the laboratory. The laboratory does a preliminary (screening) test that separates the samples into three groups:

- samples that are clearly positive,

- samples that might be positive, and

- samples that are negative.

All samples that might be positive receive a more specific (confirmatory) test to find those that are truly positive. All the clearly positives from the preliminary test and the truly positives from the more specific test are reported to you as positive.

You should note that a positive result does not mean that you are infected with HCV. If you receive a positive result from this test, you should see your doctor for further testing and information.

Chapter 64

HIV Home Test

Human Immunodeficiency Virus (HIV)

What does this test do? This is a home-use collection kit to detect whether or not you have antibodies to HIV (human immunodeficiency virus). HIV is the virus that causes AIDS (acquired immunodeficiency syndrome).

What type of test is this? This is a qualitative test—you find out whether or not you have this infection, not how advanced your disease is.

Why should you do this test? You should do this test to find out if you have an HIV infection. If you know that you have an HIV infection,

- you can obtain medical treatment that helps slow the course of the disease, and

- you can take precautions to keep from infecting others.

Untreated, HIV destroys your immune system. The most advanced stage of HIV infection is AIDS, an often-fatal disease.

When should you do this test? You should do this test if you believe there is a chance you may have an HIV infection. You are at greatest risk for HIV if you:

This chapter includes "Home Use Tests: Human Immunodeficiency Virus (HIV)," U.S. Food and Drug Administration (FDA), March 17, 2010; and "Vital Facts about HIV Home Test Kits," FDA, March 19, 2011.

- have ever shared injection drug needles and syringes or "works;"
- have ever had sex without a condom with someone who had HIV;
- have ever had a sexually transmitted disease, like chlamydia or gonorrhea;
- received a blood transfusion or a blood-clotting factor between 1978 and 1985;
- have ever had sex with someone who has done any of those things.

If you use this test, no one but you will know you were tested for HIV or what the results showed.

How accurate is this test? This test is similar to the test your doctor would use. Researchers have found that about 90 of 100 home users were able to obtain acceptable samples for sending to the laboratory. After the laboratory got these 90 samples, they could get results for about 81 of 100 of them. Of these 81 samples, the laboratory almost always shows whether or not the person tested had HIV infection.

Does a positive test mean you have HIV? If you test positive in this test, you are infected with the HIV virus. You should take precautions so you do not spread this infection to your sexual partners or others who might be at risk. You should not donate blood because this infection could spread to others. Having HIV infection does not necessarily mean you have AIDS. You should see your doctor so you can learn the status of your disease and decide what therapy, if any, you need.

If your results are negative, can you be sure that you do not have HIV infection? If you test negative for HIV, it means you did not have antibodies to HIV at the time of the test. However, if you are newly infected, it will take time for you to make antibodies. It is uncertain how long it may take you to develop antibodies—it may take more than three months. So, although you may be infected, the results of your testing will not verify that you are infected for several months. If you think you were exposed to the virus and might be infected, you should test yourself again in a few months.

How do you do this test? The test comes with sterile lancets, an alcohol pad, gauze pads, a blood specimen collection card, a bandage, a lancet disposal container, a shipping pouch, and instructions. To do the test, you:

- call a specified telephone number;
- register a code number that is included with the specimen collection kit;

- prick your finger with a lancet to get a drop of blood;
- place drops of blood on the card;
- send the shipping pouch by express courier service to the central testing laboratory;
- receive results by phone after 3–7 business days; and
- if you test positive for HIV, you get counseling on what to do about your infection.

Vital Facts about HIV Home Test Kits

Privacy and confidentiality are main factors that lead people to choose home testing kits to find out if they are infected with human immunodeficiency virus (HIV), which causes AIDS.

It is important that consumers know there is only one product currently approved by FDA and legally sold in the United States as a home testing system for HIV. This product is a kit marketed as either *The Home Access HIV-1 Test System* or *The Home Access Express HIV-1 Test System*. The kit is a home collection-test system that requires users to collect a blood specimen, and then mail it to a laboratory for professional testing. No test kits allow consumers to interpret the results at home.

Beware of False Claims

Numerous HIV home test systems that have not been approved by FDA are currently being marketed online and in newspapers and magazines. Manufacturers of unapproved systems have falsely claimed that their products can detect antibodies to HIV in blood or saliva samples, and that they can provide results in the home in 15 minutes or less. Some have even claimed that their systems are approved by FDA or are manufactured in a facility that is registered with FDA. FDA takes appropriate action against people or firms that sell unapproved and ineffective tests.

About the Approved Product

The FDA-approved Home Access System kits allow people to collect a blood sample. Using a personal identification number (PIN), they then mail the sample anonymously to a laboratory for testing. The PIN can then be used to obtain results.

The kits, manufactured by Illinois-based Home Access Health Corporation, can be purchased at pharmacies, by mail order, or online. They only allow testing for the presence of antibodies of the virus known as HIV-1. They do not provide the ability to test for HIV-2, a less common cause of AIDS.

The Home Access System offers users pre- and post-test, anonymous and confidential counseling through both printed material and telephone interaction. It also provides the user with an interpretation of the test result.

Checking for Antibodies to HIV

Like most HIV tests, the approved Home Access testing system checks for the presence of antibodies to HIV that are produced once the virus enters the body. The rate at which individuals infected with HIV produce these antibodies differs. There's a "window period" between the time someone is infected with HIV and the time the body produces enough antibodies to be detected through testing. During this time, an HIV-infected person will still get a negative test result.

According to FDA's Center for Biologics and Research (CBER), which regulates all HIV tests, detectable antibodies usually develop within two to eight weeks. The average is about 22 days. Still, some people take longer to develop detectable antibodies. Most will develop antibodies within three months following infection. In very rare cases, it can take up to six months to develop detectable antibodies to HIV.

Rapid Tests: A Clinical Option

Consumers do have the option of taking a rapid test, some of which test for both HIV-1 and HIV-2. These tests are run where the sample is collected, and produce results within 20 minutes. Because HIV testing requires interpretation and confirmation, rapid antibody tests are only approved and available in a professional health care setting, such as doctors' offices, clinics, and outreach testing sites.

To Find FDA-Approved HIV Tests

FDA Center for Biologics Evaluation and Research
1401 Rockville Pike
Suite 200N, HFM-47
Rockville, MD 20852
Toll-Free: 800-835-4709
Phone: 301-827-1800
Website: http://www.fda.gov/BiologicsBloodVaccines
E-mail: ocod@fda.hhs.gov

Chapter 65

Prothrombin Home Test

Home Use Prothrombin Test

What does this test do? This is a home-use test kit to measure how long it takes for your blood to clot.

Why should you do this test? If you take blood-thinning drugs such as Coumadin or Warfarin, you may need to test your blood regularly to make sure it clots properly. Doctors often prescribe these drugs to prevent blood clots in patients who have artificial heart valves, irregular heartbeats or inherited clotting tendencies. Your doctor will prescribe this test for you if you need to do it.

How often should you do this test? You should follow your doctor's instructions about how often you do this test. Your doctor may ask you to use the results to adjust the amount of drugs you take to control your blood clotting. Never change the drugs you take without your doctor's permission.

How do you do this test? You prick your finger with a lancet to get a drop of blood. Place the drop of blood on a test strip or cartridge, and insert it into your test meter. Your meter will measure how long it takes for the blood to form a clot and how much anticoagulant effect there is.

This chapter includes "Home Use Tests: Prothrombin," U.S. Food and Drug Administration (FDA), March 17, 2010; and an excerpt from "Pub 100–04 Medicare Claims Processing," Centers for Medicare and Medicaid Services (CMS), January 8, 2009.

How can you make sure your meter works properly? Your meter has some built-in features that allow it to test itself and detect problems in its operation. Your meter comes with sample solutions to use instead of your blood to assure that it is working properly. Look in your meter's operator manual to see how to check on its accuracy.

Take your meter with you to your doctor's office. Have your doctor watch you do your testing. Your doctor may want to take a sample of your blood and compare the clotting time of that sample with the time your meter gives. The value you get should match your doctor's value.

Prothrombin Time Monitoring for Home Anticoagulation Management Covered by Medicare and Medicaid Services

Background: The prothrombin time (PT) test is an in-vitro test to assess coagulation. PT testing and its normalized correlate, the international normalized ratio (INR), are the standard measurements for therapeutic effectiveness of warfarin therapy. Warfarin, Coumadin®, and others, are self-administered, oral anticoagulant, or blood thinner, medications that affect a person's vitamin K-dependent clotting factors.

Policy: Effective for claims with dates of service on and after March 19, 2008, Centers for Medicare and Medicaid Services (CMS) revised its national coverage determination on prothrombin time (PT/INR) monitoring for home anticoagulation management.

Medicare will cover the use of home PT/INR monitoring for chronic, oral anticoagulation management for patients with mechanical heart valves, chronic atrial fibrillation, or venous thromboembolism (inclusive of deep venous thrombosis and pulmonary embolism) on warfarin. The monitor and the home testing must be prescribed by a treating physician as provided at 42 CFR 410.32(a) and all of the following requirements must be met:

1. The patient must have been anticoagulated for at least three months prior to use of the home INR device; and,

2. The patient must undergo a face-to-face educational program on anticoagulation management and must have demonstrated the correct use of the device prior to its use in the home; and,

3. The patient continues to correctly use the device in the context of the management of the anticoagulation therapy following the initiation of home monitoring; and,

4. Self-testing with the device should not occur more frequently than once a week.

Part Seven

Additional Help
and Information

Chapter 66

Glossary of Terms Related to Medical Tests

auditory brainstem response (ABR) test: A test used to detect some types of hearing loss, such as hearing loss caused by injury or tumors that affect nerves involved in hearing. Also called BAER test, and brainstem auditory evoked response test.

angiography: A procedure to x-ray blood vessels. The blood vessels can be seen because of an injection of a dye that shows up in the x-ray.

assessment: In health care, a process used to learn about a patient's condition. This may include a complete medical history, medical tests, a physical exam, a test of learning skills, tests to find out if the patient is able to carry out the tasks of daily living, a mental health evaluation, and a review of social support and community resources available to the patient.

barium swallow: The process of getting x-ray pictures of the esophagus or the upper gastrointestinal (GI) tract (esophagus, stomach, and duodenum). The x-ray pictures are taken after the patient drinks a liquid that contains barium sulfate (a form of the silver-white metallic element barium). The barium sulfate coats and outlines the inner walls of the esophagus and the upper GI tract so that they can be seen on the x-ray pictures.

Excerpted from "Dictionary of Cancer Terms," National Cancer Institute (NCI), available at http://www.cancer.gov/dictionary.

biopsy: The removal of cells or tissues for examination by a pathologist. The pathologist may study the tissue under a microscope or perform other tests on the cells or tissue. There are many different types of biopsy procedures. The most common types include: (1) incisional biopsy, in which only a sample of tissue is removed; (2) excisional biopsy, in which an entire lump or suspicious area is removed; and (3) needle biopsy, in which a sample of tissue or fluid is removed with a needle. When a wide needle is used, the procedure is called a core biopsy. When a thin needle is used, the procedure is called a fine-needle aspiration biopsy.

body mass index (BMI): A measure that relates body weight to height. BMI is sometimes used to measure total body fat and whether a person is a healthy weight. Excess body fat is linked to an increased risk of some diseases including heart disease and some cancers.

bone mineral density scan: see DEXA scan.

bone scan: A technique to create images of bones on a computer screen or on film. A small amount of radioactive material is injected into a blood vessel and travels through the bloodstream; it collects in the bones and is detected by a scanner.

bronchoscopy: A procedure that uses a bronchoscope to examine the inside of the trachea, bronchi (air passages that lead to the lungs), and lungs. A bronchoscope is a thin, tube-like instrument with a light and a lens for viewing. It may also have a tool to remove tissue to be checked under a microscope for signs of disease.

capsule endoscope: A device used to look at tissues in the esophagus, stomach, and intestines. It is a capsule with a lens, a light, a camera, a radio transmitter, and a battery inside. The patient swallows the capsule and it takes video pictures of the inner walls of the esophagus, stomach, and intestines as it travels through the digestive tract. The pictures are sent to a small wireless receiver that is worn on the waist of the patient and are later viewed on a computer. The capsule endoscope is passed from the body in the stool. Also called wireless capsule endoscope.

cardiopulmonary: Having to do with the heart and lungs.

cardiovascular: Having to do with the heart and blood vessels.

complete blood count (CBC): A test to check the number of red blood cells, white blood cells, and platelets in a sample of blood.

colonoscopy: Examination of the inside of the colon using a colonoscope, inserted into the rectum. A colonoscope is a thin, tube-like instrument with a light and a lens for viewing. It may also have a tool to remove tissue to be checked under a microscope for signs of disease.

computed tomography scan (CT): A series of detailed pictures of areas inside the body taken from different angles. The pictures are created by a computer linked to an x-ray machine. Also called computerized axial tomography (CAT) scan.

contrast material: A dye or other substance that helps show abnormal areas inside the body. It is given by injection into a vein, by enema, or by mouth. Contrast material may be used with x-rays, CT scans, magnetic resonance imaging (MRI), or other imaging tests.

cystoscopy: Examination of the bladder and urethra using a cystoscope, inserted into the urethra. A cystoscope is a thin, tube-like instrument with a light and a lens for viewing. It may also have a tool to remove tissue to be checked under a microscope for signs of disease.

deoxyribonucleic acid (DNA): The molecules inside cells that carry genetic information and pass it from one generation to the next.

DEXA scan: An imaging test that measures bone density (the amount of bone mineral contained in a certain volume of bone) by passing x-rays with two different energy levels through the bone. It is used to diagnose osteoporosis (decrease in bone mass and density). Also, called BMD scan, bone mineral density scan, DEXA, dual energy x-ray absorptiometric scan, dual x-ray absorptiometry, and DXA.

diagnostic technique: A type of method or test used to help diagnose a disease or condition. Imaging tests and tests to measure blood pressure, pulse, and temperature are examples of diagnostic techniques.

digital image analysis: A method in which an image or other type of data is changed into a series of dots or numbers so that it can be viewed and studied on a computer. In medicine, this type of image analysis is being used to study organs or tissues, and in the diagnosis and treatment of disease.

electrocardiogram (EKG): A line graph that shows changes in the electrical activity of the heart over time. It is made by an instrument called an electrocardiograph. The graph can show that there are abnormal conditions, such as blocked arteries, changes in electrolytes (particles with electrical charges), and changes in the way electrical currents pass through the heart tissue.

electroencephalogram (EEG): A recording of electrical activity in the brain. It is made by placing electrodes on the scalp (the skin covering the top of the head), and impulses are sent to a special machine. An EEG may be used to diagnose brain and sleep disorders.

electronic medical record: A collection of a patient's medical information in a digital (electronic) form that can be viewed on a computer and easily shared by people taking care of the patient.

endoscopic retrograde cholangiopancreatography (ERCP): A procedure that uses an endoscope to examine and x-ray the pancreatic duct, hepatic duct, common bile duct, duodenal papilla, and gallbladder. An endoscope is a thin, tube-like instrument with a light and a lens for viewing.

endoscopy: A procedure that uses an endoscope to examine the inside of the body. An endoscope is a thin, tube-like instrument with a light and a lens for viewing. It may also have a tool to remove tissue to be checked under a microscope for signs of disease.

erythrocyte sedimentation rate (ESR): See sedimentation rate.

false-negative test result: A test result that indicates that a person does not have a specific disease or condition when the person actually does have the disease or condition.

false-positive test result: A test result that indicates that a person has a specific disease or condition when the person actually does not have the disease or condition.

fine-needle aspiration (FNA) biopsy: The removal of tissue or fluid with a thin needle for examination under a microscope.

fluoroscopy: An x-ray procedure that makes it possible to see internal organs in motion.

gallium scan: A procedure to detect areas of the body where cells are dividing rapidly. It is used to locate cancer cells or areas of inflammation. A very small amount of radioactive gallium is injected into a vein and travels through the bloodstream. The gallium is taken up by rapidly dividing cells in the bones, tissues, and organs and is detected by a scanner.

genetic counseling: A communication process between a specially trained health professional and a person concerned about the genetic risk of disease. The person's family and personal medical history may be discussed, and counseling may lead to genetic testing.

genetic testing: Analyzing DNA to look for a genetic alteration that may indicate an increased risk for developing a specific disease or disorder.

imaging: In medicine, a process that makes pictures of areas inside the body. Imaging uses methods such as x-rays (high-energy radiation), ultrasound (high-energy sound waves), and radio waves.

intravenous pyelogram: An x-ray image of the kidneys, ureters, and bladder. It is made after a substance that shows up on x-rays is injected into a blood vessel. The substance outlines the kidneys, ureters, and bladder as it flows through the system and collects in the urine. An intravenous pyelogram is usually made to look for a block in the flow of urine.

kidney function test: A test in which blood or urine samples are checked for the amounts of certain substances released by the kidneys. A higher- or lower-than-normal amount of a substance can be a sign that the kidneys are not working the way they should. Also, called renal function test.

laboratory test: A medical procedure that involves testing a sample of blood, urine, or other substance from the body. Tests can help determine a diagnosis, plan treatment, check to see if treatment is working, or monitor the disease over time.

lower gastrointestinal (GI) series: X-rays of the colon and rectum that are taken after a person is given a barium enema.

lumbar puncture: A procedure in which a thin needle called a spinal needle is put into the lower part of the spinal column to collect cerebrospinal fluid or to give drugs. Also, called spinal tap.

lung function test: See pulmonary function test.

magnetic resonance imaging: A procedure in which radio waves and a powerful magnet linked to a computer are used to create detailed pictures of areas inside the body. These pictures can show the difference between normal and diseased tissue. Magnetic resonance imaging makes better images of organs and soft tissue than other scanning techniques, such as computed tomography (CT) or x-ray. Magnetic resonance imaging is especially useful for imaging the brain, the spine, the soft tissue of joints, and the inside of bones. Also, called MRI, NMRI, and nuclear magnetic resonance imaging.

magnetic resonance perfusion imaging: A special type of magnetic resonance imaging (MRI) that uses an injected dye in order to see blood flow through tissues. Also called perfusion magnetic resonance imaging.

magnetic resonance spectroscopic imaging: A noninvasive imaging method that provides information about cellular activity (metabolic information). It is used along with magnetic resonance imaging (MRI) which provides information about the shape and size of the tumor (spatial information).

monitor: In medicine, to regularly watch and check a person or condition to see if there is any change. Also refers to a device that records and/or displays patient data, such as for an electrocardiogram (EKG).

myelogram: An x-ray of the spinal cord after an injection of dye into the space between the lining of the spinal cord and brain.

nuclear magnetic resonance imaging: A procedure in which radio waves and a powerful magnet linked to a computer are used to create detailed pictures of areas inside the body. These pictures can show the difference between normal and diseased tissue. Nuclear magnetic resonance imaging is especially useful for imaging the brain, the spine, the soft tissue of joints, and the inside of bones.

optical coherence tomography: A procedure that uses infrared light waves to give three-dimensional (3-D) pictures of structures inside tissues and organs. The pictures are made by a computer linked to the light source.

oxygen saturation test: A test that measures the amount of oxygen being carried by red blood cells.

pancreatic function test: A test used to help diagnose problems in the pancreas, such as gastrinomas and pancreatitis. It measures the ability of the pancreas to respond to the hormone secretin (a hormone that causes other substances to be released by the stomach, liver, and pancreas).

Pap test: A procedure in which cells are scraped from the cervix for examination under a microscope. It is used to detect cancer and changes that may lead to cancer. Also, called Pap smear and Papanicolaou test.

pathology report: The description of cells and tissues made by a pathologist based on microscopic evidence, and sometimes used to make a diagnosis of a disease.

pelvic examination: A physical examination in which the health care professional will feel for lumps or changes in the shape of the vagina, cervix, uterus, fallopian tubes, ovaries, and rectum. The health care professional will also use a speculum to open the vagina to look at the cervix and take samples for a Pap test. Also, called internal examination.

personal medical history: A collection of information about a person's health. It may include information about allergies, illnesses and surgeries, and dates and results of physical exams, tests, screenings, and immunizations. It may also include information about medicines taken and about diet and exercise. Also, called personal health record and personal history.

positron emission tomography (PET) scan: A procedure in which a small amount of radioactive glucose (sugar) is injected into a vein, and a scanner is used to make detailed, computerized pictures of areas inside the body where the glucose is used. Because cancer cells often use more glucose than normal cells, the pictures can be used to find cancer cells in the body.

positive test result: A test result that reveals the presence of a specific disease or condition for which the test is being done.

pulmonary function test: A test used to measure how well the lungs work. It measures how much air the lungs can hold and how quickly air is moved into and out of the lungs. It also measures how much oxygen is used and how much carbon dioxide is given off during breathing. A pulmonary function test can be used to diagnose a lung disease and to see how well treatment for the disease is working. Also, called lung function test and PFT.

radioimaging: A method that uses radioactive substances to make pictures of areas inside the body. The radioactive substance is injected into the body, and locates and binds to specific cells or tissues, including cancer cells. Images are made using a special machine that detects the radioactive substance.

radiology: The use of radiation (such as x-rays) or other imaging technologies (such as ultrasound and magnetic resonance imaging) to diagnose or treat disease.

radionuclide scanning: Procedure that produces pictures (scans) of structures inside the body, including areas where there are cancer cells. Radionuclide scanning is used to diagnose, stage, and monitor disease. A small amount of a radioactive chemical (radionuclide) is injected into a vein or swallowed. A computer forms an image of the areas where the radionuclide builds up. These areas may contain cancer cells. Also called scintigraphy.

reference range: In medicine, a set of values that a doctor uses to interpret a patient's test results. The reference range for a given test is based on test results for 95% of the healthy population. The reference range for a test may be different for different groups of people (for example, men and women). Also, called normal range, reference interval, and reference values.

scintimammography: A type of breast imaging test that is used to detect cancer cells in the breasts of some women who have had abnormal mammograms, or who have dense breast tissue. It is not used for screening or in place of a mammogram. Also, called Miraluma test and sestamibi breast imaging.

sigmoidoscopy: Examination of the lower colon using a sigmoidoscope, inserted into the rectum. A sigmoidoscope is a thin, tube-like instrument with a light and a lens for viewing. It may also have a tool to remove tissue to be checked under a microscope for signs of disease.

screening: Checking for disease when there are no symptoms. Since screening may find diseases at an early stage, there may be a better chance of curing the disease. Examples of cancer screening tests are the mammogram (breast), colonoscopy (colon), Pap smear (cervix), and PSA blood level and digital rectal exam (prostate). Screening can also include checking for a person's risk of developing an inherited disease by doing a genetic test.

sedimentation rate: The distance red blood cells travel in one hour in a sample of blood as they settle to the bottom of a test tube. The sedimentation rate is increased in inflammation, infection, cancer, rheumatic diseases, and diseases of the blood and bone marrow. Also, called erythrocyte sedimentation rate and ESR.

sentinel lymph node biopsy: Removal and examination of the sentinel node(s) (the first lymph node(s) to which cancer cells are likely to spread from a primary tumor).

sestamibi scan: An imaging test used to find overactive parathyroid glands (four pea-sized glands found on the thyroid) and breast cancer cells, and to diagnose heart disease.

single photon emission computed tomography (SPECT): A special type of computed tomography (CT) scan in which a small amount of a radioactive drug is injected into a vein and a scanner is used to make detailed images of areas inside the body where the radioactive material is taken up by the cells. Single-photon emission computed tomography can give information about blood flow to tissues and chemical reactions (metabolism) in the body.

skin test: A test for an immune response to a compound by placing it on or under the skin.

slit-lamp eye exam: An eye exam using an instrument that combines a low-power microscope with a light source that makes a narrow beam of light. The instrument may be used to examine the retina, optic nerve, and other parts of the eye. Also, called slit-lamp biomicroscopy.

sonogram: See ultrasound.

spiral CT scan: detailed picture of areas inside the body. The pictures are created by a computer linked to an x-ray machine that scans the body in a spiral path. Also, called helical computed tomography.

symptom: An indication that a person has a condition or disease. Some examples of symptoms are headache, fever, fatigue, nausea, vomiting, and pain.

tethered capsule endoscope: A device used to look at tissues in the esophagus. It is a tiny capsule with a laser scanner inside and a very thin cord attached to it. The patient swallows the capsule and the thin cord helps keep the capsule in a specific area in the esophagus. The cord is also used to remove the capsule. Pictures are taken by the laser scanner and sent to a computer for viewing. A tethered capsule endoscope is used to find early cancers of the esophagus and other parts of the body. Also, called TCE.

ultrasound: A procedure in which high-energy sound waves are bounced off internal tissues or organs and make echoes. The echo patterns are shown on the screen of an ultrasound machine, forming a picture of body tissues called a sonogram. Also, called ultrasonography.

upper endoscopy: Examination of the inside of the stomach using an endoscope, passed through the mouth and esophagus. An endoscope is a thin, tube-like instrument with a light and a lens for viewing. It may also have a tool to remove tissue to be checked under a microscope for signs of disease. Also, called gastroscopy.

upper gastrointestinal (GI) series: A series of x-ray pictures of the esophagus, stomach, and duodenum (the first part of the small intestine). The x-ray pictures are taken after the patient drinks a liquid containing barium sulfate (a form of the silver-white metallic element barium). The barium sulfate coats and outlines the inner walls of the upper gastrointestinal tract so that they can be seen on the x-ray pictures.

ureteroscopy: Examination of the inside of the kidney and ureter, using a ureteroscope. A ureteroscope is a thin, tube-like instrument with a light and a lens for viewing. It may also have a tool to remove tissue to be checked under a microscope for signs of disease. The ureteroscope is passed through the urethra into the bladder, ureter, and renal pelvis (part of the kidney that collects, holds, and drains urine).

urinalysis: A test that determines the content of the urine.

venipuncture: The puncture of a vein with a needle for the purpose of drawing blood. Also, called phlebotomy.

venography: A procedure in which an x-ray of the veins is taken after a special dye is injected into the bone marrow or veins.

venous sampling: A procedure in which a sample of blood is taken from a certain vein and checked for specific substances released by nearby organs and tissues.

virtual colonoscopy: A method to examine the inside of the colon by taking a series of x-rays. A computer is used to make 2-dimensional (2-D) and 3-D pictures of the colon from these x-rays. The pictures can be saved, changed to give better viewing angles, and reviewed after the procedure, even years later. Also, called computed tomographic colonography, computed tomography colonography, CT colonography, and CTC.

x-ray: A type of high-energy radiation. In low doses, x-rays are used to diagnose diseases by making pictures of the inside of the body. In high doses, x-rays are used to treat cancer.

Chapter 67

Online Health Screening Tools

Alcoholism, Drug Dependence, and Addictions

About My Drinking and Other Drug Use
Hazelden
Website: http://www.aboutmydrinking.org

Drug Abuse Screening Test (DAST)
Project Cork Online
Website: http://www.projectcork.org/clinical_tools/html/DAST.html

Food Addiction
Addicted.com
Website: http://www.addicted.com/addiction-resources/self-tests/
food-addiction-quiz

Tobacco Dependence
Addicted.com
Website: http://www.addicted.com/addiction-resources/self-tests/
tobacco-addiction-quiz

Resources in this chapter were compiled from several sources deemed reliable; all contact information was verified and updated in April 2011. Inclusion does not imply endorsement. This list is not comprehensive, it is intended as a starting point for gathering of information. Discuss findings and questions with your health care provider.

Auditory

Hearing Test, Environmental Sounds, and Simulated Hearing Loss
Freehearingtest.com
Website: http://www.freehearingtest.com/test.shtml

Sensitivity, equal loudness contours and audiometry
University New South Wales
Website: http://www.freehearingtest.com/test.shtml

Autism

Quick Test
Iautistic
Website: http://iautistic.com/free-autism-tests.php

Milestone Checklist
Centers for Disease Control and Prevention
Website: http://www.cdc.gov/ncbddd/actearly/milestones

AQ Test (Adult Autism)
Autism Research Centre
Website: http://www.wired.com/wired/archive/9.12/aqtest.html

Bone and Joint Risk Assessments

Osteoporosis Risk Questionnaire
Washington University School of Medicine: Your Disease Risk
Website: http://www.yourdiseaserisk.wustl.edu/hccpquiz.pl?lang=eng
lish&func=home&quiz=osteoporosis

Back Pain and Joint Disorders Risk Assessment
Trinity Iowa Health System
Website: https://www.healthawareservices.com/nahrs/index.htm?hosp
ID=21&moduleName=jointAware

Spine and Back Risk Assessment
Trinity Iowa Health System
Website: https://www.healthawareservices.com/nahrs/index.htm?hosp
ID=21&moduleName=spineAware

Cancer Risk Assessments

Risk for Developing Bladder Cancer
Washington University School of Medicine: Your Disease Risk
Website: http://www.yourdiseaserisk.wustl.edu/hccpquiz.pl?lang=eng
lish&func=home&quiz=bladder

Risk Assessment for Developing Breast Cancer
Washington University School of Medicine: Your Disease Risk
Website: http://www.yourdiseaserisk.wustl.edu/hccpquiz.pl?lang=eng
lish&func=home&quiz=breast

Breast Cancer Risk Assessment Tool
National Cancer Institute
Website: http://www.cancer.gov/bcrisktool/Default.aspx

Risk Assessment for Developing Cervical Cancer
Washington University School of Medicine: Your Disease Risk
Website: http://www.yourdiseaserisk.wustl.edu/hccpquiz.pl?lang=eng
lish&func=home&quiz=cervical

Risk Assessment for Developing Colon Cancer
Washington University School of Medicine: Your Disease Risk
Website: http://www.yourdiseaserisk.wustl.edu/hccpquiz.pl?lang=eng
lish&func=home&quiz=colon

Risk Assessment for Developing Kidney Cancer
Washington University School of Medicine: Your Disease Risk
Website: http://www.yourdiseaserisk.wustl.edu/hccpquiz.pl?lang=eng
lish&func=home&quiz=kidney

Risk Assessment for Developing Lung Cancer
Washington University School of Medicine: Your Disease Risk
Website: http://www.yourdiseaserisk.wustl.edu/hccpquiz.pl?lang=eng
lish&func=home&quiz=lung

Lung Cancer Prediction Tool for Long-Term Smokers
Memorial Sloan-Kettering Cancer Center
Website: http://www.mskcc.org/mskcc/html/12463.cfm

Risk Assessment for Developing Melanoma Cancer
Washington University School of Medicine: Your Disease Risk
Website: http://www.yourdiseaserisk.wustl.edu/hccpquiz.pl?lang=eng
lish&func=home&quiz=melanoma

Risk Assessment for Developing Ovarian Cancer
Washington University School of Medicine: Your Disease Risk
Website: http://www.yourdiseaserisk.wustl.edu/hccpquiz.pl?lang=eng
lish&func=home&quiz=ovarian

Risk Assessment for Developing Pancreatic Cancer
Washington University School of Medicine: Your Disease Risk
Website: http://www.yourdiseaserisk.wustl.edu/hccpquiz.pl?lang=eng
lish&func=home&quiz=pancreatic

Prostate Cancer Prevention Trial Prostate Cancer Risk Calculator (PCPTRC)
UT Health Science Center–San Antonio
Website: http://deb.uthscsa.edu/URORiskCalc/Pages/uroriskcalc.jsp

Risk Assessment for Developing Stomach Cancer
Washington University School of Medicine: Your Disease Risk
Website: http://www.yourdiseaserisk.wustl.edu/hccpquiz.pl?lang=eng
lish&func=home&quiz=stomach

Risk Assessment for Developing Uterine Cancer
Washington University School of Medicine: Your Disease Risk
Website: http://www.yourdiseaserisk.wustl.edu/hccpquiz.pl?lang=eng
lish&func=home&quiz=uterine

Diabetes and Kidney Disease Risk

Risk Assessment for Developing Diabetes
Washington University School of Medicine: Your Disease Risk
Website: http://www.yourdiseaserisk.wustl.edu/hccpquiz.pl?lang=eng
lish&func=home&quiz=diabetes

Diabetes Risk Test
American Diabetes Association
Website: http://www.diabetes.org/diabetes-basics/prevention/
diabetes-risk-test

Diabetes Risk Score
Diabetes UK
Website: http://www.diabetes.org.uk/riskscore

GFR Calculators for Adults and Children
National Kidney Disease Educational Program
Website: http://www.nkdep.nih.gov/professionals/gfr_calculators

Heart Attack Risk, Heart Disease Risk, and Arterial Age Risk

Heart Disease Risk Questionnaire
Washington University School of Medicine: Your Disease Risk
Website: http://www.yourdiseaserisk.wustl.edu/hccpquiz.pl?lang=eng
lish&func=home&quiz=heart

Heart Disease Risk Calculator
American College of Cardiology
Website: http://www.cardiosmart.org/CardioSmart/Default
.aspx?id=298

Heart Attack Risk Assessment
American Heart Association
Website: http://www.heart.org/HEARTORG/Conditions/HeartAttack/
HeartAttackToolsResources/Heart-Attack-Risk-Assessment_
UCM_303944_Article.jsp

My Life Check: State of Your Heart
American Heart Association
Website: http://mylifecheck.heart.org/PledgePage.aspx?NavID
=5&CultureCode=en-US

Risk Assessment Tool for Estimating Your 10-Year Risk of Having a Heart Attack
National Cholesterol Education Program
Website: http://hp2010.nhlbihin.net/atpiii/calculator.asp

Coronary Artery Calcium (CAC) Score Reference Values
University of Washington
Website: http://www.mesa-nhlbi.org/CACReference.aspx

Infectious Disease Risk Assessment

Assess Your Risk for HIV and Other Similarly Transmitted Diseases
Body Health Resources Foundation
Website: http://www.thebody.com/surveys/sexsurvey.html

Malaria Risk Assessment
Centers for Disease Control and Prevention (CDC)
Website: http://www.cdc.gov/malaria/travelers/risk_assessment.html

Mental Health Risk Assessments

Adult Self-Report Scale-V1.1 (ASRS-V1.1) Screener for ADHD
World Health Organization (WHO)
Website: http://webdoc.nyumc.org/nyumc/files/psych/attachments/
psych_adhd_screener.pdf

Adult ADHD Self-Report Scale (ASRS-v1.1)
New York University Medical Center
Website: http://webdoc.nyumc.org/nyumc/files/psych/attachments/
psych_adhd_checklist.pdf

Anxiety Screening Test
New York University (NYU) Langone Medical Center
Website: http://psych.med.nyu.edu/patient-care/anxiety-screening-test

Goldburg Bipolar Screening Quiz
Psych Central
Website: http://psychcentral.com/quizzes/bipolarquiz.htm

Depression Screener
Mental Health America
Website: http://www.depression-screening.org/depression_screen.cfm

Depression Screening Test
New York University (NYU) Langone Medical Center
Website: http://psych.med.nyu.edu/patient-care/depression-screening-test

Mood Monitor for Anxiety, Depression, Post-Traumatic Stress Disorder (PTSD), and Bipolar Disorder
M-3 Information
Website: http://www.mymoodmonitor.com/User/DiagnosisQues.aspx

Personality Disorders Screening Test
New York University (NYU) Langone Medical Center
Website: http://psych.med.nyu.edu/patient-care/personality
-disorders-screening-test

Stress Screener
Mental Health America
Website: http://www.mentalhealthamerica.net/llw/stressquiz.html

Pregnancy

Online Pregnancy Test
Live Pregnancy Test
Website: http://www.livepregnancytest.com/pregnancytest

Online Pregnancy Due Date Calculator
Live Pregnancy Test
Website: http://www.livepregnancytest.com/duedate

Ovulation Calendar
Live Pregnancy Test
Website: http://www.livepregnancytest.com/ovulation

Radiation Exposure Risk

RADAR Medical Procedure Radiation Dose Calculator
doseinfo-radar
Website: http://www.doseinfo-radar.com/RADARDoseRiskCalc.html

Sexual Health

Sexual Disorders Screening Test for Men
New York University (NYU) Langone Medical Center
Website: http://psych.med.nyu.edu/patient-care/sexual-disorders
-screening-test-men

Sexual Disorders Screening Test for Women
New York University (NYU) Langone Medical Center
Website: http://psych.med.nyu.edu/patient-care/sexual-disorders
-screening-test-women

Sleep

Sleep Risk Assessment
Trinity Iowa Health System
Website: https://www.healthawareservices.com/nahrs/index.htm?hosp
ID=21&moduleName=sleepAware

Stroke

Stroke Risk Questionnaire
Washington University School of Medicine: Your Disease Risk
Website: http://www.yourdiseaserisk.wustl.edu/hccpquiz.pl?lang=eng
lish&func=home&quiz=stroke

Visual Tests

Adult Vision Risk Assessment
Prevent Blindness America
Website: http://www.preventblindness.net/site/Survey?ACTION_
REQUIRED=URI_ACTION_USER_REQUESTS&SURVEY_ID=1240

Color Vision Tests
Sight and Hearing Association
Website: http://www.freevisiontest.com/colortest.php

Near Vision Test for Adults
Prevent Blindness America
Website: http://www.preventblindness.org/eye_tests/near_vision
_test.html

Distance Vision Test for Adults
Prevent Blindness America
Website: http://www.preventblindness.org/eye_tests/Adult_distance
_test.html

Self Vision Screening Tests
Sight and Hearing Association
Website: http://www.freevisiontest.com/selfvision.php

Weight Risk

Weight Assessment
Trinity Iowa Health System
Website: https://www.healthawareservices.com/nahrs/index.htm?hosp
ID=21&moduleName=spineAware

Body Mass Index Calculator
National Heart, Lung, and Blood Institute (NHLBI)
Website: http://www.nhlbisupport.com/bmi/bmicalc.htm
Mobile application: http://apps.usa.gov/bmi-app

Chapter 68

Directory of Breast and Cervical Cancer Early Detection Programs

Alabama
Breast and Cervical Cancer
Early Detection Program
Bureau of Family Health
Services
AL Dept. of Public Health
P.O. Box 303017
Montgomery, AL 36130
Toll-Free: 877-252-3324
Phone: 334-206-5851
Fax: 334-206-2950
Website: http://www.adph.org/
earlydetection

Alaska
Breast and Cervical Health
Check
Div. of Public Health
Women's, Children's, and Family
Health
4701 Business Pk. Blvd.
Bldg. J, Suite 20
Anchorage, AK 99503
Toll-Free in AK: 800-410-6266
Phone: 907-269-3491
Fax: 907-269-3414
Website: http://www.hss.state
.ak.us/dph/wcfh/BCHC

Resources in this chapter were excerpted from: "National Breast and Cervical Cancer Early Detection Program: State, U.S. Territory and Organization Program Contacts," Centers for Disease Control and Prevention (CDC). All contact information was verified and updated in April 2011.

American Samoa
Breast and Cervical Cancer
Early Detection Program
Dept. of Health
American Samoa Government
Territory of American Samoa
Pago Pago, AS 96799
Phone: 011 684-633-2135
Fax: 011 684-633-2136

Arizona
Well Woman Healthcheck
Program
Bureau of Chronic Disease
Prevention and Control
AZ Dept. of Health Services
1740 W. Adams, No. 205
Phoenix, AZ 85007
Toll-Free: 888-257-8502
Fax: 602-542-7520
Website: http://
wellwomanhealthcheck.org

Arkansas
BreastCare
AR Dept. of Health
4815 W. Markham St., Slot 11
Little Rock, AR 72205
Toll-Free: 877-670-2273
Website: http://www.healthy
.arkansas.gov/programsServices/
chronicDisease/ArBreastCare

California
Cancer Detection Programs:
Every Woman Counts
CA Dept. of Public Health
MS 7203
P.O. Box 997377
Sacramento, CA 95899
Toll-Free: 800-511-2300
Phone: 916-449-5300
Fax: 916-449-5310
Website: http://www.cdph.ca.gov/
programs/CancerDetection/Pages/
CancerDetectionProgramsEvery
WomanCounts.aspx
E-mail: cancerdetection
@cdph.ca.gov

Colorado
Women's Wellness Connection
CO Dept. of Public Health and
Environment
PSD-WWC-A5
4300 Cherry Crk. Dr. S.
Denver, CO 80246
Toll-Free: 866-951-9355
Toll-Free in CO: 800-886-7689
Phone: 303-692-2000
Website: http://www
.womenswellnessconnection.org

Commonwealth of Northern Mariana Islands
Dept. of Public Health
Breast and Cervical Cancer
Screening Program
P.O. Box 500409 CK
Saipan, MP 96950
Phone: 670-236-8703
Website:
http://www.dphsaipan.com

Connecticut

Breast and Cervical Cancer
Program
CT Dept. of Public Health
410 Capitol Ave., MS #11CCS
Hartford, CT 06106
Phone: 860-509-7804;
or 860-509-8000
Website: http://www.ct.gov/dph/
cwp/view.asp?a=3124&q=388824
&dphPNavCtr=|47735|#47737

Delaware

Screening for Life
Div. of Public Health
DE Dept. of Health and Social
Services
417 Federal St.
Jesse Cooper Bldg.
Dover, DE 19901
Toll-Free: 800-464-4357
Phone: 302-744-4700
Fax: 302-739-6659
Website: http://www.dhss
.delaware.gov/dph/dpc/sfl.html

District of Columbia

Breast and Cervical Cancer
Early Detection Program
DC Dept. of Health
899 N. Capitol St., NE
Washington, DC 20002
Phone: 202-442-5900
Website: http://doh
.dc.gov/doh/cwp/
view,a,1373,q,582368,dohNav
_GID,1801,dohNav,|33183|
33184|,.asp

Florida

Breast and Cervical Cancer
Early Detection Program
Bureau of Chronic Disease
Prevention
FL Dept. of Health
4052 Bald Cypress Way,
Bin #A-18
Tallahassee, FL 32399
Phone: 850-245-4444
Fax: 850-414-6625
Website: http://www.doh.state
.fl.us/Family/cancer/bcc

Georgia

GA Dept. of Human Resources
Div. of Public Health
2 Peachtree St., NW, 13th Fl.
Atlanta, GA 30303
Phone: 404-657-3156
Website: http://health.state
.ga.us/programs/bccp

Guam

Breast and Cervical Cancer
Early Detection Program
Div. of Public Health
Dept. of Public Health and
Social Services
123 Chalan Kareta, Rm. 160
Mangilao, GU 96913
Phone: 671-735-0671
Fax: 671-734-7626

Hawaii

Hawaii Breast and Cervical
Cancer Program
HI State Dept. of Health
601 Kamokila Blvd., #344
Kapolei, HI 96707
Phone: 808-692-7480
Fax: 808-692-7478
Website: http://hawaii.gov/
health/family-child-health/
chronic-disease/bcccp

Idaho

Women's Health Check
Division of Health
ID Dept. of Health and Welfare
450 W. State St., 4th Fl.
P.O. Box 83720
Boise, ID 83720
Toll-Free in ID: 800-926-2588
ID Care Line: 211
Phone: 208-332-7311
Fax: 208-334-0657
Website: http://
healthandwelfare.idaho.gov/
Health/DiseasesConditions/
Cancer/WomensHealthCheck/
tabid/255/Default.aspx

Illinois

Illinois Breast and Cervical
Cancer Program
Office of Women's Health
Services
IL Dept. of Public Health
535 W. Jefferson S., 1st Fl.
Springfield, IL 62761
Women's Health Line:
888-522-1282
Toll-Free TTY: 800-547-0466
Website: http://cancerscreening
.illinois.gov
E-mail:
DPH.OWHLine@Illinois.gov

Indiana

Breast and Cervical Cancer
Early Detection Program
IN State Dept. of Health
2 N. Meridian St.
Mailstop 6B-F4
Indianapolis, IN 46204
Toll-Free: 800-433-0746
Phone: 317-233-7405
Fax: 317-234-2275
Website: http://www.in.gov/
isdh/24967.htm

Iowa

Care for Yourself
Iowa Breast and Cervical Cancer
Early Detection Program
IA Dept. of Public Health
321 E. 12th St.
Des Moines, IA 50319
Toll-Free: 800-369-2229
Toll-Free TTY: 800-735-2942
Phone: 515-281-7689
Website: http://www.idph.state
.ia.us/careforyourself

Kansas

Early Detection Works
KS Dept. of Health and
Environment
State Office Bldg.
1000 SW Jackson, Suite 230
Topeka, KS 66612
Toll-Free: 877-277-1368
Phone: 785-296-1207
Fax: 785-368-7287
Website:
http://www.kdheks.gov/edw

Kentucky

Women's Cancer Screening
Program
275 E. Main St., HS1WF
Frankfort, KY 40621
Toll-Free: 800-422-6237
Phone: 502-564-3236
Fax: 502-564-1552
Website: http://chfs.ky.gov/dph/
info/dwh/cancerscreening.htm

Louisiana

LSUHSC School of Public
Health
Louisiana Breast and Cervical
Health Program
1615 Poydras St., Ste. 1400
New Orleans, LA 70112
Toll-Free: 888-599-1073
Fax: 504-568-5838
Website: http://labchp.lsuhsc.edu

Maine

Breast and Cervical Health
Program
11 State House Station
Augusta, ME 04333
Toll-Free in ME: 800-350-5180
Toll-Free TTY: 800-438-5514
Phone: 207-287-8068
Fax: 207-287-4100 not
confidential
Fax: 800-325-5760 confidential
Website: http://www.maine.gov/
dhhs/bohdcfh/bcp

Maryland

Breast and Cervical Cancer
Screening Program
201 W. Preston St., Rm. 306
Baltimore, MD 21201
Toll-Free: 800-477-9774
Phone: 410-767-5300
Fax: 410-333-7106
Website: http://fha.maryland
.gov/cancer/bccp_home.cfm

Massachusetts

Women's Health Network
Bureau of Community Health
Access and Promotion
250 Washington St.
Boston, MA 02108
Toll-Free: 877-414-4447
Phone: 617-624-5434
TTY: 617-624-5992
Fax: 617-624-5055
Website: http://www.mass.gov/
dph/whn

Michigan

Breast and Cervical Cancer
Control Program
MI Dept. of Community Health
Capitol View Bldg.
201 Townsend St.
Lansing, MI 48913
Toll-Free: 800-922-6266
Phone: 517-373-3740
Toll-Free TTY: 800-649-3777
Website: http://www.michigan
.gov/mdch/1,1607,7-132-
2940_2955-13487--,00.html

Minnesota

SAGE Screening Program
MN Dept. of Health
85 E. Seventh Pl.
P.O. Box 64882
St. Paul, MN 55164
Toll-Free: 888-643-2584
Phone: 651-201-5000
TTY: 651-201-5797
Website:
http://www.health.state.mn.us/
divs/hpcd/ccs/screening/sage

Mississippi

Breast and Cervical Cancer
Early Detection Program
MS State Dept. of Health
570 E. Woodrow Wilson
P.O. Box 1700
Jackson, MS 39215
Toll-Free: 800-721-7222
Phone: 601-576-7466
Fax: 601-576-8030
Website: http://msdh.ms.gov/
msdhsite/_static/41,0,103.html

Missouri

Show Me Healthy Women
Program
MO Dept. of Health and Senior
Services
P.O. Box 570
Jefferson City, MO 65102
Phone: 573-522-2845
Fax: 573-522-2899
Website: http://health.mo.gov/
living/healthcondiseases/chronic/
showmehealthywomen
E-mail: info@health.mo.gov

Montana

Breast and Cervical Health
Program
1400 Broadway, C-317
P.O. Box 202951
Helena, MT 59620
Toll-Free: 888-803-9343
Phone: 406-444-0063
Fax: 406-444-7465
Website: http://www.dphhs
.mt.gov/PHSD/cancer-control/
Breast&Cerv-index.shtml

Nebraska

Every Woman Matters Program
Office of Women's Health
301 Centennial Mall S., 3rd Fl.
P.O. Box 94817
Lincoln, NE 68509
Toll-Free: 800-532-2227
Toll-Free TDD: 800-833-7352
Phone: 402-471-0929
Fax: 402-471-0913
Website: http://www.hhs.state
.ne.us/womenshealth/ewm
E-mail: dhhs.ewm@nebraska.gov

Nevada
Women's Health Connection
4150 Technology Way, Ste. 101
Carson City, NV 89706
Toll-Free: 888-463-8942
Phone: 775-684-4285
Fax: 775-684-4031
Website: http://health.nv.gov/
CD_WHC_BreastCervical_
Cancer.htm

New Hampshire
Breast and Cervical Cancer
Program
NH Dept. of Health and Human
Services
129 Pleasant St.
Concord, NH 03301
Toll-Free in NH: 800-852-3345
ext. 4931
Phone: 603-271-4886
Fax: 603-271-0539
Website: http://www.dhhs.nh.gov/
dphs/cdpc/bccp

New Jersey
Cancer Education and Early
Detection Program
NJ Dept. of Health and Senior
Services
50 E. State St., 6th Fl.
P.O. Box 364
Trenton, NJ 08625
Toll-Free: 800-328-3838
Phone: 609-292-8540
Fax: 609-588-3638
Website: http://www.state.nj.us/
health/cancer/njceed

New Mexico
Breast and Cervical Cancer
Early Detection Program
NM Dept. of Health
5301 Central Ave. NE, Suite 800
Albuquerque, NM 87108
Toll-Free: 877-852-2585
Phone: 505-841-5860
Fax: 505-222-8602
Website: http://www.cancernm
.org/bcc

New York
Cancer Services Program
Bureau of Chronic Disease
Services
NY State Dept. of Health
Riverview Ctr., Suite 350
Albany, NY 12204
Toll-Free: 866-442-2262
Phone: 518-474-1222
Fax: 518-473-0642
Website: http://www.health
.ny.gov/diseases/cancer/services
E-mail: canserv@health.state
.ny.us

North Carolina
Breast and Cervical Cancer
Control Program
1922 Mail Service Ctr.
Raleigh, NC 27699
Phone: 919-707-5300
Fax: 919-870-4812
Website: http://www.bcccp
.ncdhhs.gov

North Dakota

Women's Way
Div. of Cancer Prevention and
Control
ND Dept. of Health
600 E. Blvd. Ave., Dept. 301
Bismarck, ND 58505
Toll-Free in ND: 800-449-6636
Phone: 701-328-2333
Fax: 701-328-2036
Website: http://www.ndhealth
.gov/womensway
E-mail: womensway@nd.gov

Ohio

Breast and Cervical Cancer Project
OH Dept. of Health
246 N. High St.
Columbus, OH 43215
Phone: 614-728-2177
Fax: 614-564-2409
Website: http://www.odh.ohio
.gov/odhPrograms/hprr/bc_canc/
bcanc1.aspx
E-mail: BHPRR@odh.ohio.gov

Oklahoma

Breast and Cervical Cancer
Early Detection Program
OK State Dept. of Health
1000 NE 10th
Oklahoma City, OK 73117
Toll-Free (all ages): 888-669-5934
Phone (age 50 and older):
405-271-4072
Website:
http://www.ok.gov/health/
County_Health_Departments/
Carter_County_Health_
Department/Take_Charge!

Oregon

Oregon Breast and Cervical
Cancer Program
800 NE Oregon St., Suite 360
Portland, OR 97232
Toll-Free: 877-255-7070
Phone: 971-673-0581
Fax: 971-673-0997
TTY: 971-673-0372
Website:
http://public.health.oregon.gov/
PHD/OFH/WRH/BCC

Pennsylvania

Healthy Woman Program
PA Dept. of Health
625 Forster St., 8th Fl. W.
Harrisburg, PA 17120
Toll-Free: 800-215-7494
Toll-Free TTY: 800-332-8615
Fax: 717-772-0608
Website: http://
www.pahealthywoman.org

Puerto Rico

Breast and Cervical Cancer
Early Detection Program
Univ. of Puerto Rico
Comprehensive Cancer Center
Medical Sciences Campus
P.O. Box 70344 PMB 371
San Juan, PR 00936
Phone: 787-772-8300 ext. 1122
Fax: 787-767-8008

Rhode Island

Women's Cancer Screening
Program
RI Cancer Control Program
RI Dept. of Health
3 Capitol Hill
Providence, RI 02908
Health Information Line:
401-222-4324
Website: http://
www.health.ri.gov/programs/
womenscancerscreening

South Carolina

Best Chance Network
Div. of Cancer Prevention and
Control
Bureau of Chronic Disease
Prevention
1800 St. Julian Pl.
Columbia, SC 29204
Toll-Free: 800-227-2345
Website: http://www.scdhec.gov/
health/chcdp/cancer/bcn.htm

South Dakota

All Women Count!
SD Dept. of Health
615 E. Fourth St.
Pierre, SD 57501
Toll-Free in SD: 800-738-2301
Phone: 605-773-5728
Fax: 605-773-5509
Website: http://getscreened
.sd.gov/count

Tennessee

Breast and Cervical Cancer
Early Detection Program
TN Dept. of Health
Cordell Hull Bldg., 3rd Fl.
425 Fifth Ave. N.
Nashville, TN 37247
Toll-Free: 877-969-6636 (leave
a message, a nurse will return
your call)
Phone: 615-741-3111
Fax: 615-741-3806
Website: http://health.state
.tn.us/BCC
E-mail: tn.health@tn.gov

Texas

Breast and Cervical Cancer
Services
TX Dept. of State Health
Services
Preventive and Primary Care
Unit
1100 W. 49th St., MC 1923
P.O. Box 149347
Austin, TX 78714
Phone: 512-458-7796
Fax: 512-458-7203
Website: http://www.dshs.state
.tx.us/bcccs
E-mail: BCCSprogram
@dshs.state.tx.us

Utah

Utah Cancer Control Program
Bureau of Health Promotion
UT Dept. of Health
288 N. 1460 W.
P.O. Box 141010
Salt Lake City, UT 84114
Toll-Free: 800-717-1811
Phone: 801-538-6101
Website:
http://www.cancerutah.org

Vermont

Ladies First
VT Dept. of Health
108 Cherry St.
P.O. Box 70, Drawer 38 (LF)
Burlington, VT 05402
Toll-Free: 800-508-2222
Toll-Free TDD: 800-319-3141
Phone: 802-863-7330
Website: http://healthvermont
.gov/prevent/ladies_first.aspx
E-mail: vdhco@ahs.state.vt.us

Virginia

Every Woman's Life
109 Governor St., 8th Fl.
Richmond, VA 23219
Toll-Free in VA: 866-395-4968
Phone: 804-864-8204
Fax: 804-864-7763
Website:
http://www.vahealth.org/ewl

Washington

Breast, Cervical, and Colon
Health Program
WA State Dept. of Health
111 Israel Rd., Twn Cntr 2, 3rd Fl.
Tumwater, WA 98501
Toll-Free: 888-438-2247
Phone: 360-236-3672
Fax: 360-664-2619
Website:
http://www.doh.wa.gov/cfh/bcchp
E-mail: cancer@doh.wa.gov

West Virginia

Breast and Cervical Cancer
Screening Program
WV Dept. of Health and Human
Resources
350 Capital St., Rm. 427
Charleston, WV 25301
Toll-Free in WV: 800-642-8522
Phone: 304-558-5388
Fax: 304-558-7164
Website:
http://www.wvdhhr.org/bccsp

Wisconsin

Well Woman Program
Div. of Public Health
WI Dept. of Health Services
1 W. Wilson St., Rm. 218
P.O. Box 2659
Madison, WI 53701
Phone: 608-261-6872
TTY: 888-701-1251
Website:
http://www.dhs.wisconsin.gov/
womenshealth/wwwp

Wyoming

Breast and Cervical Cancer
Early Detection Program
Preventive Health and Safety Div.
WY Dept. of Health
6101 Yellowstone Rd., Ste. 510
Cheyenne, WY 82002
Toll-Free: 800-264-1296
Phone: 307-777-7172
Fax: 307-777-5402
Website:
http://www.health.wyo.gov/
PHSD/bccedp

Chapter 69

Organizations with Resources for People Undergoing Medical Tests

Government Organizations

Agency for Healthcare Research and Quality (AHRQ)
540 Gaither Rd.
Rockville, MD 20850
Toll-Free: 800-358-9295
Phone: 301-427-1364
Website: http://www.ahrq.gov

Center for Biologics Evaluation and Research (CBER)
Consumer Affairs Branch (CBER)
1401 Rockville Pike
Suite 200N/HFM-47
Rockville, MD 20852
Toll-Free: 800-835-4709
Phone: 301-827-1800
Website:
http://www.fda.gov/
BiologicsBloodVaccines/default
.htm
E-mail: ocod@fda.hhs.gov

Resources in this chapter were compiled from several sources deemed reliable; all contact information was verified and updated in April 2011. Inclusion does not imply endorsement. This list is not comprehensive, it is intended as a starting point for gathering of information.

Centers for Disease Control and Prevention (CDC)
1600 Clifton Rd.
Atlanta, GA 30333
Toll-Free: 800-CDC-INFO
(232-4636)
Toll-Free TTY: 888-232-6348
Website: http://www.cdc.gov
E-mail: cdcinfo@cdc.gov

Centers for Medicare and Medicaid Services
7500 Security Blvd.
Baltimore, MD 21244
Toll-Free: 800-633-4227
Toll-Free TTY: 877-486-2048
Website: http://www.cms.hhs.gov

Federal Trade Commission (FTC)
Consumer Response Center
600 Pennsylvania Ave., NW
Washington, DC 20850
Toll-Free: 877-FTC-HELP
(382-4357)
Toll-Free TTY: 866-653-4261
Phone: 202-326-2222
Website: http://www.ftc.gov

National Breast and Cervical Cancer Early Detection Program
Toll-Free: 800-232-4636
Toll-Free TTY: 888-232-6348
Website: http://www.cdc.gov/
cancer/nbccedp

National Cancer Institute (NCI)
NCI Public Inquiries Office
6116 Executive Blvd.
Room 3036A
Bethesda, MD 20892
Toll-Free: 800-4-CANCER
(800-422-6237)
Website: http://www.cancer.gov

National Diabetes Education Program
1 Diabetes Way
Bethesda, MD 20814
Toll-Free: 888-693-NDEP (6337)
Toll-Free TTY: 866-569-1162
Fax: 703-738-4929
Website: http://www.ndep.nih
.gov
E-mail: ndep@mail.nih.gov

National Digestive Diseases Information Clearinghouse
2 Information Way
Bethesda, MD 20892
Toll-Free: 800-891-5389
Toll-Free TTY: 866-569-1162
Fax: 703-738-4929
Website: http://digestive.niddk
.nih.gov
E-mail: nddic@info.niddk.nih.gov

National Eye Institute
31 Center Dr., MSC 2510
Bethesda, MD 20892
Phone: 301-496-5248
Website: http://www.nei.nih.gov/
index.asp
E-mail: 2020@nei.nih.gov

National Heart, Lung, and Blood Institute (NHLBI)
Health Information Center
P.O. Box 30105
Bethesda, MD 20824
Phone: 301-592-8573
TTY: 240-629-3255
Fax: 240-629-3246
Website: http://nhlbi.nih.gov
E-mail: nhlbiinfo@nhlbi.nih.gov

National Institute of Diabetes and Digestive and Kidney Diseases (NIDDK)
Bldg. 31, Rm. 9A06
31 Center Dr., MSC 2560
Bethesda, MD 20892
Phone: 301-496-3583
Website: http://www2.niddk.nih.gov

National Institute of Mental Health (NIMH)
6001 Executive Blvd.
Rm. 8184, MSC 9663
Bethesda, MD 20892
Toll-Free: 866-615-6464
Toll-Free TTY: 866-415-8051
Phone: 301-443-4513
TTY: 301-443-8431
Fax: 301-443-4279
Website: http://www.nimh.nih.gov
E-mail: nimhinfo@nih.gov

National Institute of Neurological Disorders and Stroke (NINDS)
P.O. Box 5801
Bethesda, MD 20824
Toll-Free: 800-352-9424
Phone: 301-496-5751
TTY: 301-468-5981
Website: http://www.ninds.nih.gov

National Institute on Aging (NIA)
Bldg. 31, Rm. 5C27
31 Center Dr., MSC 2292
Bethesda, MD 20892
Toll-Free: 800-222-2225
Toll-Free TTY: 800-222-4225
Phone: 301-496-1752
Fax: 301-496-1072
Website: http://www.nia.nih.gov

National Institute on Deafness and Other Communication Disorders (NIDCD)
Information Clearinghouse
1 Communication Ave.
Bethesda, MD 20892
Toll-Free: 800-241-1044
Toll-Free TTY: 800-241-1055
Fax: 301-770-8977
Website: http://www.nidcd.nih.gov
E-mail: nidcdinfo@nidcd.nih.gov

National Library of Medicine (NLM)
8600 Rockville Pike
Bethesda, MD 20894
Toll-Free: 888-346-3656
Phone: 301-594-5983
Fax: 301-402-1384
Website: http://www.nlm.nih.gov

National Prevention Information Network
P.O. Box 6003
Rockville, MD 20849
Toll-Free: 800-458-5231
Phone: 404-679-3860
Fax: 888-282-7681
Website: http://www.cdcnpin.org
E-mail: info@cdcnpin.org

National Women's Health Information Center
Office on Women's Health
200 Independence Ave. SW
Rm. 712E
Washington, DC 20201
Toll-Free: 800-994-9662
Toll-Free TDD: 888-220-5446
Phone: 202-690-7650
Fax: 202-205-2631
Website: http://www.4woman.gov

Substance Abuse and Mental Health Services Administration (SAMHSA)
P.O. Box 2345
Rockville, MD 20847
Toll-Free: 877-SAMHSA-7
(877-726-4727)
Toll-Free TTY: 800-487-4889
Fax: 240-221-4292
Website: http://www.samhsa.gov
E-mail: SAMHSAinfo@samhsa
.hhs.gov

U.S. Department of Health and Human Services
200 Independence Ave., SW
Washington, DC 20201
Toll-Free: 877-696-6775
Website: http://www.hhs.gov

U.S. Food and Drug Administration (FDA)
10903 New Hampshire Ave.
Silver Spring, MD 20993
Toll-Free: 888-INFO-FDA
(463-6332)
Website: http://www.fda.gov

FDA Center for Devices and Radiological Health (CDRH)
Website: http://www.fda.gov/
MedicalDevices/default.htm

FDA MedWatch
Toll-Free: 800-FDA-1088
Website: http://www.fda.gov/
Safety/MedWatch

U.S. Preventive Services Task Force (USPSTF)
540 Gaither Road
Rockville, MD 20850
Website:
http://www.
uspreventiveservicestaskforce
.org

Private Organizations

American Academy of Allergy, Asthma, and Immunology
555 E. Wells St., Suite 1100
Milwaukee, WI 53202
Toll-Free: 800-822-2762
Phone: 414-272-6071
Website: http://www.aaaai.org
E-mail: info@aaaai.org

American Academy of Family Physicians
11400 Tomahawk Crk. Pkwy.
Leawood, KS 66211
Toll-Free: 800-274-2237
Phone: 913-906-6000
Fax: 913-906-6075
Website: http://www.aafp.org
E-mail: contactcenter@aafp.org

American Academy of Pediatrics
141 NW Point Blvd.
Elk Grove Village, IL 60007
Phone: 847-434-4000
Fax: 847-434-8000
Website: http://www.aap.org
E-mail: kidsdocs@aap.org

American Association for Clinical Chemistry
Lab Tests Online
1850 K St. NW, Suite 625
Washington, DC 20006
Toll-Free: 800-892-1400
Phone: 202-857-0717
Website: http://www.
labtestsonline.org
E-mail: 2labtestsonline@aacc.org

American College of Physicians
American Society of Internal Medicine
190 N. Independence Mall W.
Philadelphia, PA 19106
Toll-Free: 800-523-1546
Phone: 215-351-2600
Website: http://www.acponline.org

American Association of Neurological Surgeons
5550 Meadowbrook Dr.
Rolling Meadows, IL 60008
Toll-Free: 888-566-AANS (2267)
Phone: 847-378-0500
Fax: 847-378-0600
Website: http://www.aans.org
E-mail: info@aans.org

American Cancer Society
Toll-Free: 800-227-2345
Toll-Free TTY: 866-228-4327
Website: http://www.cancer.org

American College of Gastroenterology
P.O. Box 342260
Bethesda, MD 20827
Phone: 301-263-9000
Fax: 301-263-9025
Website: http://www.acg.gi.org
E-mail: info@acg.gi.org

American College of Radiology
1891 Preston White Dr.
Reston, VA 20191
Toll-Free: 800-227-5463
Phone: 703-648-8900
Fax: 703-295-6773
Website: http://www.acr.org
E-mail: info@acr.org

American Diabetes Association
1701 N. Beauregard St.
Alexandria, VA 22311
Toll-Free: 800-DIABETES
(342-2383)
Website: http://www.diabetes.org
E-mail: AskADA@diabetes.org

American Gastroenterological Association
4930 Del Ray Ave.
Bethesda, MD 20814
Phone: 301-654-2055
Fax: 301-654-5920
Website: http://www.gastro.org
E-mail: member@gastro.org

American Heart Association
7272 Greenville Ave.
Dallas, TX 75231
Toll-Free: 800-242-8721
Website: http://www.heart.org

American Kidney Fund
6110 Executive Blvd., Suite 1010
Rockville, MD 20852
Toll-Free: 800-638-8299
Website:
http://www.kidneyfund.org
E-mail: helpline@kidneyfund.org

American Society of Echocardiography
2100 Gateway Centre Blvd., Ste. 310
Morrisville, NC 27560
Phone: 919-861-5574
Fax: 919-882-9900
Website: http://www.asecho.org

American Society of Radiologic Technologists
15000 Central Ave. SE
Albuquerque, NM 87123
Toll-Free: 800-444-2778
Phone: 505-298-4500
Fax: 505-298-5063
Website: http://www.asrt.org
E-mail: memberservices@asrt.org

American Speech-Language-Hearing Association

2200 Research Blvd.
Rockville, MD 20850
Toll-Free: 800-638-8255
Phone: 301-296-5700
TTY: 301-296-5650
Fax: 301-296-8580
Website: http://www.asha.org
E-mail: actioncenter@asha.org

American Stroke Association

7272 Greenville Ave.
Dallas, TX 75231
Toll-Free: 888-478-7653
Website: http://www.
strokeassociation.org

Breast Health Access for Women with Disabilities

Alta Bates Summit Medical
Center
Herrick Campus
Rehabilitation Services
2001 Dwight Way, 2nd Fl.
Berkeley, CA 94704
Phone: 510-204-4866
TDD: 510-204-4574
Fax: 510-204-5892
Website: http://www.bhawd.org

Glaucoma Research Foundation

251 Post St., Ste. 600
San Francisco, CA 94108
Toll-Free: 800-826-6693
Phone: 415-986-3162
Fax: 415-986-3763
Website: http://www.glaucoma
.org
E-mail: grf@glaucoma.org

Health Physics Society

1313 Dolley Madison Blvd.
Suite 402
McLean, VA 22101
Phone: 703-790-1745
Fax: 703-790-2672
Website: http://www.hps.org
E-mail: HPS@BurkInc.com

Healthline

Healthline Networks, Inc.
660 Third St.
San Francisco, CA 94107
Phone: 415-281-3100
Fax: 415-281-3199
Website: http://www.healthline
.com

Imaginis Corporation

Women's Health Information
5 E. Court St., Suite 301
Greenville, SC 29601
Phone: 864-209-1139
Website: http://www.imaginis
.com
E-mail: learnmore@imaginis.com

International Foundation for Functional Gastrointestinal Disorders
P.O. Box 170864
Milwaukee, WI 53217
Toll-Free: 888-964-2001
Phone: 414-964-1799
Fax: 414-964-7176
Website: http://www.iffgd.org
E-mail: iffgd@iffgd.org

The Joint Commission
One Renaissance Blvd.
Oakbrook Terrace, IL 60181
Phone: 630-792-5000
Fax: 630-792-5000
Website: http://www.jointcommission.org

Juvenile Diabetes Research Foundation International
26 Broadway, 14th Fl.
New York, NY 10004
Toll-Free: 800-533-CURE (2873)
Fax: 212-785-9595
Website: http://www.jdrf.org
E-mail: info@jdrf.org

March of Dimes
1275 Mamaroneck Ave.
White Plains, NY 10605
Toll-Free: 888-MODIMES (663-4637)
Phone: 914-997-4488
Website: http://www.marchofdimes.com
E-mail: askus@marchofdimes.com

MedicineNet.com
Website: http://www.medicinenet.com

Mental Health America
2000 N. Beauregard St., 6th Fl.
Alexandria, VA 22311
Toll-Free: 800-969-6642
Phone: 703-684-7722
Fax: 703-684-5968
Website: http://www.mentalhealthamerica.net

Muscular Dystrophy Association–USA
National Headquarters
3300 E. Sunrise Dr.
Tucson, AZ 85718
Toll-Free: 800-572-1717
Website: http://www.mdausa.org

National Kidney Foundation
30 East 33rd St.
New York, NY 10016
Toll-Free: 800-622-9010
Phone: 212-889-2210
Website: http://www.kidney.org

National Newborn Screening and Genetics Resource Center
1912 W. Anderson Ln., Ste. 210
Austin, TX 78757
Phone: 512-454-6419
Fax: 512-454-6509
Website: http://genes-r-us.uthscsa.edu

National Sleep Foundation
1010 N. Glebe Road, Ste. 310
Arlington, VA 22201
Phone: 703-243-1697
Website: http://www.sleepfoundation.org
E-mail: nsf@sleepfoundation.org

National Stroke Association
9707 E. Easter Ln., Ste. B
Centennial, CO 80112
Toll-Free: 800-STROKES
(787-6537)
Fax: 303-649-1328
Website: http://www.stroke.org
E-mail: info@stroke.org

Nemours Foundation
1600 Rockland Rd.
Wilmington, DE 19803
Phone: 302-651-4000
Website: http://www.kidshealth
.org
E-mail: info@kidshealth.org

*Radiological Society of
North America (RSNA)*
820 Jorie Blvd.
Oak Brook, IL 60523
Toll-Free: 800-381-6660
Phone: 630-571-2670
Fax: 630-571-7837
Website: http://www.rsna.org
E-mail: webmaster@rsna.org

RESOLVE
The National Infertility
Association
1760 Old Meadow Rd., Ste. 500
McLean, VA 22102
Phone: 703-556-7172
Fax: 703-506-3266
Website: http://www.resolve.org
E-mail: info@resolve.org

*Society of American
Gastrointestinal Endoscopic
Surgeons (SAGES)*
11300 W. Olympic Blvd., Ste. 600
Los Angeles, CA 90064
Phone: 310-437-0544
Fax: 310-437-0585
Website: http://www.sages.org
E-mail: sagesweb@sages.org

Society of Nuclear Medicine
1850 Samuel Morse Dr.
Reston, VA 20190
Phone: 703-708-9000
Fax: 703-708-9015
Website: http://www.snm.org

*Susan G. Komen for the
Cure*
5005 LBJ Fwy., Ste. 250
Dallas, TX 75244
Toll-Free: 877-465-6636
Website: http://www.komen.org

*University of Maryland
Medical Center*
22 S. Greene St.
Baltimore, MD 21201
Toll-Free: 800-492-5538
Toll-Free TDD: 800-735-2258
Physician Referral:
800-373-4111
Phone: 410-328-8667
Website: http://www.umm.edu

WebMD
Website: http://www.webmd.com

Index

Index

W

waist circumference,
body mass index (BMI) 55
Waldenström's macroglobulinemia,
tumor marker *421*
Washington, DC
see District of Columbia
Washington state
breast and cervical cancer early
detection program 606
newborn screening
conditions *20–21, 24–25, 30–31*
WebMD, website address 617
weight management
body mass index (BMI) 39–42
online screening tests 596
Weigl, Bernhard 90
West Virginia
breast and cervical cancer early
detection program 606
newborn screening
conditions *20–21, 24–25, 30–31*
"What is breast thermography?"
(American College of
Clinical Thermology) 281n
"What Is Computed
Tomography?" (FDA) 224n
"What is Molecular Imaging"
(Society of Nuclear Medicine) 256n
"What You Need to Know
about Angiography"
(American Society of
Radiological Technologists) 182n
"What You Need to Know
about Myelography"
(American Society of
Radiological Technologists) 197n
white blood cells
described 94, 123
normal range results *97*
"Why does my eye care
professional ask me to read
the letters on an eye chart?"
(Cukras) 516n
"Why I Might Need a
Circulation Ultrasound"
(American Society
of Echocardiography) 209n

Wisconsin
breast and cervical cancer early
detection program 606
newborn screening
conditions *20–21, 24–25, 30–31*
"With Home Testing, Consumers
Take Charge of Their Health: Buyer
Beware" (American Association for
Clinical Chemistry) 534n
"With Home Testing, Consumers
Take Charge of Their Health:
Introduction, Types of Tests,
and Avoiding Errors"
(American Association for
Clinical Chemistry) 530n
"Women: Stay Healthy at
Any Age" (AHRQ) 50n
Wyoming
breast and cervical cancer early
detection program 607
newborn screening
conditions *20–21, 24–25, 30–31*

X

x-rays
angiography 182–84
cardiomyopathy 455
chest 171–73
congenital heart defects 460
cystograms 185
defined 588
dental care 174–76
gastrointestinal tract 187
intravenous pyelogram 199–200
lung cancer 409–10
mammograms 285–89
medical usage 170–71
myelography 197–98
osteoporosis 486
radiation exposure 166–68
see also radiation exposure

Y

"Your Kidney Test Results"
(NKDEP) 93n

Z

Z-score, bone mineral density test 178